Allergy in a Nutshell
A Handbook

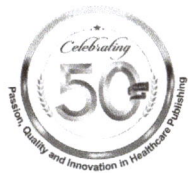

Allergy in a Nutshell
A Handbook

Neeraj Gupta
MBBS (UCMS, Delhi) DCH (MAMC, Delhi)
DNB Pediatrics (St. Stephens Hospital, Delhi)
Fellowship Pediatric Critical Care (GOSH, UK)
IDPCCM (CPCC, India), DAA (CMC, Vellore & IAS, USA)

Pediatric Intensivist and Allergy Specialist
Consultant
Division of Pediatric Emergency, Critical Care,
Pulmonology and Allergic Disorders
Sir Ganga Ram Hospital
New Delhi, India

Forewords

Harsh Vardhan MS
Anil Sachdev MD
Pudupakkam K Vedanthan MD

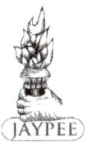

JAYPEE BROTHERS MEDICAL PUBLISHERS
The Health Sciences Publisher
New Delhi | London | Panama

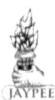

Jaypee Brothers Medical Publishers (P) Ltd

Headquarters
Jaypee Brothers Medical Publishers (P) Ltd
4838/24, Ansari Road, Daryaganj
New Delhi 110 002, India
Phone: +91-11-43574357
Fax: +91-11-43574314
E-mail: jaypee@jaypeebrothers.com

Overseas Offices

JP Medical Ltd
83 Victoria Street, London
SW1H 0HW (UK)
Phone: +44 20 3170 8910
Fax: +44 (0)20 3008 6180
E-mail: info@jpmedpub.com

Jaypee-Highlights Medical Publishers Inc
City of Knowledge, Bld. 235, 2nd Floor
Clayton, Panama City, Panama
Phone: +1 507-301-0496
Fax: +1 507-301-0499
E-mail: cservice@jphmedical.com

Jaypee Brothers Medical Publishers (P) Ltd
Bhotahity, Kathmandu, Nepal
Phone: +977-9741283608
E-mail: kathmandu@jaypeebrothers.com

Website: www.jaypeebrothers.com
Website: www.jaypeedigital.com

© 2019, Jaypee Brothers Medical Publishers

The views and opinions expressed in this book are solely those of the original contributor(s)/author(s) and do not necessarily represent those of editor(s) of the book.

All rights reserved. No part of this publication may be reproduced, stored or transmitted in any form or by any means, electronic, mechanical, photocopying, recording or otherwise, without the prior permission in writing of the publishers.

All brand names and product names used in this book are trade names, service marks, trademarks or registered trademarks of their respective owners. The publisher is not associated with any product or vendor mentioned in this book.

Medical knowledge and practice change constantly. This book is designed to provide accurate, authoritative information about the subject matter in question. However, readers are advised to check the most current information available on procedures included and check information from the manufacturer of each product to be administered, to verify the recommended dose, formula, method and duration of administration, adverse effects and contraindications. It is the responsibility of the practitioner to take all appropriate safety precautions. Neither the publisher nor the author(s)/editor(s) assume any liability for any injury and/or damage to persons or property arising from or related to use of material in this book.

This book is sold on the understanding that the publisher is not engaged in providing professional medical services. If such advice or services are required, the services of a competent medical professional should be sought.

Every effort has been made where necessary to contact holders of copyright to obtain permission to reproduce copyright material. If any have been inadvertently overlooked, the publisher will be pleased to make the necessary arrangements at the first opportunity. The **CD/DVD-ROM** (if any) provided in the sealed envelope with this book is complimentary and free of cost. **Not meant for sale.**

Inquiries for bulk sales may be solicited at: jaypee@jaypeebrothers.com

Allergy in a Nutshell: A Handbook
First Edition: **2019**

ISBN 978-93-5270-899-4

Dedicated to
*My parents, Mr Ram Avtar Gupta and Mrs Kamlesh Gupta,
whose values, love, support and unfading belief in me have helped
me become the compassionate person that I am today.
I am extremely appreciative of my wife, Poojan, for being
the pillar of strength on every step of the way.*

Foreword

डॉ हर्ष वर्धन
DR. HARSH VARDHAN

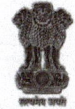

मंत्री
विज्ञान और प्रौद्योगिकी एवं पृथ्वी विज्ञान;
पर्यावरण, वन और जलवायु परिवर्तन
भारत सरकार
नई दिल्ली - 110001
MINISTER
SCIENCE & TECHNOLOGY AND EARTH SCIENCE;
ENVIRONMENT, FOREST AND CLIMATE CHANGE
GOVERNMENT OF INDIA
NEW DELHI - 110001

Allergic diseases are a major concern worldwide and India is no exception. India is a land of diverse climates, flora, fauna, populace and food habits. People are sensitized with broad range of allergens starting from inhalants, ingestants to contactants. Allergic symptoms can range from mild rhinitis to severe asthma and even life-threatening anaphylaxis.

It is my pleasure to introduce "*Allergy in a Nutshell: A Handbook*" to the dedicated and hardworking medical fraternity. Only a well-prepared and well-trained mind can face challenges of the changing health paradigms in the society. This concise book on allergies has been written with the view to recognize, treat and manage most allergic disorders, especially in the budding pediatric population. The author has reviewed the International literature as well as penned down his own experiences in managing people with allergic disorders. I hope this written text adds onto the existing literature on allergic diseases and benefits in the betterment of my fellow countrymen.

My good wishes to Dr. Neeraj Gupta and his team for this new venture. I hope they will continue the hard work and strive for excellence in patient care.

Harsh Vardhan MS
Minister, Government of India

Foreword

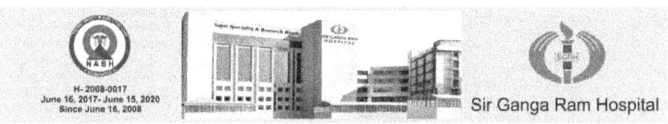

It is with a great degree of pleasure and pride, I write this foreword for *Allergy in a Nutshell: A Handbook* written by my colleague Neeraj Gupta. In my over 30 years of practice in the field of pulmonology, I have envisaged the need of knowledge dissemination. The key lies in better training and education. This concise book is a devout attempt for improving reader understanding of the field of Allergy, Asthma and Immunology. It covers allergies from basic pathophysiology to new management techniques and will likely prove beneficial for physicians, pediatricians and residents in training. The book also covers core points in respiratory allergies including role of diagnostic nasal endoscopy, bronchoscopy and impulse oscillometry. Other unique features included colored plates describing the local flora and fauna responsible for the environment biological changes, discussion on all forms of allergies and specifically designed algorithms to approach and manage a child with allergic symptoms. It definitely adds onto the existing literature on allergic diseases.

A lot of labor has gone into penning of this book and I am sure those who read it, will reap the benefits from the author's literary research and consolidation of data under one umbrella.

Anil Sachdev MD
Director
Division of Pediatric Emergency, Critical Care,
Pulmonology and Allergic Disorders
Institute of Child Health
Sir Ganga Ram Hospital
New Delhi, India

Foreword

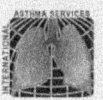 **GLOBAL CHEST INITIATIVES**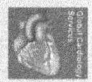

International Asthma Services   Global Cardiology Services

(A Registered Non-Profit Organization Helping the Needy around the World)

When Dr Neeraj Gupta (Neeraj) requested me to write the foreword for his book, "*Allergy in a Nutshell: A Handbook*", I was overwhelmed. I really needed to read and digest the contents of the book before writing the foreword. This took more effort and time than I anticipated. I found the book, not in a 'nutshell' (which means 'summing up in a few words'), but actually 'more descriptive and specific'. This book could be used in several ways: as a quick reference, bedside guide, futuristic, evidence and guideline based. The topics that have been covered are quite comprehensive at the same time concise. The various tables and figures that have been inserted are self descriptive, but surely needs close study. One of the interesting and very useful chapters was regarding the 'Myths and Beliefs about allergies'. Practically all possible queries that are raised during the clinical practice of allergy have been covered. Some of the recent and unusual topics for this size of a book include, Impulse Oscillometry, Component Resolved Diagnosis, Nasal Endoscopy, Nasal and Bronchial inhalation tests as well as extensive coverage of the Aerobiology for practically whole of India. I was particularly impressed by the coverage of the topic of Anaphylaxis, especially regarding the management and descriptive presentation regarding administration of IM Adrenaline with figures and text. This is the most essential part of the knowledge regarding allergy management anyone should be aware of, not restricting to the allergy specialists. Hence, I strongly feel this book should appeal to the cross-section of health professionals: medical students, residents and fellows in training, consultants in the field of Pediatrics, ENT, Pulmonary Medicine, General Medicine, Surgery, as well as nurses and allied health professionals. I truly wish this book which is backed by evidence and experience will serve as a very useful tool in any health care setting.

I again congratulate Dr Neeraj for his unrelenting determination, hard work, focus, and accuracy to bring out this very useful book to our armamentarium of knowledge to face and manage various allergic conditions.

Pudupakkam K Vedanthan MD
Clinical Professor of Medicine
University of Colorado, Denver, USA
Program Co-Director
Diploma in Allergy and Asthma (DAA),
Christian Medical College
Vellore, Tamil Nadu, India

Preface

Put your heart, mind and soul into even smallest of acts.
This is the secret of success.
—**Swami Sivananda**

I am delighted to write the preface for the first-ever book on allergies, namely *"Allergy in a Nutshell: A Handbook"*. For long, there was the need of a book that covers basic allergy pathophysiology, management, and diagnostic modalities available in the Indian scenario. This book has 16 dedicated chapters on allergy epidemiology, immunology, aerobiology, systemic allergies, modalities in allergy testing, and immunotherapy. Each chapter carries explanatory diagrams and tables with recent updated international guidelines to help understand allergic disorders better. Also, at the end of every chapter, several article titles have been suggested for further reading and learning. The highlights of this book are the consolidated algorithms at the end. These have been prepared with an aim to provide practical approach in managing an allergic child in the office. This book also discusses common myths regarding allergies in the general population. Managing allergies correctly is the key to provide better quality-of-life and eventually cure majority of patients. Being an avid reader, I believe in continuous training of mind to better understand a subject. Keeping in view with the Indian sensibilities, rising trend of allergic disorders in the country and my own experience in regularly dealing with allergic patients, this book has been compiled. This book will be beneficial for general practitioners, pediatricians, allergologists, and residents to better manage their patients. As has been said, "Knowledge is of no value until put to practice", the aim of this book is to provide practical tips for managing patients on a daily basis.

I received wide encouragement and support from my esteemed colleagues at Sir Ganga Ram Hospital, New Delhi, India and also from M/s Jaypee Brothers Medical Publishers, in putting tremendous effort to compile the chapters in due time. It is my hope and expectation that this book will provide an effective learning experience and serve as a reference resource for all health professionals leading to improved patient care.

Neeraj Gupta

Acknowledgments

I am extremely grateful to my colleagues and seniors at the Institute of Child Health, Sir Ganga Ram Hospital (SGRH), New Delhi, India, and its board of management for inspiring me to develop the field of Pediatric Allergies at the SGRH. Most importantly, it is due to the constant motivation and challenges posed by my patients that I am pushed to train further, work harder and treat better. This book is an offshoot of my journey in the field of allergies.

I appreciate the contribution of M/s Jaypee Brothers Medical Publishers (P) Ltd, New Delhi, India, for tireless follow-up and finishing the book within the timeline.

Contents

1. **Allergy: Public Health Issue** — 1
2. **Allergy Immunology** — 16
3. **Aerobiology** — 31
4. **Respiratory Allergies** — 77
   - 4.1 *Allergic rhinitis* 78
   - 4.2 *Sinusitis* 92
   - 4.3 *Otitis media* 104
   - 4.4 *Asthma* 112
5. **Anaphylaxis** — 143
6. **Gastrointestinal Allergies** — 160
   - 6.1 *Milk allergy* 160
   - 6.2 *Food allergy* 167
7. **Skin Allergies** — 179
8. **Other Allergies** — 213
9. **Approach to an Allergic Patient** — 248
10. **Allergy Testing: Allergen Identification** — 255
11. **Allergy Testing: Supportive Investigations** — 272
12. **Newer Allergy Tests** — 291
13. **Management of Allergies** — 297
14. **Complementary Medicine in Allergy** — 306
15. **Myths and Beliefs about Allergies** — 313
16. **Allergy: Future Perspectives** — 335

Annexure I: Algorithmic Approaches
- *Multi-model approach for allergic disorders* 337
- *Approach to a child with allergic symptoms* 338
- *Approach to a child with suspected milk allergy* 339
- *Approach to a patient with suspected adverse food reaction* 340
- *Immunotherapy (IT) algorithm* 341
- *Approach to a child with hypereosinophilia* 342
- *Approach to a child with atopic dermatitis* 343
- *Approach to a patient with suspected insect hypersensitivity* 344
- *High total IgE levels—differentials* 345
- *Approach to a child with anaphylaxis* 346
- *Approach to a patient with chronic urticaria* 347

Annexure II: Pharmacotherapy
- *Allergic rhinoconjunctivitis* 348
- *Angioedema* 349
- *Asthma* 350
- *Topical steroid potency chart* 352
- *Urticaria* 353

Index *355*

Plate 1

COMMON AEROALLERGENS (WITH LOCAL NAME)

1. *Acacia arabica* (*Gursoonder*, Babool, *Kikar*)

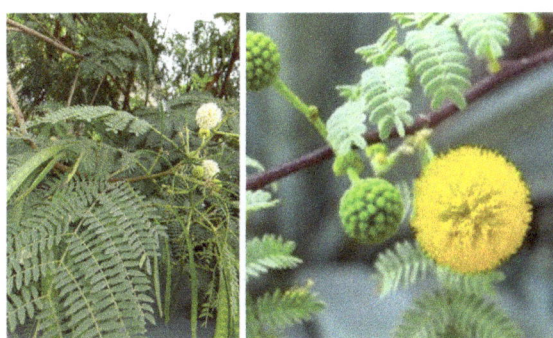

2. *Ageratum conyzoides* (*Nilam*, Billy goat weed)

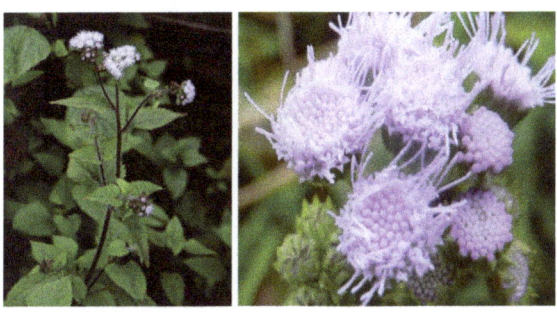

3. *Ailanthus excelsa* (*Urru, Aralu,* Indian tree of Heaven, *Neem*)

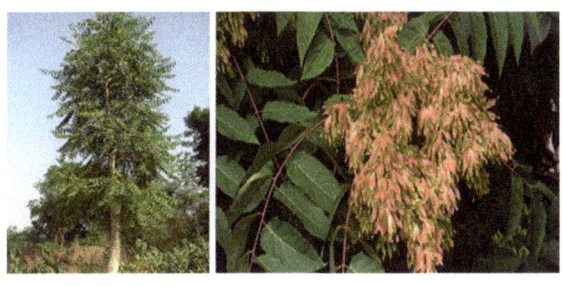

Plate 2

4. *Albizia lebbeck* (*Siras*, Woman's tongue tree)

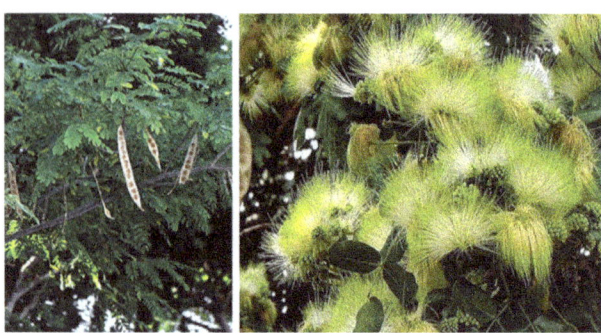

5. *Alnus nitida* (Grey alder)

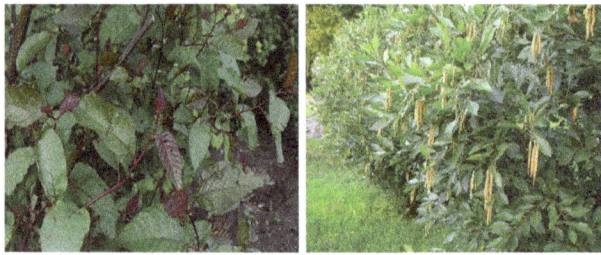

6. *Amaranthus spinosus* (*Kantewali chaulai*, Needle burr)

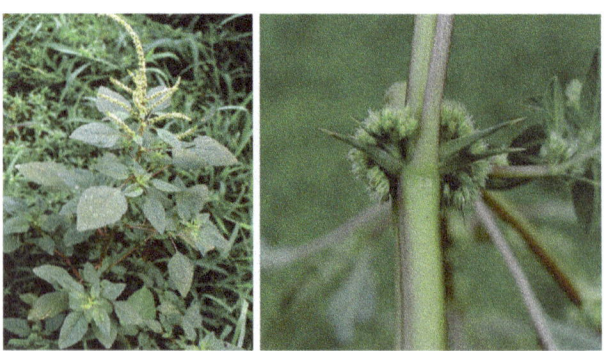

Plate 3

7. *Argemone mexicana* (*Siyal-kanta, Satyanashi*)

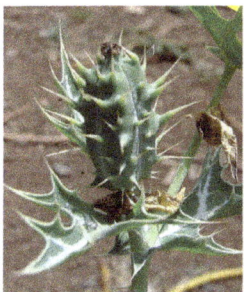
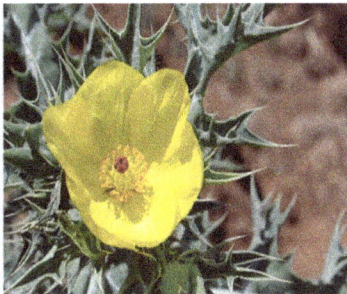

8. *Artemisia vulgaris* (Mugwort, Nagdona, Common wormwood)

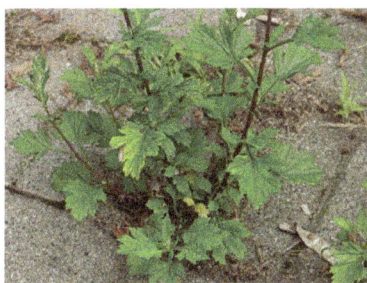
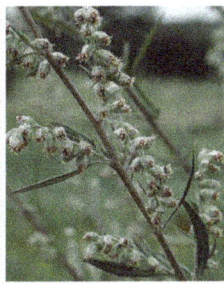

9. *Asphodelus tenuifolius* (*Jungle piyaz*)

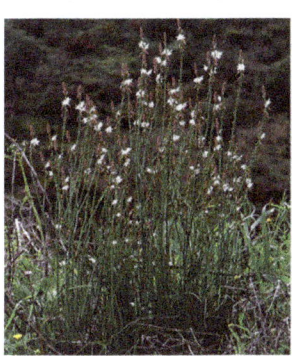
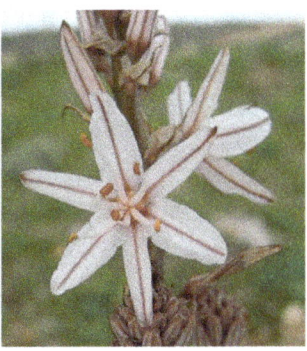

Plate 4

10. *Azadirachta indica* (*Neem*)

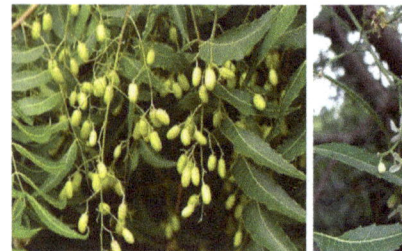
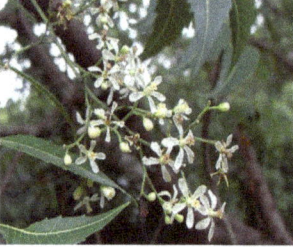

11. *Betula utilis* (Silver birch, *Bhojpatra*)

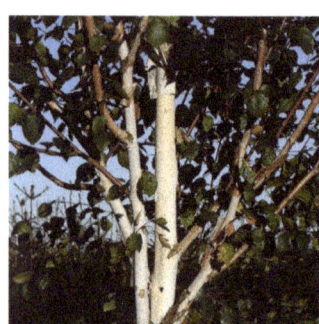
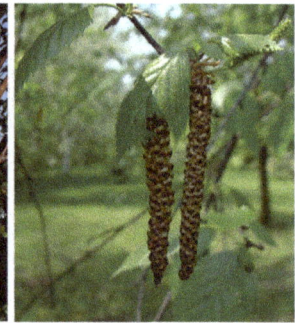

12. *Borassus flabellifer* (*Tal, Taad*)

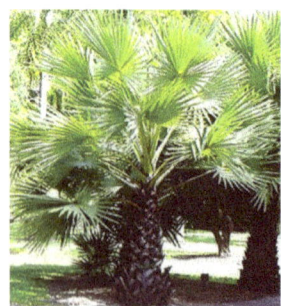
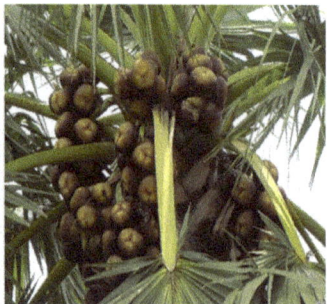

Plate 5

13. *Brassica campestris* (*Sarson*, Mustard)

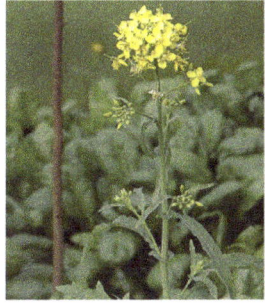
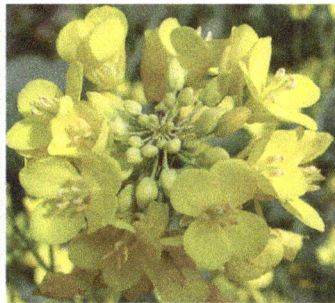

14. *Cannabis sativa* (*Ganja, Bhang*)

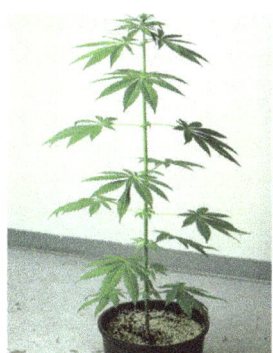
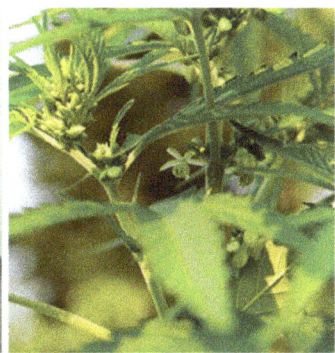

15. *Cassia fistula* (*Sonali, Ahilla,* Golden shower tree)

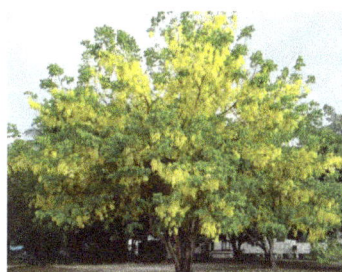
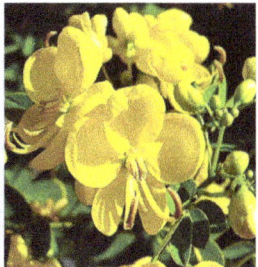

Plate 6

16. *Casuarina equisetifolia* (*Kasagaha*, Beefwood tree)

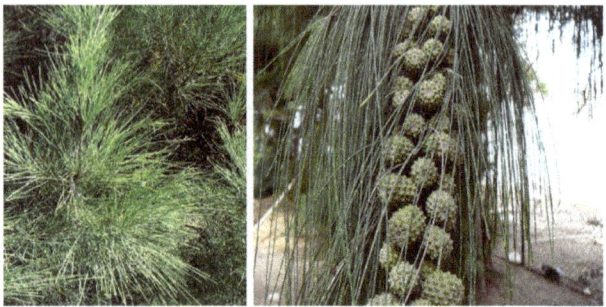

17. *Cenchrus ciliaris* (*Anjhan, Anjan*)

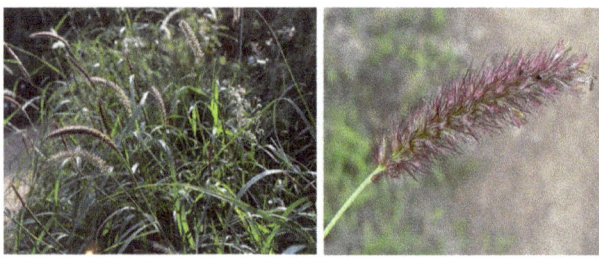

18. *Cedrus deodara* (*Devdar*)

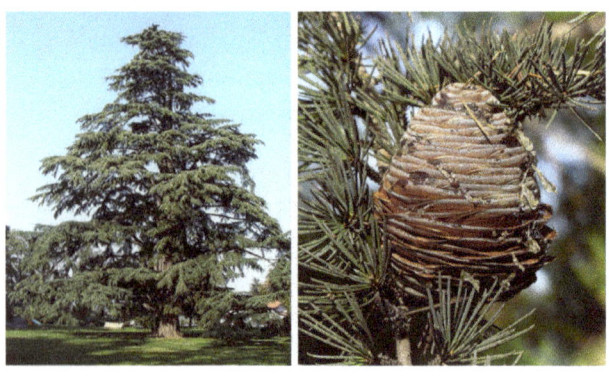

Plate 7

19. *Chenopodium album* (*Bathua*)

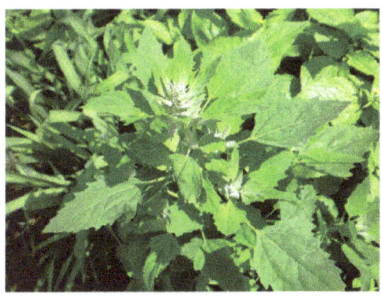
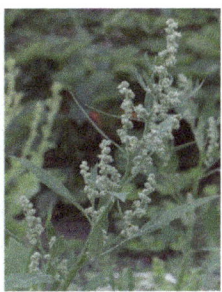

20. *Cocos nucifera* (*Narikel, Nariyal*)

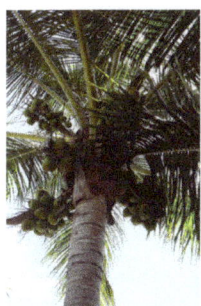
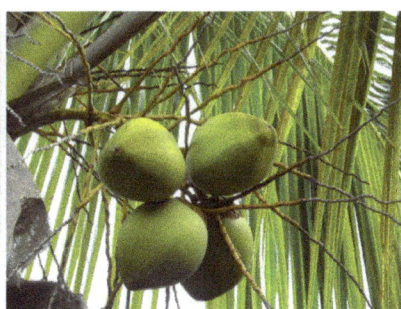

21. *Coriandrum sativum* (*Dhania*)

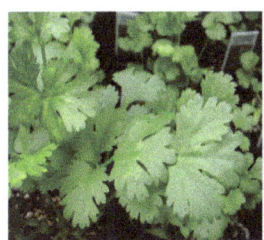
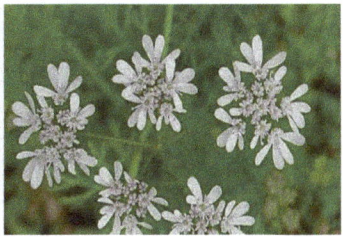

Plate 8

22. *Cynodon dactylon* (Bermuda grass, *Doob ghash*)

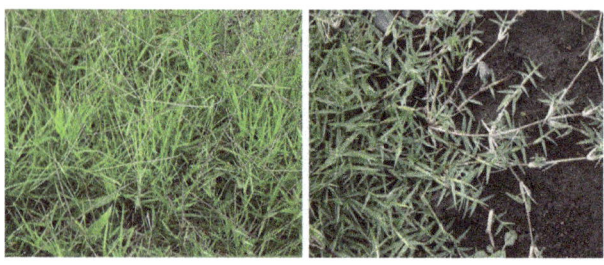

23. *Dodonaea viscosa* (*Vilayati mehndi*)

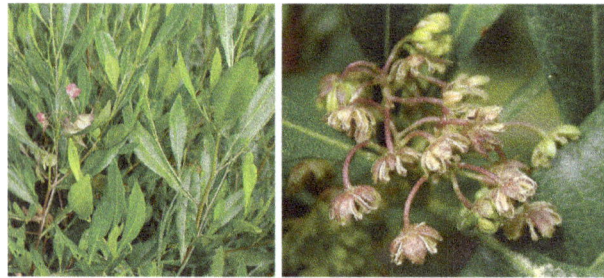

24. *Eucalyptus sp.* (Blue gum, *Safeda*)

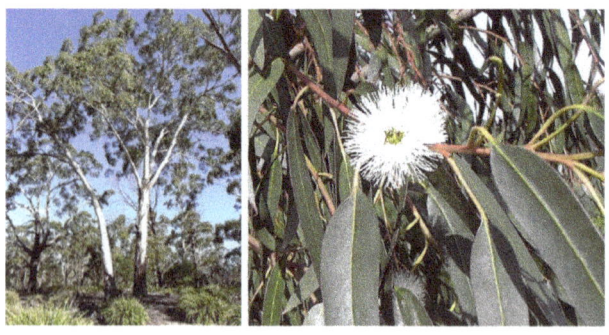

Plate 9

25. *Gynandropsis gynandra* (*Hulhul, Kathal*)

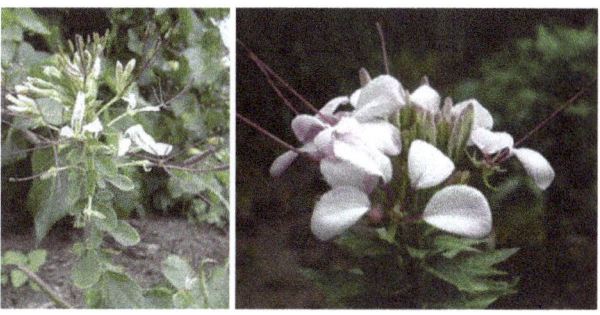

26. *Holoptelea integrifolia* (Chilbil, *Papri*, Indian Elm)

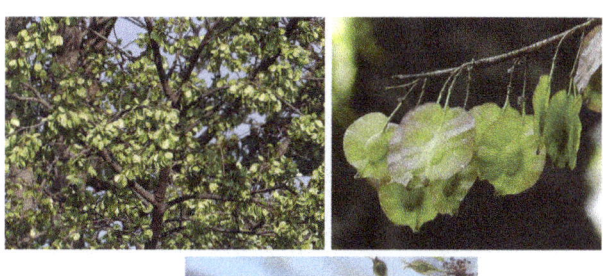

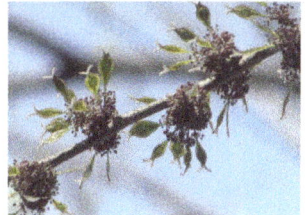

Plate 10

27. *Imperata cylindrica* (*Bhurighash*)

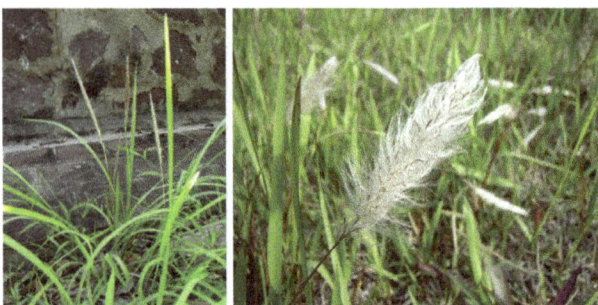

28. *Lolium perenne* (*Rye grass*)

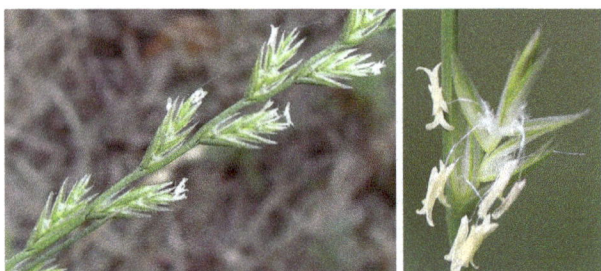

29. *Mallotus philippensis* (Kamala tree)

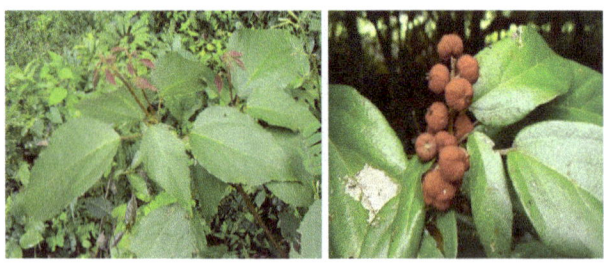

Plate 11

30. *Mangifera indica* (*Aam*, Mango)

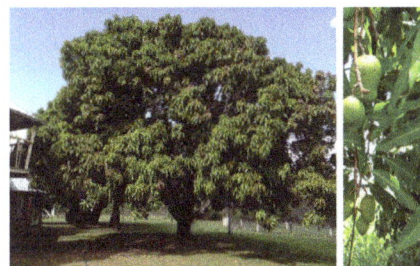
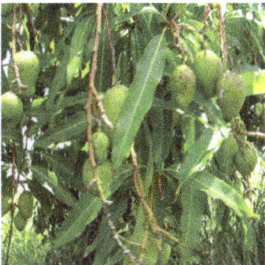

31. *Melia azedarach* (*Dek, Nim*)

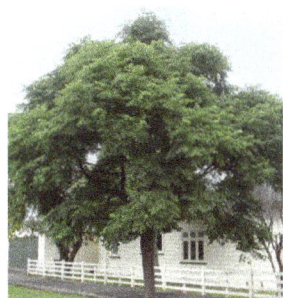
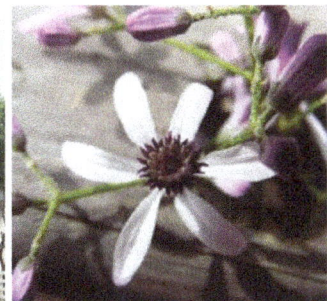

32. *Morus alba* (*Sehtoot*, Mulberry)

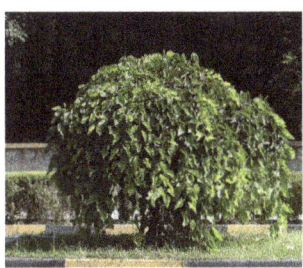
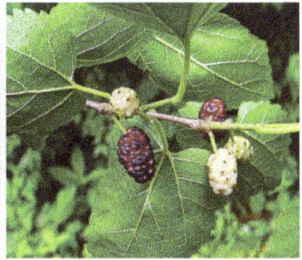

Plate 12

33. *Parthenium hysterophorus* (*Congress grass*)

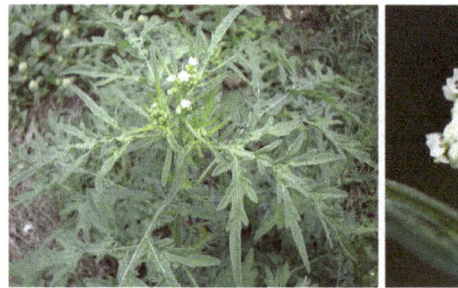
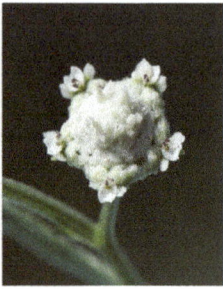

34. *Pennisetum typhoides* (*Bajra*)

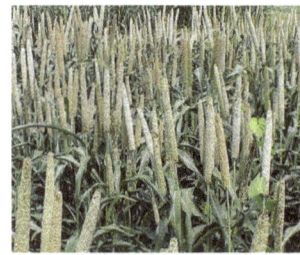
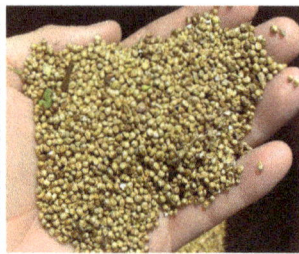

35. *Phoenix sylvestris* (Wild date palm, *Khajoor*)

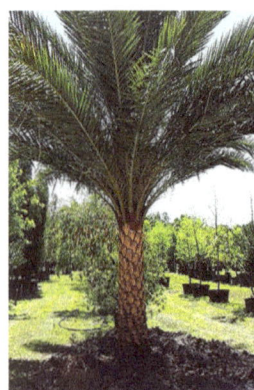
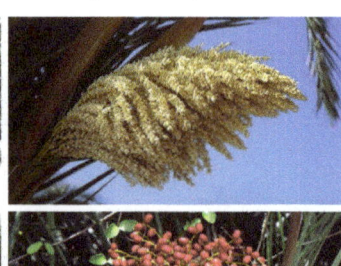
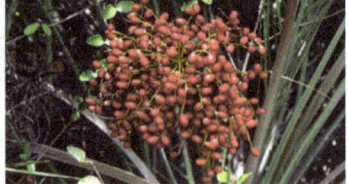

Plate 13

36. *Pinus strobus* (White pine)

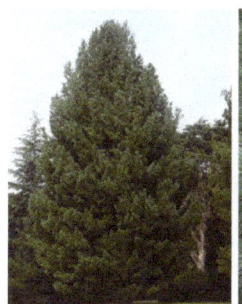
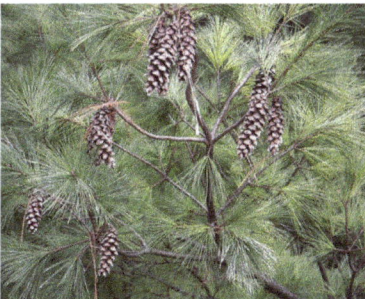

37. *Poa annua* (*Ghas*)

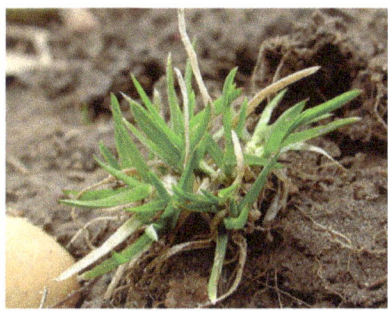
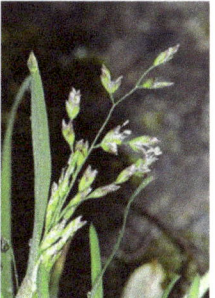

38. *Prosopis juliflora* (*Kabuli kikar*)

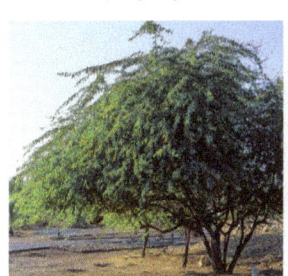
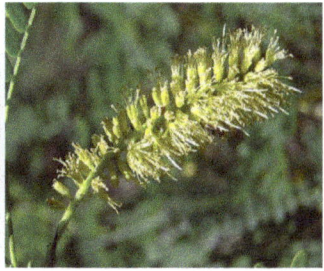

Plate 14

39. *Ricinus communis* (Castor, Castor bean, African coffee bean)

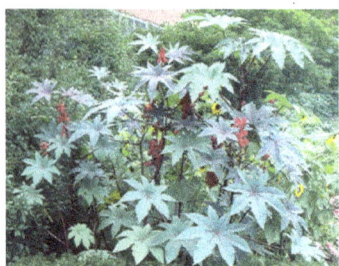
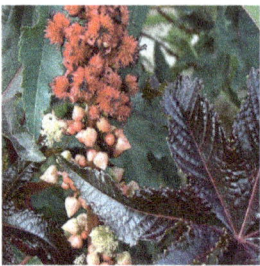

40. *Salix caprea* (Goat willow, Pussy willow)

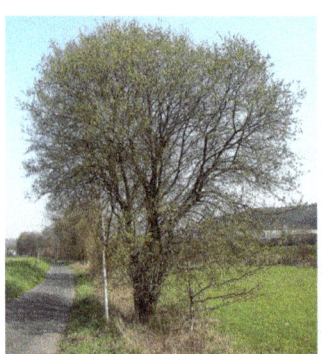
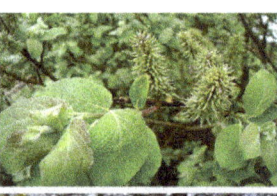
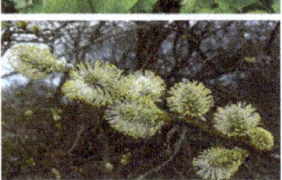

41. *Sorghum vulgare* (*Jowar, Karbi*)

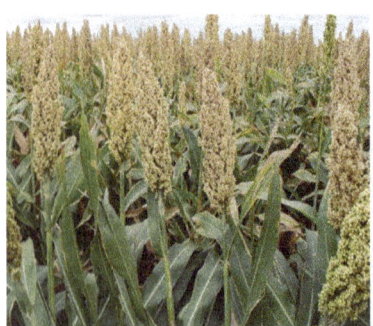
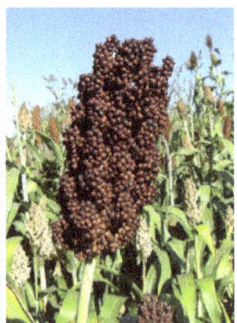

Plate 15

42. *Suaeda fruticosa* (Shrubby seablight, Lonia)

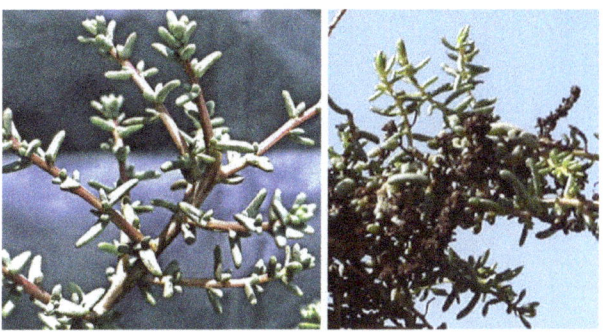

43. *Syzygium cumini* (Jamun, Black plum, Indian blackberry)

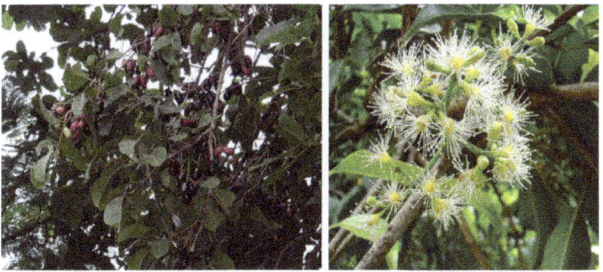

44. *Xanthium strumarium* (Adhisishi, *Chota dhatura*)

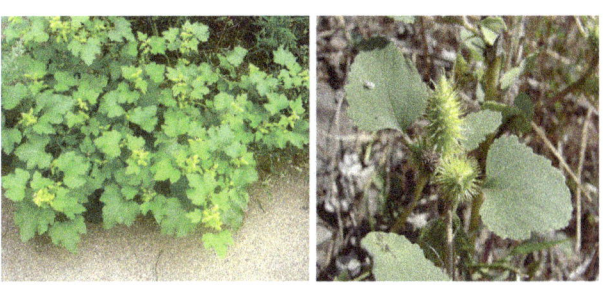

Plate 16

45. *Zea mays* (*Mokka, Bhutta, Makki*)

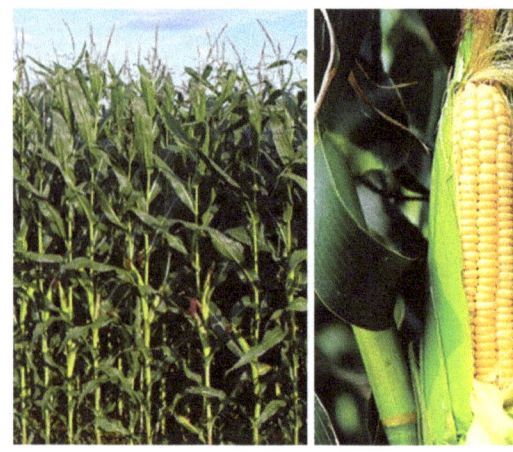

Plate 17

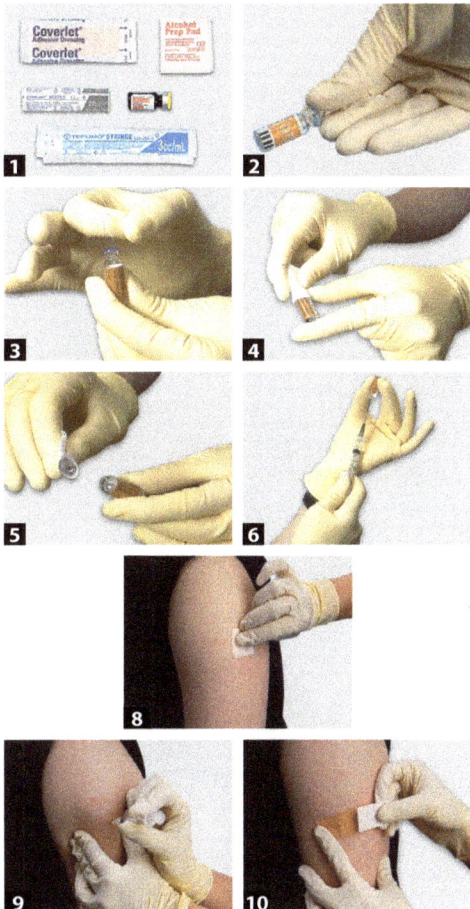

Fig. 3: Technique of administering intramuscular epinephrine. 1. Prepare the equipment; 2. Check the medication for expiry date; 3. Wear the gloves, hold the ampule upright and tap its top to dislodge any trapped solution; 4. Place gauze around the thin neck; 5. Snap it off with your thumb; 6. Draw up the medications, holding syringe with needle up, expel any air from the syringe; 9. Insert the needle at 90° angle, aspirate for blood, if none, then inject the required dose; 10. Remove the needle and cover the site.

Plate 18

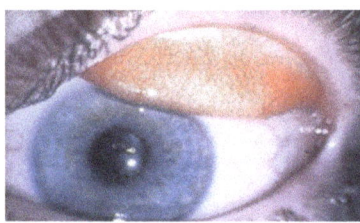

Fig. 1: Conjunctival swelling and chemosis in seasonal allergic conjunctivitis.

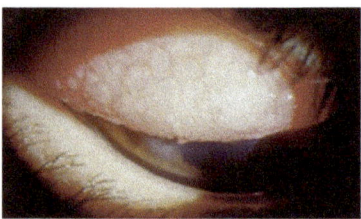

Fig. 2: Cobblestone-like appearance in vernal conjunctivitis.

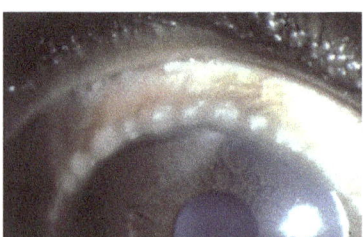

Fig. 3: Horner-Trantas dots.

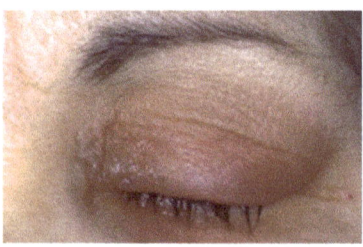

Fig. 4: Sandpaper-like texture of eyelid skin.

Plate 19

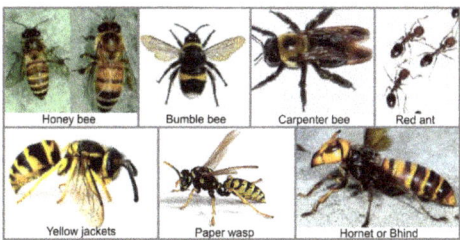

Fig. 5: Images of culprit insects.

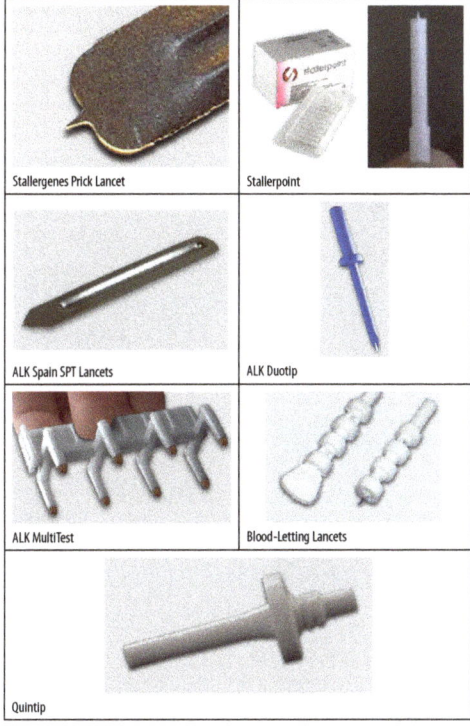

Fig 2: Lancet to be used for allergy skin testing (AST).

Plate 20

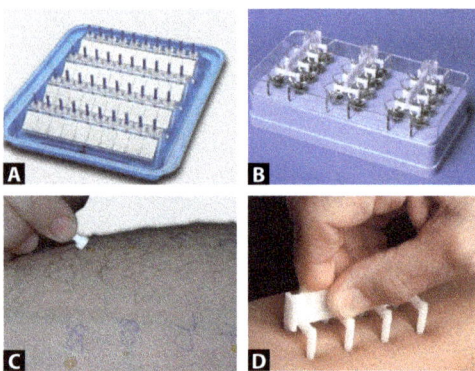

Figs. 3A to D: Lancets and multi-test devices for allergy skin testing (AST): (A) Duotips in tray containing extracts, waiting for use; (B) Multi-test devices in tray containing extracts, waiting for use (C) Drops applied to skin being pricked with a blood lancet (prick and lift technique); (D) Multi-test device applied to skin.

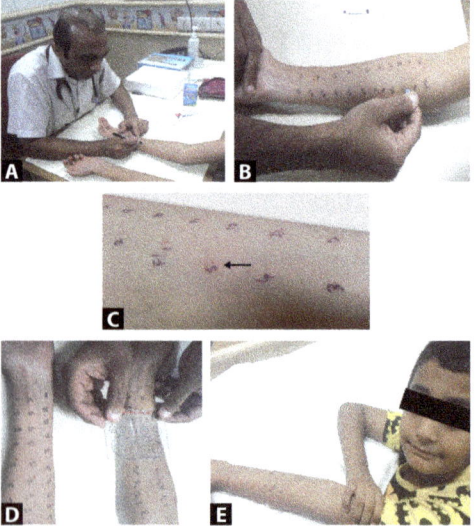

Figs. 4A to E: Skin prick test or skin touch test (STT) at an allergy clinic. (A) Marking on forearm for allergen identification; (B) STT with lancet; (C) Wheal and flare reaction (marked by arrow); (D) Measurement of allergic reaction and (E) Child after STT (a blood less pain less procedure).

Allergy: Public Health Issue

BURDEN OF DISEASE

Allergic diseases are a nuisance worldwide with rising trends witnessed over the last few decades (Fig. 1). Children bear the greatest burden of these disorders. An allergy can affect any body system, the most common being nose, sinus, eye, respiratory system, skin, and gastrointestinal tract. As per the recent estimates, 300 million people suffer from asthma and about 200–250 million people suffer from food allergies across the world at a given time.

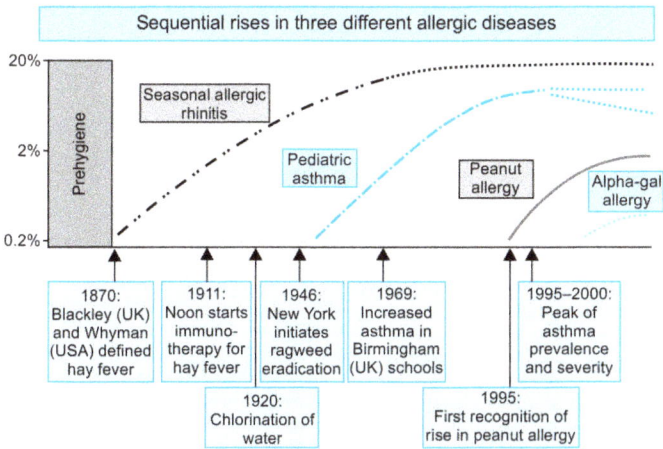

Fig. 1: Burden of allergic diseases over last five decades.
Source: Bloomfield SF, Rook GA, Scott EA, et al. Time to abondon the hygiene hypothesis: new perspectives on allergic disease, the human microbiome, infectious disease prevention and the role of trageted hygiene. Perpect Public Health. 2016;136:213-24.

Another 400 million have rhinitis, at least once, in their lifetime and 10% suffered from drug allergies. Allergic rhinitis (AR) affects 10–25% of population globally and it contributes to about 55% of all types of allergies. In spite of this quantum of allergic disorders, allergy services are still fragmented and far from ideal even in developed world.

India is a rich country in terms of flora and fauna, which means more number of allergens exist in the environment, hence, more chances of allergies. As per the recent literature, approximately 20–30% of the Indian population is suffering from one or other types of allergy at a given time. AR alone contributes to 20–30% of all allergic patients, whereas asthma shares 15% and the numbers are continuously rising (Fig. 2). Socioeconomic status affects childhood asthma with prevalence of 9.4% in lower class, 7.3% in middle class, 9.4% in upper class in urban Delhi area and 3.9% in rural Delhi.

Food allergens are identified as culprit for 4.5% of adolescents and adult asthmatic patients. True food allergy is reported in 1–2% of adult population and 6–8% of children. The numbers of perceived food allergies are much higher than the actual cases as any noticeable adverse effect to food whether intolerance or true

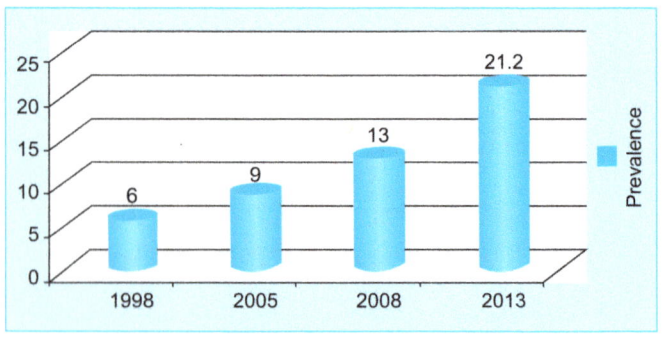

Fig. 2: Prevalence of allergic rhinitis (in percentage in community).
Source: Chandrika D. Allergic rhinitis in India: an overview. Int J Otorhinolaryngol Head Neck Surg. 2017;3(1):1-6.

allergy is misinterpreted as food allergy by both physicians and patients.

Allergic disorders, though of milder severity as compared to any infectious etiology, still significantly affect quality of life. As per World Health Organization (WHO) estimate, asthma alone is responsible for 250,000 deaths annually. These can have negative impact on the physical, psychological, and social aspects of an individual. AR and asthma can adversely change behavior, work performance, and lifestyle of affected people. It imparts a huge burden on nation's economy. Table 1 depicts latest global

Table 1: Global economic burden of asthma and rhinitis.

Country	Year costs calculated	Population (2010)	Disease	Direct costs*	Indirect costs**	Total costs estimated
Australia	2007	23 million	All allergies	A$ 1.1 billion	A$ 8.3 billion	A$9.4 billion
Finland	2005	5.3 million	All allergies	€A68 million	€51.7 million	€519.7 million
South Korea	2005	50 million	Asthma	–	–	US$1.78 billion
			Allergic rhinitis			US$266 million
Israel		7.5 million	Asthma	–	–	US250 million
Mexico	2007	103 million	Asthma			US$35 million
USA	2007	310.2 million	Asthma	US$14.7 billion	US$5 billion	US$19.7 billion
	2005		Allergic rhinitis	US$11.2 billion	Up to US$ 9.7 billion	Up to $20.9 billion

*Direct costs: Expenditure on medications and healthcare provision
**Indirect costs: Cost to society from loss of work, social support, loss of taxation income, home modifications, lower productivity at work, etc.
Source: Pawankar R. Allergic diseases and asthma: a global public health concern and a call to action. World Allergy Organization J. 2014;7:12.

economic figures for two common allergic diseases, viz. asthma and rhinitis. Atopic dermatitis, urticaria, drug and insect allergies are underestimated, because of absence of robust criteria for diagnosis and reporting.

HISTORY OF ALLERGY

Though the term "allergy" is relatively new, these disorders date back to ancient times. Various hypothesis, for their origin, have been postulated over time depending on the latest understanding and observations (Flowchart 1).

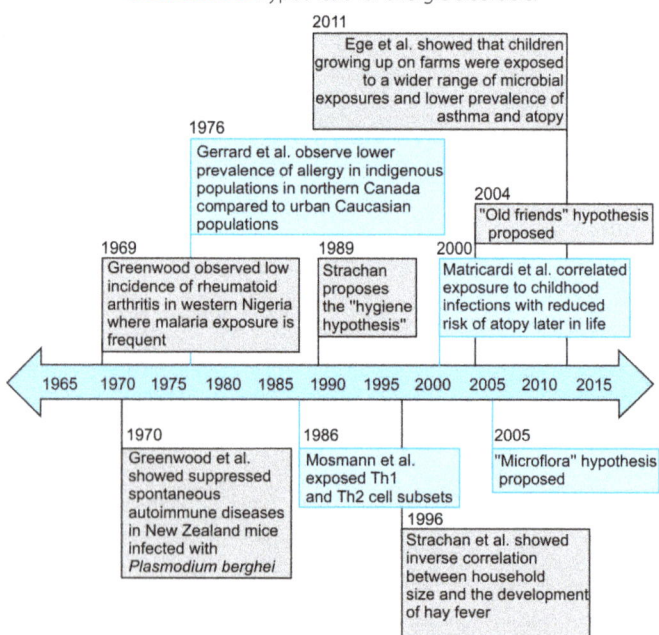

Flowchart 1: Hypothesis for allergic disorders.

Source: Stiemsma LT, Reynolds LA, Turvey SE, et al. The hygiene hypothesis: current perspectives and future therapies. Immunotargets Ther. 2015;4:143-57.

Hygiene hypothesis: Strachan, in 1989, proposed that increased microbial exposure in early life could protect children from hypersensitivity reactions later in life. This concept leads to a belief that "nonhygienic conditions invite infections on one hand, whereas more hygiene bring allergies with them on the other hand". This was well supported by observations like atopic patients had lower prevalence of *Toxoplasma gondii*, *Helicobacter pylori*, and hepatitis A; and children grown in rural area have lower incidence of allergic diseases compared to their urban counterparts. It is up to the individual what to choose among allergy or infections?—to be clean or not to be.

Old friends hypothesis: Hygiene hypothesis was soon challenged by observations noticed about reduction in allergic disorders due to exposure of certain microorganisms early in life. This has led to "old friend" concept in 2004. Human race has grown up along with many commensals since early paleolithic era. These microorganisms have stimulated the immune system in favorable way reducing the chances of allergic or autoimmune processes. During first epidemiological transition, newer microbiota (many viruses) invaded the human body but "old friends" continued to protect us. However, there was a phase of rapid decline in commensal or protective microbes with the onset of second or current epidemiological transition (Flowchart 2). This epidemiological shift has left the immune system partially trained leading to surge of Th2-mediated allergic and Th1-/Th17-mediated autoimmune disorders (Flowchart 3). This hypothesis was the basis of supplementing probiotics in early part of life, which might be potentially beneficial for prevention of immune-mediated (atopic and autoimmune) diseases.

Microflora hypothesis: In extension of "old friend hypothesis", it was observed that early life perturbations (driven by antibiotic use, infection or diet) to the microorganisms, residing in the human intestine disrupts the normal microbiota-mediated mechanisms promoting immunological tolerance and consequently bias the immune system toward hypersensitive disorders (Figs. 3 and 4).

Flowchart 2: Epidemiological transition and loss of protective microbiota.

History	Lifestyle	Microorganisms
Paleolithic >10,000 BCE	Small groups (<100), hunter/gatherer/scavenger	**Organisms implicated in the "Old Friends Hypothesis" that will have been present in early humans:** Helminths, saprophytic myobacteria, tuberculosis, hepatitis A virus, gut microbiota, *Helicobacter pylori*, *Salmonella*, *Toxoplasma*, Lactobacilli
First epidemiological transition		
Neolithic 3300 BCE **Bronze age** 1300 BCE **Iron age to preindustrial** 1800 CE	Large social groups. Animal husbandry. Domesticated cats, dogs. Increased orofecal. 97% still in rural environment; farms, animals, feces mud, untreated water	**Major microbial changes at 1st epidemiological transition** 1. More settled lifestyle, so more helminths and orofecal 2. Novel sporadic infections that epidemiology suggests are not relevant to "Old Friends Hypothesis":- Calici-, rota-, corona-, paramyxo-, orthomyxoviruses, (influenza B,C) measles, mumps, parainfluenza, smallpox. Cholera, plague, typhus.
Second epidemiological transition		
Modern	Cities, concrete, tarmac (less mud), soap detergents, washed food, less orofecal transmission. Chlorinated water. Less animal contact. Antibiotics. De-worming	**Less** Helminths, **Less** *Toxoplasma*, **Less** *Helicobacter pylori*, *Salmonella*, TB, **Less** Hepatitis A virus (HAV) **Less** "Pseudocommensals" from mud and water. **Disturbes** and less varied gut microbiota

Source: Modified from Rook GA, A Darwinian view of the Hygiene or 'Old Friends' Hypothesis. Microbe. 2012;7:173-80.

Antibiotic's usage in the first 2 years of life has been associated with the development of asthma at 7.5 years of age in a dose-dependent manner in a prospective observational study. Breastfeeding promotes colonization and reduces the risk of allergic diseases like atopic dermatitis, recurrent wheezing, and urticaria.

Any one hypothesis alone cannot explain the entire spectrum of allergic and autoimmune disorders. "Targeted hygiene" seems more appropriate than absolute hygiene or no hygiene.

EVOLUTION OF TERMINOLOGY

The phenomenon of allergy and anaphylaxis has been known to human race for thousands of years, much before the birth of modern science. The term "immune system" came into existence

Flowchart 3: Old friend hypothesis. Heavy loads of immunoregulatory organisms leading to accumulation of single nucleotide polymorphisms (SNP), which controls inflammation. The imbalance created, due to depletion of old friends, causes rise in chronic inflammatory disorders which are further aggravated by obesity and vitamin D deficiency.

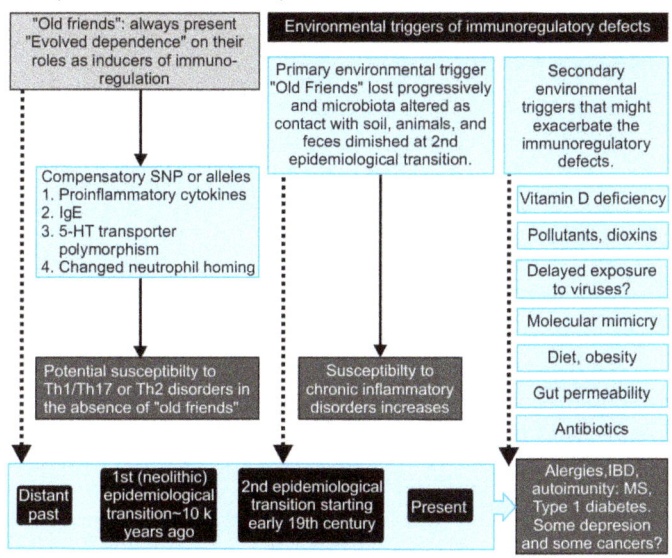

(IBD: inflammatory bowel disease; MS: multiple sclerosis)

Source: Modified from Rook GA, A Darwinian view of the Hygiene or 'Old Friends' Hypothesis. Microbe. 2012;7:173-80.

since late 19th and early 20th centuries, when it was first referred as a novel system which defends the body from microorganisms. The term "aphylaxis" was coined in 1902 by Charles Richet, which was later changed to "anaphylaxis" due to sweeter pronunciation. Richet demonstrated fatal reaction in a dog on re-exposure of sea anemone (*Actinia*) toxin. Body's reactions to certain antitoxins and vaccines, which were unexplained for long, came into limelight by Viennese pediatrician Clemens von Pirquet Freiher (Fig. 5) in April 1903.

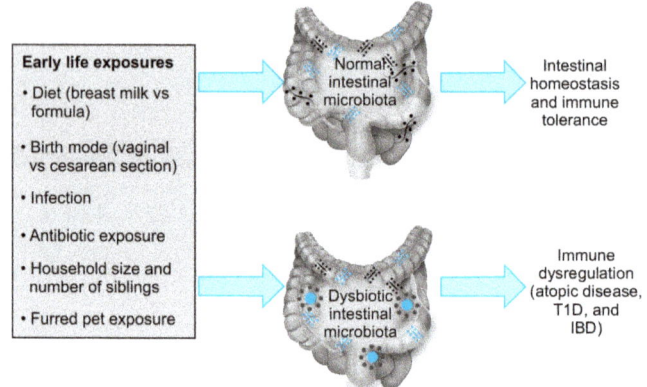

Fig. 3: Correlation of intestinal microbiota with immunological tolerance or dysregulation.
(IBD: inflammatory bowel disease)
Source: Stiemsma LT, Reynolds LA, Turvey SE, et al. The hygiene hypothesis: current perspectives and future therapies. Immunotargets Ther. 2015;4:143-57.

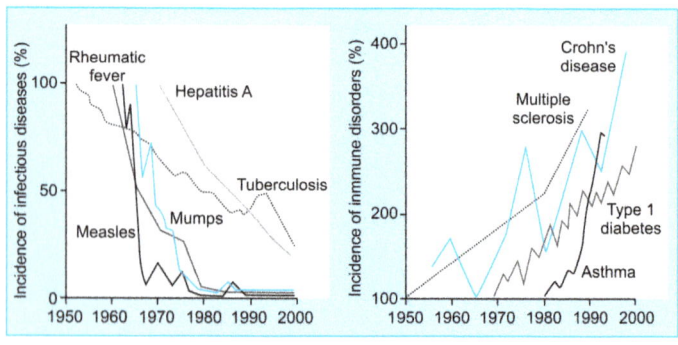

Fig. 4: Decline in infections and rise in immune-mediated disorders due to dysbiotic microflora.
Source: Bach JF. The effect of infections on susceptibility to autoimmune and allergic diseases. N Engl J Med. 2002;347(12):911-20.

In 1906, for the first time, Pirquet coined the term "allergy", which he defined as a change in reactivity whenever an individual comes in contact with an antigen, which could be protective, named immunity or harmful, named as hypersensitivity (Fig. 6).

The idea of allergy gained popularity over first half of 20th century with perverted meaning to represent the dark side of immunity only (Fig. 7).

Thereafter, prevalence of allergy and anaphylaxis has seen a steady rise over last century (Fig. 8).

Field of "allergy and immunology" entered its golden era when Teruko and Kimishige Ishizaka, from La Jolla (California) in 1966, and Gunnar Johansson and Hans Bennich, from Uppsala-Karolinska (Suecia) in 1967, independently discovered an unclassified immunoglobulin (Ig) relevant to allergies, which

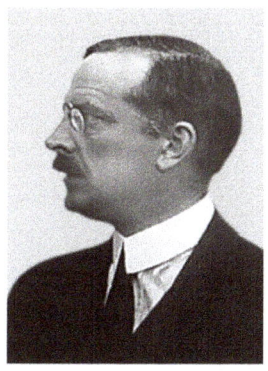

Fig. 5: Clemens von Pirquet (1874–1929), creator of the idea of allergy.
Source: Igea JM. The history of the idea of allergy. Allergy. 2013;68: 966-73.

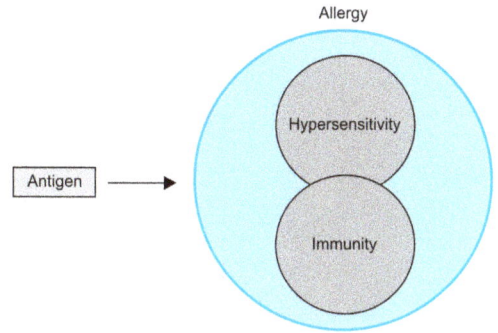

Fig. 6: Original idea of allergy.
Source: Igea JM. The history of the idea of allergy. Allergy. 2013;68:966-73.

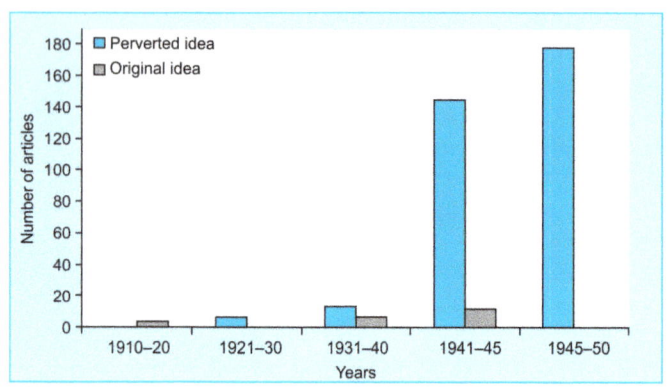

Fig. 7: Scientific literature with "original" and "perverted" idea of allergy.
Source: Igea JM. The history of the idea of allergy. Allergy. 2013;68:966-73.

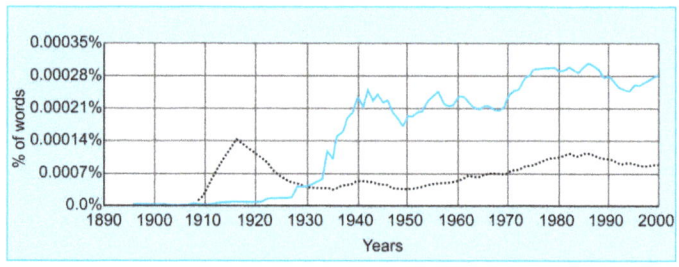

Fig. 8: Prevalence of "allergy" and "anaphylaxis" over last century. Solid line—allergy (with perverted meaning); Dotted line—anaphylaxis.
Source: Igea JM. The history of the idea of allergy. Allergy. 2013;68:966-73.

was later named as IgE by WHO in 1968. Philip Gell and Robin Coombs classified adverse allergic reactions into types I-IV, based on initiating immune mechanisms in 1963, in which IgE was involved in type I hypersensitivity reaction.

At the end of 20th century, the word "allergy" was used as an umbrella term covering various immunological and nonimmunological reactions, including side effects of drugs, psychological reactions, and adverse reactions to food and others.

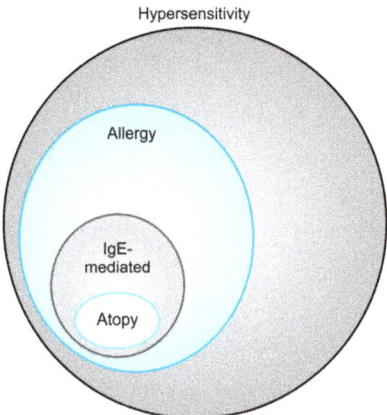

Fig. 9: Current concept of "allergy". Hypersensitivity is an abnormal response to a stimulus in physiological doses in susceptible individual. This response could be mediated by various immunological processes, called "allergy" among which immunoglobulin E (IgE)-mediated type I hypersensitivity plays significant role. There are "atopic" individuals with personal or familial tendencies for various types of hypersensitivities.

The current understanding, as per World Allergy Organization (WAO) and European Academy of Allergology and Clinical Immunology (EAACI), for hypersensitivity is "objectively reproducible symptoms or signs initiated by exposure to a defined stimulus at a dose tolerated by normal persons". The hypersensitivity reactions mediated by immunological mechanisms are known as "allergy". Figure 9 defines current concept of allergy. The concept also highlights the importance of various nonimmunological causes of hypersensitivity and non-IgE-mediated mechanisms of allergy.

ALLERGY SPECTRUM

Allergic disorders include food allergies, asthma, rhinitis, conjunctivitis, anaphylaxis, angioedema, urticaria, atopic dermatitis, eosinophilic disorders, including eosinophilic esophagitis, and drug, insect and occupational allergies under a huge umbrella (Fig. 10).

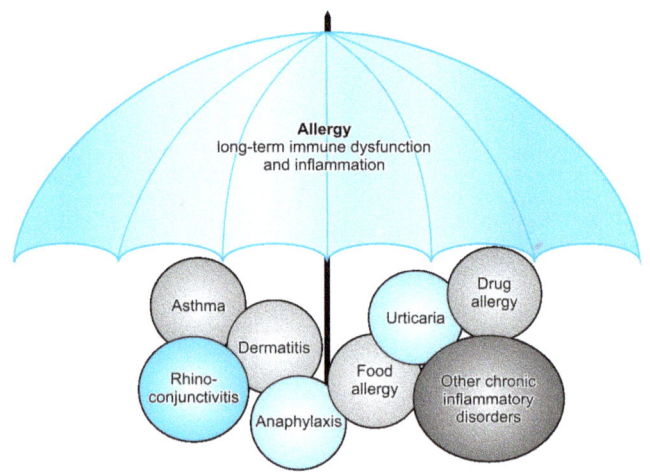

Fig. 10: Allergy—an umbrella term.
Source: Haahtela T, Holgate S, Pawankar R, et al. The biodiversity hypothesis and allergic disease: World Allergy Organization position statement. World Allergy Organization Journal; 2013.

RISK FACTORS

- *Genetic factors*: Epigenetic influences involve multiple mechanisms, which play key role in gene-environmental interactions. Some of the pathways could be methylation of CpG islands in gene promoters, histone acetylation, phosphorylation and methylation and a large number of micro-RNAs, can potentially explain transgenerational effects.
- *Allergens*: IgE antibody response (sensitization) to foreign proteins in the environment (derived from pollens, molds, dust mites, and cockroaches) is present in up to 40% of the population. Grass pollen are strongly associated with seasonal symptoms of hay fever.
- *Environmental risk factors*: Both indoor and outdoor pollution significantly affect respiratory health, including an increased prevalence of new onset and frequent exacerbations of asthma,

rhinitis, rhinoconjunctivitis, acute respiratory infections, and hospital admissions for respiratory symptoms. Indoor pollution alone (largely contributed by biomass fuel usage), may be responsible for almost 2 million deaths per annum in developing countries.
- *Climate change and migration*: Global warming coupled with air pollutant exposures may have serious adverse consequences for human health, especially in urban and polluted regions. Climatic factors (temperature, wind speed, humidity, thunderstorms, etc.) can affect both biological and chemical components of air pollution and respiratory allergies. Thunderstorms may induce hydration of pollen grains with fragmentation leading to release of biological aerosols and causing asthma outbreaks. Migration from one place to another may expose sensitized individuals to new allergens.
- *Socioeconomic factors*: There is an inverse relationship of asthma morbidity and mortality to social and economic status (SES) as people with lower SES face suboptimal, unhealthy environmental conditions (e.g. physical, social, and psychological conditions).

ADULT VS PEDIATRIC ALLERGY

Most of the allergic diseases start in childhood. Many children outgrow from milk and egg allergies by 3rd and 5th birthday, respectively. Other food allergens cause lifelong sensitivity which could be clinically relevant. Respiratory allergies like rhinitis and asthma, with onset in childhood, gradually settles by adolescence in two-thirds of nonatopic individuals. More than one half of all children who wheeze with viral infection during the first year of life have a transient condition that rapidly subsides during preschool and early school years.

Chronological evaluation of allergy onset is important from management aspects. A clear understanding of atopic march, a well-known phenomenon, with symptomatic involvement of various body systems in sequential manner is warranted. Diagnostic evaluation is difficult in children when compared to adults. Allergen avoidance and specific immunotherapy yield better results in children than adults, when the disease is in its naive phase.

An early suspicion, proper diagnosis, and effective management of childhood allergy are the keys for dealing with this rapidly rising allergy monster. Pediatricians and general practitioners, with an early contact with children, have to play a key role in achieving this goal.

NEED FOR AN ALLERGY SPECIALIST

There is almost negligible expertise available for allergic patients in many countries, other than organ-based specialists. Such specialists generally view allergic patients with their focused area or organ of interest, but a comprehensive care for a patient with allergic conjunctivitis, rhinitis, asthma, and atopic dermatitis can only be provided by an allergy specialist. Phenomenon of atopic march, where manifestations are changing home from organ to organ in due course of time, can only be understood by a person with comprehensive expertise in the field. An allergist can anticipate and advocate preventive steps in an atopic child or family. Specific allergen identification with source control and targeted immunotherapy services needs to be delivered to needy patients in early phase of disease. Careful interpretation of allergy tests is warranted to avoid unnecessary restrictions. Unfortunately, our medical curriculum has yet not included this very important area of concern. There is an urgent need of specialized allergy centers for better patient management, training medical students, and healthcare workers and enhancing research opportunities in the field of allergy.

SUGGESTED READING

1. Chandrika D. Allergic rhinitis in India: an overview. Int J Otorhinolaryngol Head Neck Surg. 2017;3(1):1-6
2. Pawankar R. Allergic diseases and asthma: a global public health concern and a call to action. World Allergy Organ J. 2014;7(1):12.

3. Pawankar R, Holgate ST, Canonica GW, et al. World Allergy Organization (WAO). White Book on Allergy. 2011.
4. Prasad R, Kumar R. Allergy Situation in India: What is Being Done? Indian J Chest Dis Allied Sci. 2013;55:7-8.
5. Stiemsma LT, Reynolds LA, Turvey SE, et al. The hygiene hypothesis: current perspectives and future therapies. Immuno Targets Ther. 2015;4:143-57.

CHAPTER 2

Allergy Immunology

INTRODUCTION

Modern era of allergy started two centuries ago, in 1819, with classical description of hay fever (allergic rhinitis) by John Bostock. Charles Blackley performed first skin test on himself in 1869. The 20th century witnessed major advances in diagnosis and management of allergic disorders. The word "Anaphylaxis" was coined by Richet and Portier in 1902, for the "untoward and severe systemic reaction to a suspected allergen" with detrimental outcome including death, if not recognized and managed early. The term "Allergy" was first coined in 1906 by Clemens von Pirquet, a Viennese pediatrician, who defined it as "strange or untoward reactions to harmless substances". Prausnitz and Kustner, in 1921, suggested the presence of a transferable allergenic factor by demonstrating an "allergic hive" (P-K reaction) to the same specific antigen, at the transfer site of a recipient, when the recipient (nonsensitized person) has already received the serum from a sensitized individual. Ishizaka couple (in 1966) and Johansson group (in 1967) independently identified this transferable factor, which was named as IgE immunoglobulin by the World Health Organization (WHO) in 1968. This was the beginning of the immunological basis of allergic diseases.

The discovery of IgE was actually the begining of breakthro treatment options and research for these chronic diseases. Although allergy is an 'old disease', its understanding and acceptance even in the medical community is very 'recent'.

The term "allergy" has been loosely used by physicians and patients across the globe. Any reaction which is unexplainable with the present scientific knowledge has been called allergy. As the term is often misused, the need for its appropriate management was never felt.

We need to understand the basic pathophysiology in an allergic reaction to properly manage this upcoming epidemic. Nowadays, various in vitro and in vivo allergy tests are available which create a lot of confusion among healthcare providers and receivers. A revisit to allergy immunology will help in selecting the appropriate test for patients. This will help in deciding specific allergen immunotherapy early in life, which is the only disease-modifying therapy available for combating allergies.

DEFINITIONS

Allergology: It is the science related to allergic diseases, their pathophysiology, mechanisms, and differential diagnoses.

Sensitivity: Normal host response to a defined stimulus.

Hypersensitivity: It is the altered reactivity of the body to a particular allergen. It can be immunologically or nonimmunologically mediated. The commonly available allergy tests detect hypersensitivity to particular allergen, which might not be responsible for patient's symptoms.

Allergy: It is the clinical hypersensitivity usually diagnosed by correlation of clinical presentation and allergy tests. It is mostly mediated by immunoglobulin E (IgE) production, though non-IgE pathways are also known.

Atopy: It is the genetic definition of allergy with personal or familial tendency, in an individual, for development of hypersensitivity.

Sensitizer: Sensitizer is a protein which is able to instruct the immune system to start producing IgE antibodies.

Allergen: An allergen is a protein which is able to bind specific IgE antibodies. A complete or true allergen will be having both properties as able to instruct for IgE production and will bind to specific IgE molecules; whereas, a cross-reactive allergen will be

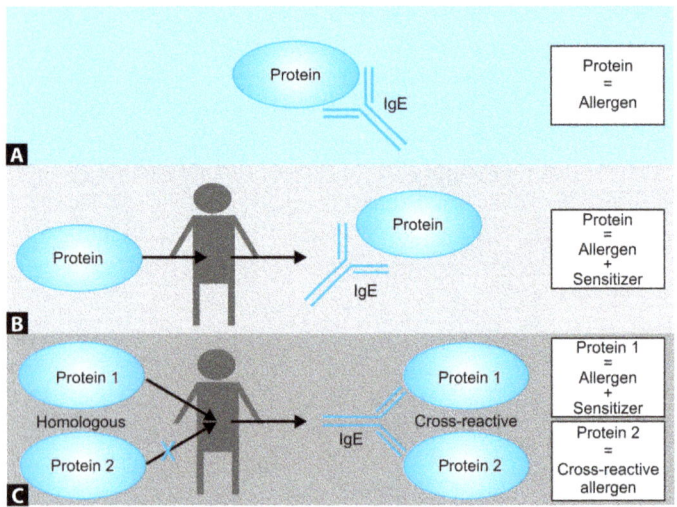

Figs. 1A to C: (A) Allergen; (B) Sensitizer; (C) Protein 1 = complete or true allergen, Protein 2 = cross-reactive allergen.
(IgE: immunoglobulin E)
Source: Akdis CA, Agache I. Global Atlas of Allergy. EAACI. 2014.

able to only bind with IgE molecules but unable to trigger for IgE production (Figs. 1A to C).

Antibody or immunoglobulin: These are Y-shaped proteins that are produced by the immune system in response to an allergen or antigen exposure. These antibodies bind to harmful allergens and mediate their destruction. There are five types of antibodies among which IgE has been linked with most of allergic manifestations.

Anaphylaxis: It is severe, generalized, life-threatening allergic reaction simultaneously affecting multiple organ systems.

ALLERGY OR TOLERANCE DEVELOPMENT

Individuals are born with genetic predisposition for allergic disorders and depending upon the dose and timing of allergenic

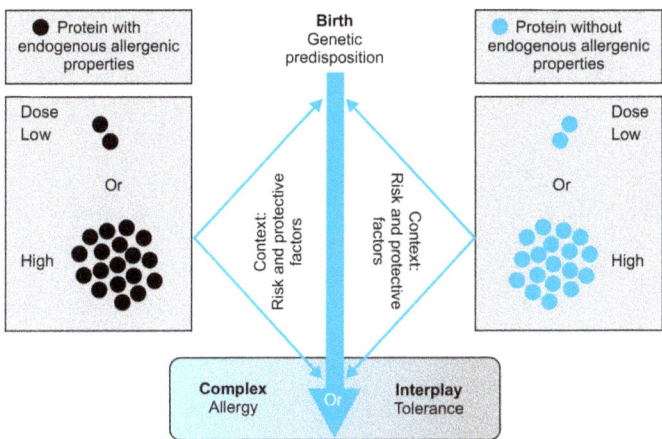

Fig. 2: Complex interplay of various factors determining onset of allergy.
Source: Akdis CA, Agache I. Global Atlas of Allergy. EAACI. 2014.

exposure, risk and protective factors later in life, either tolerance or hypersensitivity develops to that particular allergen (Fig. 2).

BASIC IMMUNOLOGY

The immune system has two components: (1) An adaptive immune system, and (2) An innate immune system. The adaptive immune system has the following advantages over the innate system:
- Specificity of antigen recognition
- Diversity of the antigen receptor repertoire
- Rapid clonal expansion
- Adaptiveness to the changing environment
- Immunological memory.

Lymphocytes are the primary cells of adaptive immunity; they include T cells, B cells, and natural killer cells.

Innate immune system: provides the first line of defense from infection in a non-specific manner. The innate responses are immediate, non-specific and lack memory. It comprises of epithelial, mucosal and enzymatic barriers. Innate immune system is found in all classes of plants and animals.

Host-Allergen Interaction

After exposure to a potentially allergenic protein, complex interaction happens at receptors on the cell surface via attachment of allergens either independently or with help of certain bacterial compounds (LPS: lipopolysaccharide, LTA: lipoteichoic acid), and the presentation to antigen-presenting cells or APCs (dendritic cells, B cells, monocytes/macrophages and their tissue counterparts) and triggering the immune response (Fig. 3).

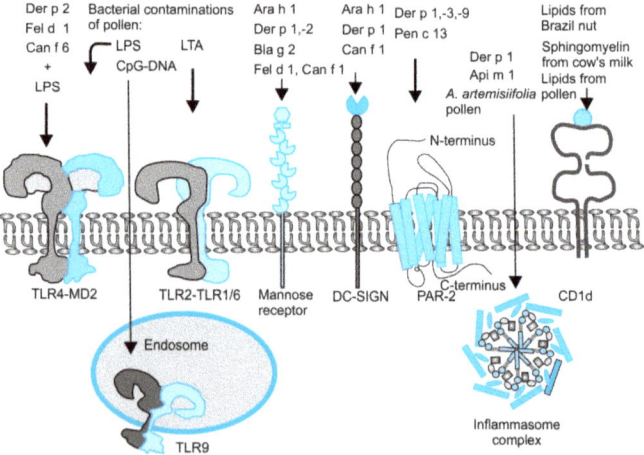

Fig. 3: Allergens acting at various receptors via several mechanisms.
(TLR: toll-like receptors; LPS: lipopolysaccharides; LTA: lipoteichoic acid; PAR: protease-activated receptor)
Various allergens viz. Der p 1, 2, -3, -9 (house-dust mite), Fel d 1 (cat), Can f 1, 6 (dog), Bla g 2 (cockroach), Ara h 1 (peanut), Pen c 13 (mold).
Source: Akdis CA, Agache I. Global Atlas of Allergy. EAACI. 2014.

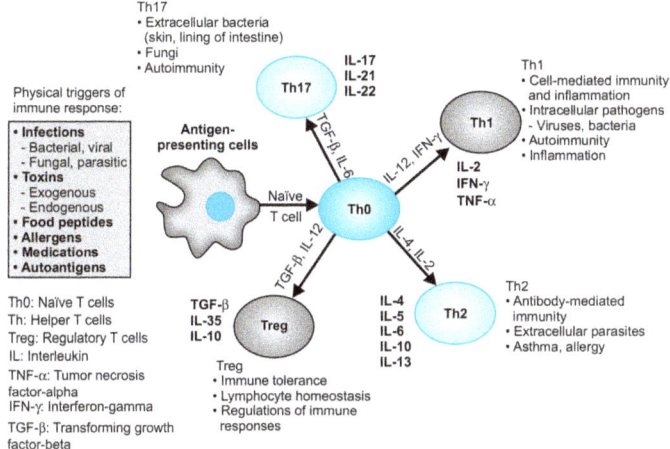

Fig. 4: CD4+ T helper cell differentiation.
Source: Modified from Zhu J, Paul WE. CD4 cells: fates, functions and faults. Blood. 2008;112:1557-69.

Selection of Allergenic Pathway

Antigen-presenting cells like dendritic cells present allergens to CD4+ T helper (Th) cells. These naïve CD4+ Th cells can differentiate into various effector helper cells with distinct capacities, viz. Th1 (induction of cellular immune responses), Th2 (antibody production and allergic response), Th17 (inflammatory responses), and Treg (regulation) cells. Depending upon the various genetic and environmental factors, either Th1 or Th2 response is decided. Th2 cells are induced by IL-4 and further produce various cytokines, which stimulates clonal proliferation of B cells producing plasma cells, leading to IgE production (Fig. 4).

TYPES OF HYPERSENSITIVITY REACTIONS

Hypersensitivity reactions can be grouped into four types depending upon mechanism involved (Fig. 5).

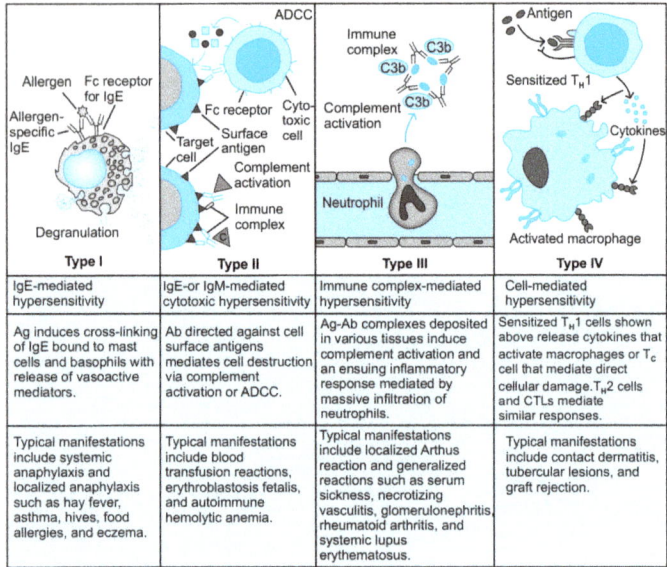

Fig. 5: Types of hypersensitivity reactions.
(ADCC: antibody-dependent cellular cytotoxicity; IgE: immunoglobulin E)
Source: Kuby Immunology, Sixth edition copyright 2007 W.H. Freeman and Company.

Type I (Immediate Type or IgE Mediated)

There are 2 phases in allergy reaction:

1st phase (Sensitization): This happens during the initial exposure of the antigen. The antigen is specially prepared for presentation to the T cell by the Antigen Presnting Cell (APC). The APC will splice up the antigen into small fragments, which then combine with special proteins called Major Histocompatibility Complex (MHC) type 2 (genetic material which helps to distinguish between self and non self). This combined complex, called Epitope, will become visible to the T lymphocyte which recognizes the antigen as 'foreign'. The T cell get activated and become an Effector T cell and produces cytokines namely Interleukin (IL) 4 and IL 13.

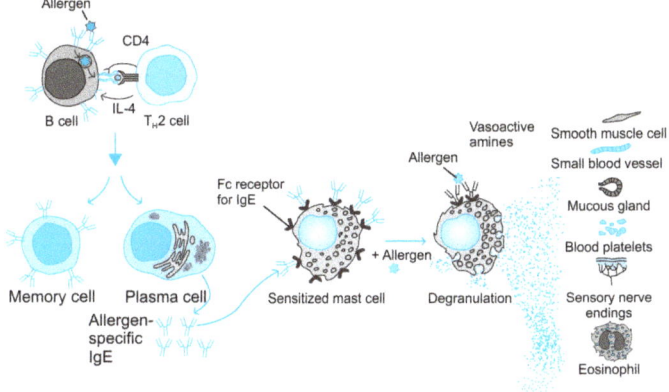

Fig. 6: Type I hypersensitivity reaction.
(IgE: immunoglobulin E)
Source: Kuby Immunology, Sixth edition copyright 2007 W.H. Freeman and Company.

IL 4 and IL 13 will stimulate the neighboring B lymphocytes to produce IgE antibodies thro class switching. The IgE antibodies are released into the circulation as free IgE and also gets bound to the high affinity IgE receptor (F Cepsilon R1) on the surface of the mast cell and basophil. This results in the mast cell being 'armed' and ready to release the mediators if coupled with the specific antigen. This is the state of 'sensitization' (Fig. 6).

2nd phase (Re-exposure): The antigen on re-exposure will be picked up thro coupling reaction by specific IgE antibodies bound on the surface of the mast cells. This reaction generally occurs with the mast cells at the site of entry of the antigen (nose, lungs, skin, eyes, GI tract) where the concentration of the mast cells are highest. The ligation of the cell bound specific IgE antibody by the specific antigen triggers the release of inflammatory lipid mediators, cytokines and chemokines to cause the allergic inflammation at the site of entry.

Type I hypersensitivity is most commonly responsible for clinically relevant allergies. Free IgE release is the basis of total or specific serum IgE testing; whereas bound IgE is responsible for skin prick test or oral and nasal challenge tests.

Common clinical effects of immediate hypersensitivity on various organs will be as:
- Lung—wheezing, dyspnea, and tachypnea
- Nose and eyes—runny nose, redness, and itching of eyes
- Skin—pruritic, vesicular or bullous lesions
- Gastrointestinal tract—vomiting and diarrhea
- Systemic—shock, hypotension, and wheezing
- Brain—behavioral disorders postulated.

Common examples include anaphylaxis, allergic rhinitis, allergic asthma, and atopic dermatitis.

Type II (Antibody-mediated Cytotoxic or Cytolytic)

Antibody reacts directly with the antigen that is bound to the cell membrane to induce cell lysis through complement activation. Hemolytic anemia, hemolytic disease of newborn, blood transfusion reactions, myasthenia gravis, and Goodpasture syndrome are the common examples.

Type III (Immune Complex Mediated)

Antigen and antibodies (IgM and IgG) bind to each other to form antigen-antibody immune complexes which get deposited in blood vessels or other tissues. This deposition causes complement activation and massive infiltration of neutrophils. Arthus reaction, serum sickness, leprosy, glomerulonephritis, necrotizing vasculitis, rheumatoid arthritis, and systemic lupus erythematosus are some of the examples of type III hypersensitivity.

Type IV (Cell-mediated or Delayed Hypersensitivity)

Initiated by T lymphocytes and mediated by Effector T cells and macrophages. The response involves the interaction of the antigens with the surface of the lymphocytes. Sensitized lymphocytes after contact with antigen, release cytokines after 48–72 hours. These cytokines are biologically active and cause inflammation. Common examples include contact dermatitis, fungal infection, tubercular lesions and graft rejection.

PHASES OF TYPE 1 ALLERGIC REACTION

Immediate Phase Reaction

Onset within minutes to initial to 2 hours due to preformed or rapidly synthesized mediators (Fig. 7). Vascular permeability and smooth muscle contraction are the most common effects noticed during this phase. The preformed mediators are:
- Histamine
- Neutral proteases (tryptase, chymase, cathepsin G, and carboxypeptidase)
- Proteoglycans (heparin and chondroitin sulfates)
- Chemotactic and activating factors [eosinophil chemotactic factor (ECF)-A and neutrophil chemotactic factor (NCF)].

Late-phase Reaction

After the chemical mediators of the acute response subside, late-phase responses can often occur (Figs. 8A to C). This is due to the migration of other leukocytes such as neutrophils, lymphocytes, eosinophils, and macrophages to the initial site. The reaction is usually seen 4–6 hours after the initial reaction. Cytokines from

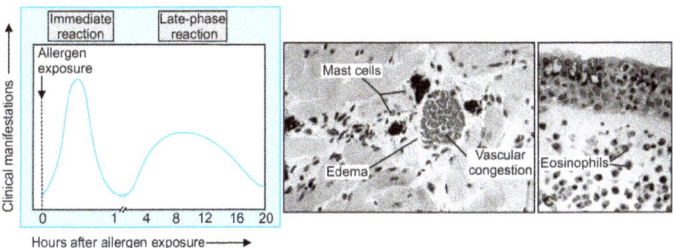

Fig. 7: Time course of allergic reaction.
Source: Downloaded from http://geoffreye-reedlife.blogspot.com/2011/02/hypersensitivity-reactions.html

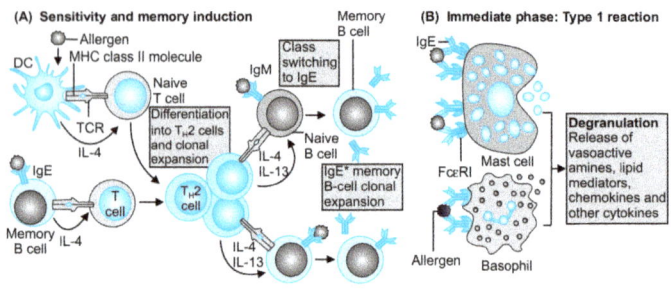

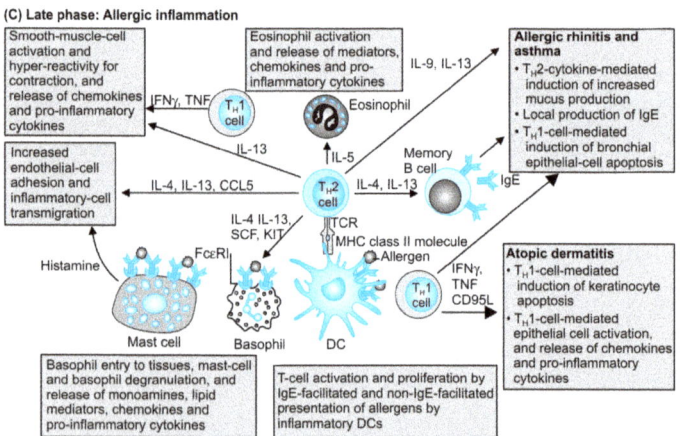

Figs. 8A to C: Various phases of allergic reaction.
(CCL: chemokine ligand; DC: dendritic cell; Ig: immunoglobulin; IL: interleukin; IFN: interferon; TNF: tumor necrosis factor; MHC: major histocompatibility complex; SCF: stem cell factor)
Source: Larche M, Akdis CA, Valenta R. Immunological mechanisms of allergen specific immunotherapy. Nature Reviews Immunol. 2006;6:761-71.

mast cells may play a role in the persistence of long-term effects. Late-phase responses seen in asthma are slightly different from those seen in other allergic responses, although they are still caused by release of mediators from eosinophils and are still dependent on activity of Th2 cells.

There are 2 types of mediators involved:
1. *Preformed*: Tryptase, Chymase, Cathepsin G, Carboxypeptidase, Histamine and Heparin.
2. *Synthesized*: Cytokines (IL 4, IL 13, IL 3, IL 5, GM-CSF, TNF-alpha), Leukotrienes (C4, D4, E4), platelet activating factor (PAF), Chemokine (MIP-1 alpha).

The early phase mediators cause acute inflammation of the allergic reaction with redness, swelling and exudation causing acute symptoms.

The late phase reactions are caused by mediators which are much more potent and cause cell infiltration, vasodilatation, tissue damage causing long term results of tissue damage, ensuing repair and continued cycle of similar events. This results in the so called 'tissue remodelling' characteristic of asthma and related conditions.

Chronic Phase

It occurs due to repetitive or persistent allergen exposure. Innate immune cells (eosinophils, basophils, neutrophils, and monocyte or macrophages) and adaptive immune cells (Th2 cells, other T cells, and B cells) take up residence in the tissues.

PRINCIPAL MEDIATORS INVOLVED IN TYPE I HYPERSENSITIVITY

Primary Mediators and Their Effects

- Histamine, heparin—increased vascular permeability, smooth muscle contraction
- Serotonin—increased vascular permeability, smooth muscle contraction
- Eosinophil chemotactic factor-A—eosinophil chemotaxis
- Neutrophil chemotactic factor-A—neutrophil chemotaxis
- Proteases—bronchial mucus secretion, degradation of blood-vessel basement membrane, generation of complement, and split products.

Secondary Mediators and Their Effects

- Platelet-activating factors—platelet aggregation and degranulation, contraction of pulmonary smooth muscles
- Leukotrienes (slow reactive substance of anaphylaxis)—increased vascular permeability, contraction of pulmonary smooth muscles
- Prostaglandins—vasodilatation, contraction of pulmonary smooth muscles, and platelet aggregation
- Bradykinin—increased vascular permeability, smooth muscle contraction
- Cytokines:
  - Interleukin-1 and tumor necrosis factor-α—systemic anaphylaxis, increased expression of cell adhesion molecules on venular endothelial cells
  - Interleukin-2(IL-2), IL-3, IL-4, IL-5, IL-6, transforming growth factor-β, and granulocyte-macrophage colony-stimulating factor—release of various mediators and direct effects.

GENETICS AND IMMUNE-MEDIATED DISORDERS

There is known association between certain genes and inflammatory disorders including allergy (Fig. 9).

UTILITY OF UNDERSTANDING INTERACTION BETWEEN IMMUNE SYSTEM AND ALLERGEN

It is very important and cucial to understand the basic allergic mechanism. Figure 10 is depicting the choices of management applicable at different levels of 'allergic cascade'.

At the bottom of the cascade, at the tissue level, the most common pharmacological agents (anti-histamines, steroids: systemic and local) are effective. The mast cell stabilisers like Cromolyn sodium and Ketotifen are working at the mast cell level, blocking the degranulation inspite of the copuling reaction of the antigen and specific IgE antibody on its surface.

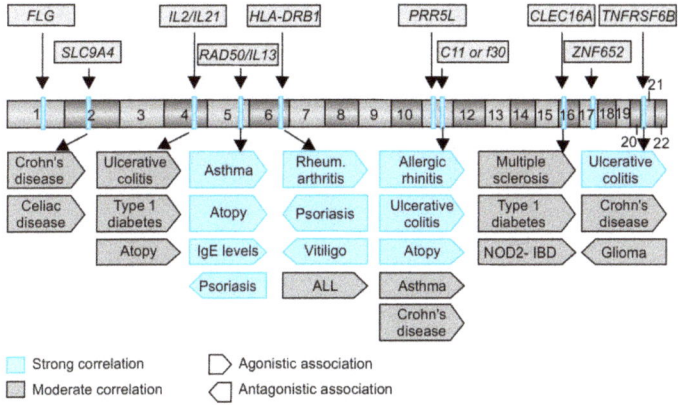

Fig. 9: Interaction between genes and environment.
Source: Akdis CA, Agache I. Global Atlas of Allergy. EAACI. 2014.

Anti-IgE (omalizumab) therapy will bind to the free IgE in circulation and brings down its level, which in turn will also reduce the numbers of F Cepsilon 1 receptors on the surface of the mast cells. Anti-IgE will also competitively block the binding of the specific IgE to the high affinity receptor. Target biologics are available against IL 4, IL 13 and IL 5, which blocks their activity.

Allergen Immunotherapy (AIT) modifies the character of the T cell itself and converts the Th2 (allergic) environment to Th1 (non-allergic). AIT is the only available treatment option that is disease modifying.

CONCLUSION

IgE plays a major role in most of the clinically relevant allergic reactions. Understanding the immunological basis of these disorders helps in allergy testing and effective management with various strategies.

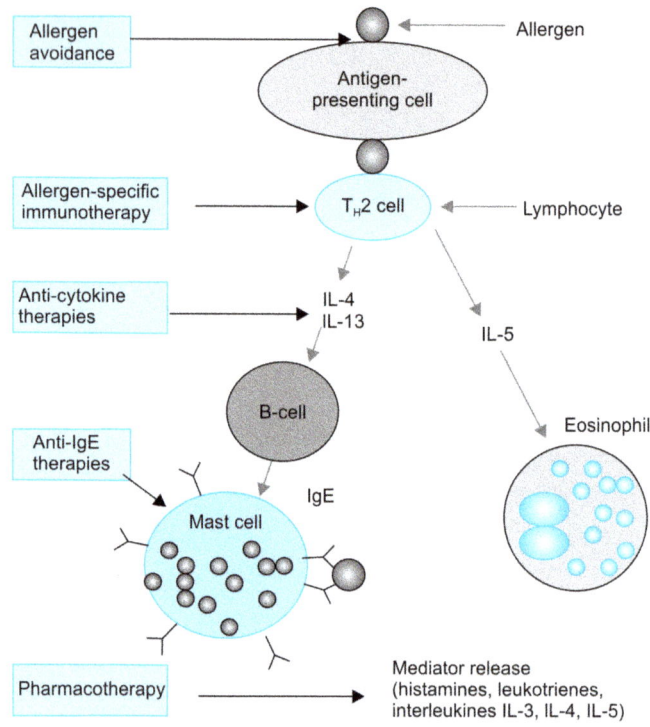

Fig. 10: Allergy immunology and therapeutic options.

SUGGESTED READING

1. Akdis CA, Agache I. Global Atlas of Allergy, EAACI. 2014.
2. Cookson W. The immunogenetics of asthma and eczema: A new focus on the epithelium. Nat Rev Immunol. 2004;4:978-88.
3. Germain RN. T-cell development and the CD4-CD8 lineage decision. Nature Rev Immunol. 2002;2:309-22.
4. Holgate S. Innate and adaptive immune responses in asthma. Nature Medicine. 2012;18:673-83.
5. Holgate ST. A brief history of asthma and its mechanisms to modern concepts of disease pathogenesis. Allergy Asthma Immunol Res. 2010;2:165-71.

Aerobiology

INTRODUCTION

Aerobiology involves the study of airborne particles of plant and animal origin. These bioparticles, when come in contact with sensitized human being, may be taken as foreign substance and thus trigger the hypersensitivity reaction. Major causative agents implicated are pollen grains, fungal spores, dust mites, insect debris, and animal epithelia. Their role in environmental pollution and disease is known for centuries but the term "aerobiology" was coined by FC Meir, a plant pathologist, in 1930. The primary objective of aerobiological studies is to monitor, determine, and detect occurrence of pollen and spores and their relative representation in the atmosphere.

Pollens are the common bioparticles released from various sources, viz. tree, grass, weed, etc. These are responsible for pollination, fertilization, seed and fruit setting, and multiplication of plants. Pollen grains have been attributed to summer catarrh and hay fever since 18th century. India is blessed with the richest flora on the earth. Pollens are proportionally more in number and variety than any other part of the world, with heterogeneous distribution across the country. Study of airborne pollen grains and fungal spores is called "Palynology". Medical palynology is concerned with the study of airborne pollen and fungal spores, responsible for causing medical diseases like allergies.

Aerobiological pathways involve five steps: Source, liberation, passive transport, deposition, and impact of pollen and spores on various substrates. Each step can be affected by surrounding environmental conditions. There could be various ways of pollen dispersal, among which wind dispersal is the most important route for causing aeroallergies.

BASIC AEROBIOLOGY

Plants can be classified as anemophilous (wind as vehicle), entomophilous (insects as vehicle), and amphiphilous (wind or insects as vehicle) based on the mode of pollination. Anemophilous plants are commonly responsible for allergic manifestations as pollens remain air borne for a longer time and can travel for long distances from the original source. The common pollen sources could be grasses, trees, and weeds. Pollen formation and liberation has a specific pattern and season for every source and a pollen calendar can be constructed for different localities based upon the knowledge of palynology.

In general, pollen production is not only controlled by its size, but also by genetic and physiologic factors. Average pollen production per flower for *Acacia mangium* is reported to be highest (16,640), followed by *Acacia auriculiformis* (15,360), *Mimosa invisa* (12,800), and *Albizia falcataria* (12,288). The pollen loss is higher for trees due to their height, so this loss is compensated by increased production, causing more allergies. Smaller the pollen size, more travel and stay time in air, more chances of allergy. Particles larger than about 5 μm diameter are deposited largely in the nose and are unlikely to penetrate in the lung. Pollen release and greater dispersal depends a lot upon weather conditions and time of the day for different species. Pollens can travel great distance depending upon their physical characteristics and environmental conditions. Pollen concentration increases with increasing wind speed. In gusty winds, these particles may be swept into the upper atmosphere and resettle toward the ground during evening hours, increasing the exposure. Pollens of *Pinus* can travel 600–1000 km from coastal areas of Greenland. *Cedrus deodara* (Cedar) pollen can travel from the Himalayan region up to Lucknow in northern India. Brisk rainfall with or without thunderstorms do not reduce the airborne pollen and spore levels, while long periods of rainfall lead to reduced allergen level in the atmosphere. The knowledge about pollination season and mode of dispersal is important for an allergist to attribute clinical features in an allergic patient to

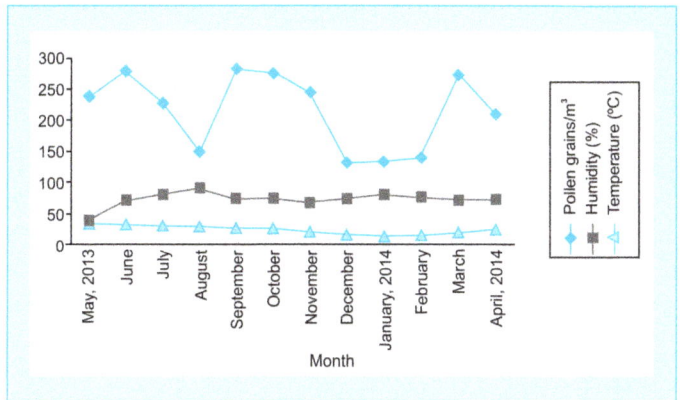

Fig. 1: Mean pollen, temperature, and humidity level variation in 1 year (May 2013 to April 2014).

Source: Kumar R, Kumar M, Robinson K, et al. Atmospheric pollen count in North Delhi region. Indian J Allergy Asthma Immunol. 2015;29:32-9.

a particular pollen. Figure 1 shows monthly variation in pollen counts along with annual changes in temperature and humidity level in Delhi.

Normally, anemophilous pollens are significant for allergy as they are predominant in the air. However, there are some entomophilus plants emitting pollen in the immediate vicinity, causing allergy. *Carica papaya* (Papaya) with heavy pollen is entomophilus. Airborne pollens of entomophilous avenue trees of *Dolichandrone platycalyx* have been reported for allergic symptoms in Mysore and Bengaluru, India.

PRINCIPAL COLLECTION METHODS

- *Passive collection*: Samples are collected from fallout on a fixed surface through gravitational force on a coated slide or open petri dish containing agar (settle plate) for a set period of time. It is simplest, least expensive but least accurate method of pollen collection. It is nonquantitative and affected by pollen size, shape, and air movement. Results are biased toward heavier and larger particles giving false-negative reports for smaller relevant pollens (like *Morus* and *Urtica*) and spores (like *Penicillium* and *Aspergillus*). Due to many fallacies, this technique is not recommended.

- *Impaction technique*: Impaction samplers use inertia of the particles to help in separating various pollens. Particles are deposited on solid or agar surface as per their inertial properties with the passage of air stream. This can be achieved by suction or rotating arm impactors. Various types of impaction sampling devices are available for indoor and outdoor sampling purpose with different pore sizes (Table 1).
- *Impingement technique*: This technique also works on the basis of inertial properties but separated particles are deposited into a liquid-collecting medium. As liquid evaporates during prolonged sampling, most samplers, like AGI-30, are only useful for shorter duration of maximum 1 hour. Newer bio-samplers (like SKC) permit longer sampling by using nonevaporating fluids.
- *Filtration technique*: Particles are trapped in a fibrous or porous substrate. These can range from small, personal-cassette samplers (for individual use) to large, high-volume samplers. Collection efficiency depends upon filter pore size and airflow.
- *Other collection methods*: Not widely used:
  - Electrostatic precipitation—charged particles are attracted to opposite charge on a collector plate
  - Thermal precipitation
  - Cyclone sampling.

SAMPLING INSTRUMENTS

- *Spore trap slit impactors*: Airborne particles (pollens and spores) are impacted, as per their inertia, on either tape or a microscope slide. Time-discriminate sampling happens over standard 7-day or an alternate 24-hour lid, which is later analyzed for daily or

Table 1: Commonly available impaction sampling devices.

Collection method	Sampler	d_{50} (μm)	Comments
Slit impaction	Burkard spore traps (Figs. 2A and B)	3.7	1-day and 7-day sampling heads available
	Lanzoni VPPS 2000	—	Wind oriented and allows time-discriminate sampling
	Burkard continuous recording sampler	5	Allows for time discrimination. Not wind oriented, so more suitable for indoors
	Allergenco MK-3	2	Programmable sampling and small particle efficiency. Not wind oriented, so more suitable for indoors
	Burkard personal sampler	2.5	Single-grab sample for total spores and pollen. Battery operated
	Air-O-Cell cassette	2.6	Single-grab sample for total spores and pollen. Easy to sample and analyze
	Cyclex-d	2	Single-grab sample for total spores and pollen
Rotating-arm impaction	Rotorod sampler (Fig. 3)	10	Independent of wind speed and direction. Easy to use and efficient for pollen sampling
Culture plate impaction	Andersen 6-stage (Fig. 4)	7.0 for stage 1 to 0.65 for stage 6	Sieve impactor. Only for culturable fungi able to grow on medium used
	Burkard sampler for agar plates	4	Sieve impactor. Only for culturable fungi able to grow on medium used. Battery operated
	SAS	1.5 to 2.0	Sieve impactor. Only for culturable fungi able to grow on medium used
	Biotest RCS	7.5	Centrifugal sampler with collection onto agar strips. Only for culturable fungi able to grow on medium used

d_{50}—cut size. This is the particle diameter at which 50% of the particles are collected. Due to a sharp cut-off, all larger particles are collected. d_{50} is one of the most commonly used parameter for sampler performance. A d_{50} of 5 μm means that sampler efficiency drops significantly for particles smaller than 5 μm.

Source: Levetin E. Methods for aeroallergen sampling. Curr Allergy Asthma Rep. 2004;4(5): 376-83.

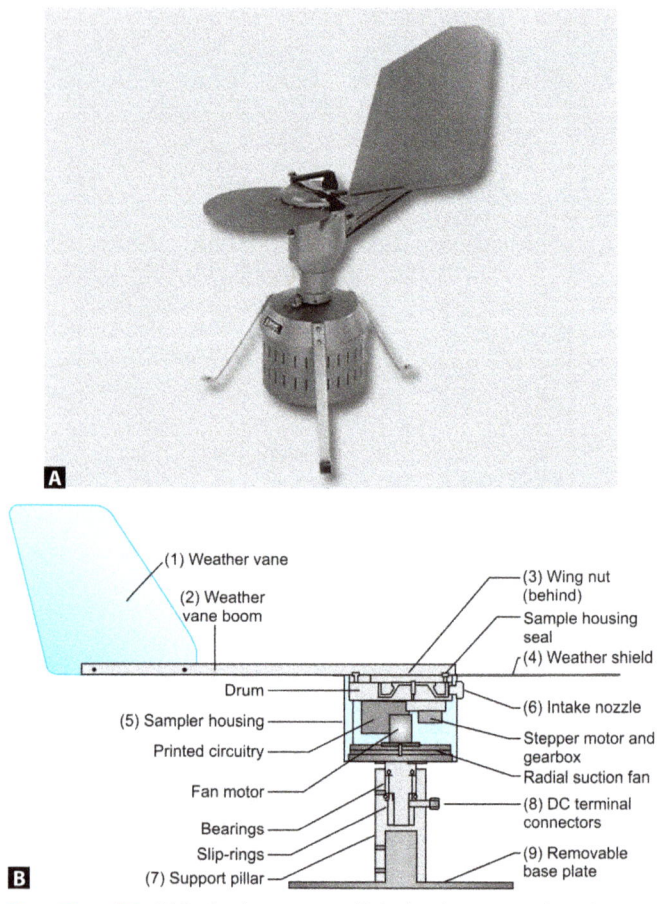

Figs. 2A and B: (A) Burkard spore trap; (B) Burkard spore trap line diagram.
Source: Kumar R, Kumar M, Robinson K, et al. Atmospheric pollen count in North Delhi region. Indian J Allergy Asthma Immunol. 2015;29:32-9.

weekly pollen report and thus pollen calendar. Burkard spore trap (Figs. 2A and B) and Air-O-Cell sampling cassettes work as slit impactors.

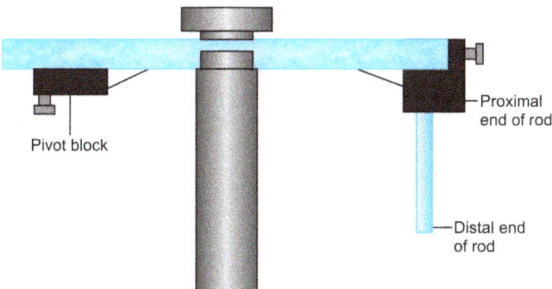

Fig. 3: Rotorod sampler model.
Source: Downloaded from internet.

- *Portable spore traps*: These are suitable for both indoor and outdoor collection purpose. This includes Allergenco (Samplair) MK-3 and Burkard continuous air sampler with d_{50} of 2.52 µm.
- *Rotating arm impactors*: These are battery driven, used for intermittent sampling (30–60 seconds every 10 minutes). This sampler is convenient to use and has good efficiency for pollen and large fungal spores of larger than 10 µm. Sampling efficiency decreases over time due to overloading of exposed rods. Rotorod samplers (Fig. 3) are commonly available in the market.
- *Sieve impactors*: These work on the basis of culture plate sampling. These can be used for airborne fungi and bacteria in both outdoor and indoor settings. Disadvantage with this technique is possibility of multiple impaction on the agar beneath a single hole, which may be counted as single colony. Andersen sampler (Fig. 4) is an example of sieve impactor.
- *Personal samplers*: These can be useful for precise estimation of one's exposure to aeroallergens. These can also be used at workplace for compliance assessment with permissible exposure limits. Personal samplers are small portable units with disposable filter, working at low flow rates of 2 L/min, which can be worn for many hours. Button aerosol sampler is wind insensitive and suitable for both indoors and outdoors. Nasal air sampler can detect particles of size 5 µm and more with minimal discomfort to patients.

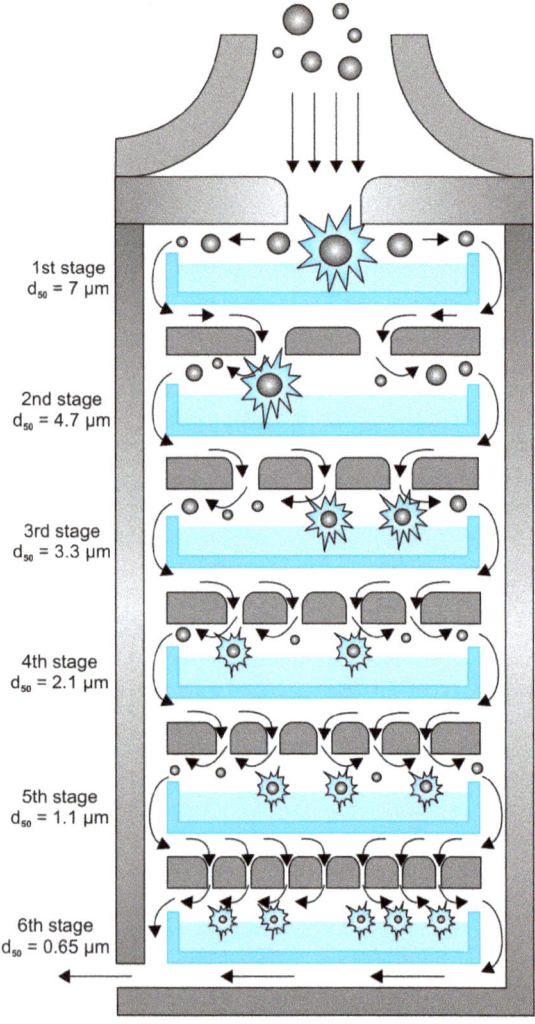

Fig. 4: Andersen 6-stage sampler.
Source: Downloaded from internet.

METHODS OF ANALYSIS

Various methods (Table 2) can be used to analyze the collected material and that helps in making pollen calendar for that area.

Pollination calendar: It indicates the characteristics of plants, which includes time, duration, and nature of flowering. It is important for a botanist or aerobiologist.

Pollen calendar: It tells us about the types of air-borne pollen and mold spores and their concentration in the atmosphere. It concerns the occurrence, abundance, and decline of pollen and

Table 2: Methods to analyze air samples.

Method	Sampler types used with	Comments
Microscopy	Slit impactors, liquid impingers, filter samples	Pollen and total spores identification. These do not permit species identification
Culturing	Sieve impactors, liquid impingers, filter samples	Allow species identification. Only for viable organisms as these can grow on culture media
Biochemistry	Slit impactors, liquid impingers, filter samples	Estimate of total fungal biomass or identification of specific mycotoxins
Immunochemistry	Slit impactors, liquid impingers, filter samples	Specific assay for allergens. Availability for limited allergens
Molecular biology (PCR)	Slit impactors, liquid impingers, filter samples	Detect specific DNA sequences. Limited use till now
Flow cytometry	Liquid impingers	Rapid analysis for quantifying total spores or pollen. Limited use in aerobiology
Image analysis	Slit impactors, liquid impingers	Rapid analysis for spore and pollen identification. It can eliminate the need for microscopy. It is still in early stage of development

Source: Levetin E. Methods for aeroallergen sampling. Curr Allergy Asthma Rep. 2004;4(5): 376-83.

spores in the atmosphere, which is compiled by aerobiologist by using pollen traps or continuous air samplers. It is important for allergist or allergologists.

Synergism between aerobiologist and allergist is essential to make customized pollen calendar for the particular region that will help in correctly identifying the offending allergen/s and implementing specific avoidance and therapeutic measures. Only relevant allergen needs to be tested on the patients, among the many, that are commercially available in allergy kits with various manufacturers. Table 3 depicts common aeroallergens across India.

Different regions of India have different pollens responsible for allergic symptoms. Tables 4 and 5 summarize important pollen and fungal allergens with geographic distribution, respectively.

LOCALIZED DISTRIBUTION OF FUNGAL ALLERGENS

- Outdoor fungal flora: *Aspergilli-Penicilli, Cladosporium, Helminthosporium, Epicoccum, Drechslera, Alternaria, Curvularia, Ascospores,* and *Nigrospora*
- Indoor fungal flora: *Aspergilli-Penicilli, Cladosporium,* and *moniliaceous* fungi
- Bakery: *Aspergilli-Penicilli* spores
- Granary: *Aspergillus, Cladosporium, Rhizopus, Curvularia, Epicoccum,* and *Alternaria*
- Poultry: *Aspergilli-penicilli, Cladosporium, Candida albicans,* and *Scopulariopsis*
- Sugar industry: *Cladosporium, Aspergillus, Epicoccum, Saccharomyces,* and smut spores
- Library: *Cladosporium, Penicillium, Paecilomyces,* and *Aspergillus*
- Cattle shed: *Aspergillus (niger* and *flavus) and Cladosporium*
- Residential houses: *Cladosporium, Aspergillus, and Rhizopus*
- Occupational setting: *Aspergillus, Cladosporium, Alternaria, Uromyces, Ustilago, Neurospora,* and *Sporotrichum*
- Crop fields: *Alternaria.*

Table 3: Common aeroallergens in different seasons in India.

Seasons		
Spring (Feb–April)	**Autumn (Sept–Oct)**	**Winter (Nov–Jan)**
Tree pollens		
Ailanthus excelsa	Anogeissus pendula	Cassia siamea
Holoptelea integrifolia	Eucalyptus sp.	Cedrus deodara
Casuarina equisetifolia	Cedrus deodara	Mallotus philippensis
Prosopis juliflora	Cocos nucifera	Salvadora persica
Mallotus philippensis	Prosopis juliflora	Quercus incana
Putranjiva roxburghii	Mallotus philippensis	
Bauhinia variegata	Phoenix sylvestris	
Quercus incana	Quercus incana	
Grass pollens		
Cynodon dactylon	Bothriochloa pertusa	Cynodon dactylon
Dichanthium annulatum	Cenchrus ciliaris	Eragrostis tenella
Imperata cylindrica	Heropogon contortus	Poa annua
Polypogon monspeliensis	Pennisetum typhoides	Phalaris minor
Paspalum distichum	Sorghum vulgare	
Poa annua		
Weed pollens		
Cannabis sativa	Amaranthus spinosus	Ageratum conyzoides
Chenopodium murale	Artemisia scoparia	Argemone mexicana
Parthenium spp.	Cassia occidentalis	Chenopodium album
Suaeda fruticosa	Ricinus communis	Asphodelus tenuifolius
Plantago major	Xanthium strumarium	Ricinus communis

Source: Gill NK, Kumar K, Rai NK. Risk assessment of outdoor airborne biological allergens in India: a review. JEZS. 2017;5(4):1069-75.

IMPORTANT CHARACTERISTICS OF RELEVANT POLLEN ALLERGENS

- *Acacia arabica*:
    - Local name: *Gursoonder, Desi babul, Babool, Kikar,* and Indian gum arabic tree

Table 4: Clinically relevant pollen allergens of different regions in India.

S. No.	Name of allergen	Habitat	North	South	East	West
1.	Ailanthus	T	+	−	−	+
2.	Alnus	T	+	−	+	−
3.	Argemone	W	+	−	−	−
4.	Artemisia	W	+	+	+	+
5.	Azadirachta	T	+	−	−	−
6.	Borassus	T	−	−	−	+
7.	Brassica	W	+	−	+	+
8.	Cassia	T	+	+	−	−
9.	Casuarina	T	−	−	+	−
10.	Cedrus	T	+	−	+	−
11.	Chenopodium album	W	+	−	+	−
12.	Cocos	T	−	+	+	−
13.	Cynodon	G	+	+	+	+
14.	Dodonaea	W	+	−	−	−
15.	Holoptelea	T	+	−	−	+
16.	Mallotus	T	+	−	−	+
17.	Morus	T	+	−	−	+
18.	Parthenium	W	−	−	+	−
19.	Pennisetum	G	+	−	+	−
20.	Phoenix	T	−	+	+	+
21.	Prosopis	T	+	−	−	−
22.	Salvadora	T	+	−	−	−
23.	Sorghum	G	+	−	−	−
24.	Syzygium	T	−	+	−	−
25.	Xanthium	W	+	−	−	+

(G: grass; T: tree; W: weed)
North India: Jammu and Kashmir, Himachal Pradesh, Haryana, Punjab, Rajasthan, Delhi, and Union Territory of Chandigarh
West India: Gujarat, Maharashtra, and Goa
South India: Andhra Pradesh, Karnataka, Kerala, Tamil Nadu, and the Union Territory of Puducherry
East India: Bihar, West Bengal, Odisha, Jharkhand, Andaman and Nicobar Islands
Source: Gill NK, Kumar K, Rai NK. Risk assessment of outdoor airborne biological allergens in India: a review. JEZS. 2017;5(4):1069-75.

Table 5: Clinically relevant fungal allergens of different regions in India.

S. No.	Name of allergen	North	South	East	West
1.	Alternaria	+	−	+	+
2.	Ascospores	−	+	−	−
3.	Aspergilli	+	+	−	+
4.	Candida	+	+	+	+
5.	Cladosporium	+	+	+	+
6.	Curvularia	+	+	+	+
7.	Helminthosporium	+	+	−	+
8.	Mucor	+	+	−	+
9.	Nigrospora	+	−	−	+
10.	Phoma	+	−	+	−
11.	Smuts	+	+	−	+
12.	Uredospores	−	+	−	−

Source: Gill NK, Kumar K, Rai NK. Risk assessment of outdoor airborne biological allergens in India: a review. JEZS. 2017;5(4):1069-75.

- Perennial shrub or tree (2.5–20 meters tall); dark black-colored stem; branchlets are purple-brown; bark is thin, rough, fissured, deep red-brown; spines (thorns) are thin, straight, light-gray in axillary pairs in young trees; mature trees are without thorns; and leaves are bipinnate
- Flowers: Golden-yellow, fragrant, in globus heads; deep sutures between the seeds giving "string of pearls" appearance; seeds deep darkish brown, smooth, subcircular
- Flowers in rainy season
- Distribution: Rajasthan, UP, Chennai, and West Bengal
- Sensitization: Mild.

- *Ageratum conyzoides*:
  - Local name: *Nilam*, *Tambakoo*, and Billygoat weed
  - Erect, hairy, branching, soft slightly aromatic annual herb (1 meter height); stems often purplish; leaves are egg shaped with broad end at base (ovate) up to 7.5 cm long
  - Flowers: Purple, blue, pinkish or white, less than 6 mm; 30–50 flowers arranged in close terminal—flower-heads

- Flowering season: January to June
- Distribution: Delhi, Punjab, UP, Bihar, West Bengal, North Eastern region, Maharashtra, Andhra Pradesh, and Karnataka
- Sensitization: Moderate.

- *Ailanthus excelsa*:
  - Local name: *Urru*, *Aralu*, Indian tree of heaven
  - Large deciduous tree (18–25 meters tall); straight trunk; light grey and smooth bark, aromatic, slightly bitter; large leaves (30–60 cm); leaflets 8–14 or more, long stalked, ovate or lance shaped, 6–10 cm long
  - Flowers: Clusters droop at leaf base, greenish yellow with ill smell, found commonly along roadsides
  - Flowering season: January to March
  - Anemophilous and Entomophilous
  - Distribution: All over India
  - Sensitization: Wild range.

- *Albizia lebbeck*:
  - Local name: Siras, Siris, and Woman's tongue tree
  - Medium or large size (18–30 meters); deciduous tree with gray trunk; leaves bi/paripinnate, 6–18 pinna on leaflet
  - Flowers: Pale yellow, fragrant
  - Flowering season: April to July
  - Distribution: Delhi, Punjab, UP, Bihar, Madhya Pradesh, Andhra Pradesh, West Bengal, and Karnataka
  - Sensitization: Moderate.

- *Alnus nitida*:
  - Local name: Gray alder
  - Deciduous tree up to 20 meters, sometimes shrubby; bark is smooth, pale gray; leaves are elliptic, velvety, and hairy
  - Flowers: Male and female flowers on same tree; male flowers set in brownish, drooping catkins
  - Flowering season: Early spring

- Distribution: Almorah, Shillong, Dehradun, UP (hilly areas), and North Eastern region
- Sensitization: Highly allergenic.
- *Amaranthus spinosus*:
  - Local name: *Kanta-nuteeya*, *Kantewali chaulai*, *Kante bhaji*, and Needle burr
  - Red tinged erect or ascending spinous herb or undershrub (30–150 cm); leaves ovate to rhombic; grows as weed in fields, gardens or on roadsides in wasteland; used in cattle fodder
  - Flowers: Green, unisexual, in dense globose or axillary clusters
  - Flowering season: During and after rainy season
  - Distribution: All over India
  - Sensitization: Wide range.
- *Argemone mexicana*:
  - Local name: *Siyal-kanta*, *Brahmadandi*, *Bharband*, *Satyanashi*, Mexican poppy, and Prickly poppy
  - Prickly, hairless, branching herb with yellow juice; leaves are thistlelike, stem-clasping, oblong, multi-cut, spiny with white veins; occurs as wasteland weed
  - Flowers: Yellow with red stigma and black seeds
  - Flowering season: October to April
  - Anemophilous
  - Distribution: All over India
  - Sensitization: Wide range.
- *Artemisia vulgaris*:
  - Local name: Mugwort, Nagdona, and common wormwood
  - Coarse perennial herb with erect, often reddish, angled stems (50–180 cm); pinnately lobed leaves, smooth and green on upper side and white and downy beneath
  - Flowers: Reddish-brownish erect heads in dense leafy structures
  - Flowering season: July to September

- Anemophilous
- Distribution: Delhi, Tirupati, Aligarh, Mumbai, and Lucknow
- Sensitization: Moderate.
- *Asphodelus tenuifolius*:
  - Local name: *Piazi*, Bokat, and *Jungle piyaz*
  - Erect glabrous herb; root yellowish in young plant and dark brown at maturity; fibrous roots twist to give a rope-like appearance; numerous leaves
  - Flowers: White with pink or purple stripe; petals 1.5 cm long in six perianth segments; stamens six; normally flowers do not open until late afternoon and unless conditions are dull and cool and will close before the next day
  - Flowering season: July to October
  - Distribution: Delhi, Punjab, and Shimla
  - Sensitization: Mild.
- *Azadirachta indica*:
  - Local name: *Neem*
  - Fast-growing tree (15–20 meters), evergreen; bark is hard, fissured or scaly, whitish-gray to reddish-brown; sapwood is greyish-white; 20–40 cm long alternate pinnate leaves, 20–31 medium to dark green leaflets
  - Flowers: White fragrant; inflorescences branch up to the third degree, bear 150–250 flowers
  - Fruits: Glabrous olive-like
  - Flowering season: March to May
  - Entomophilous
  - Distribution: State tree of Andhra Pradesh, Aurangabad, Tirupati, Lucknow, Kolkata, Jaipur, and Mumbai
  - Sensitization: Mild.
- *Betula utilis*:
  - Local name: Silver birch, *Bhojpatra*
  - Single stemmed, deciduous tree up to 25 meters; bark smooth, silvery-white above, peeling near the base of the trunk to black; ovate leaves turn yellow in autumn

- Flowers: Male and female flowers in the same tree; male flowers are in cylindrical drooping yellow-brown catkins
- Flowering season: Late spring
- Anemophilous
- Distribution: Almorah, Dehradun, and Shillong
- Sensitization: Mild to moderate.
- *Borassus flabellifer*:
  - Local name: *Tal*, *Tal-gaha*, Toddy palm, *Taalah*, *Karimpana*, *Tala*, *Taad*, and *Trinaraaj*
  - 15–30 meters height, stem unbranched; leaves 25–40, leathery, gray green, fan-shaped, 1–3 meter wide, strong stalk, are edged with hard spines
  - Flower: Big clusters of long, white string-like inflorescences
  - Fruits: Coconut-like, three sides when young, later on rounded or oval
  - Flowering season: January to May
  - Distribution: Howrah (Kolkata) and Calicut
  - Sensitization: Moderate.
- *Brassica campestris*:
  - Local name: *Sarson*, Mustard
  - Erect, tall (30–100 cm), annual herb; alternate leaves; root tuberous or fusiform
  - Flowers: Bright yellow with yellowish-brown seeds
  - Flowering season: January to April
  - Distribution: Delhi, Punjab, and UP (plains)
  - Sensitization: Highly allergenic and cross-reactive to other species.
- *Cannabis sativa*:
  - Local name: *Ganja*, *Bhang*, and *Gunjika*
  - Erect annual herb (5 meter); basal leaves opposite, upper leaves alternate, 10 cm long, 1.5 cm broad; common in waste grounds and in undergrowth of fruit orchards
  - Flowers: Monoecious or dioecious; male flowers in axillary and terminal panicles, with five yellowish petals and five

poricidal stamens; female plants crowded with leafy bracts; brown, shiny fruit
- Flowering season: In cold season
- Anemophilous
- Distribution: All over India
- Sensitization: Varied (mild to high).
- *Cassia fistula*:
  - *Sonali, Soodali, Ahilla, Cakay*, Golden shower tree, and *Kennekai*
  - Moderate size (30–40 inches) deciduous tree with thick yellowish gray bark; pinnate compound leaves with 4–8 pairs of leaflets per leaf; occurs in cultivated gardens and lawns
  - Flowers: Five-petaled, bright yellow, lightly scented flowers in long drooping
  - Flowering season: April to July
  - Entomophilous
  - Distribution: Aurangabad, Bengaluru, Tirupati, Kolkata, Bhopal, Delhi, and Aligarh
  - Sensitization: Moderate.
- *Casuarina equisetifolia*:
  - Local name: *Kasagaha*, Beefwood tree, and *Vilayati jhau*
  - Narrow, tall (30 meters), leafless, weak tree with drooping branches; reddish-brown to gray bark; branchlets resemble pine needles
  - Flowers: Cylindrical male spikes at end of branches; female flowers in globose or ovoid
  - Fruits: Contained in woody, cone-like structure
  - Flowering season: March to May
  - Distribution: Delhi and Bangalore
  - Sensitization: Moderate.
- *Cenchrus ciliaris*:
  - Local name: *Anjhan, Anjan*
  - Tufted, erect or decumbent perennial plant, 15–120 cm tall, with a knotty crown; blades are green to bluish-green

- Flowers: Racemes cylindrical, dense, pale or purplish; flowers are solitary, surrounded by numerous bristles
- Flowering season: July to September after rains
- Distribution: All over India
- Sensitization: Highly allergenic.
- *Cedrus deodara*:
  - Local name: *Dabdaru*, *Devadaru*, *Devdar*, *Babula*, *Gunduguragi*, and *Tevadaru*
  - Large evergreen coniferous tree up to 40–50 meters tall and 3-meter diameter, with spreading horizontal branches; conical crown in young and rounded in old; blue-green needles
  - Flowers: Solitary cylindrical purplish male cones at the tips of dwarf shoots; solitary, erect female cones at the terminal end of shoots, young cones are greenish, mature cones are brown, barrel-shaped
  - Flowering season: August to December
  - Distribution: Himalayas from Kashmir to Garhwal
  - Sensitization: Mild to moderate.
- *Chenopodium album*:
  - Local name: *Beto-sag*, *Bathua*
  - Erect herb (10–150 cm), variously branched, green or coated with white, mealy granular pubescence; stems are yellowish-green striated; leaves are variable in size, toothed or lobed, rhombic-oblong or deltoid-ovate
  - Flowers: Inflorescence in terminal and axillary clusters, forming compact, panicled spikes
  - Flowering season: August to December and October to January
  - Distribution: All over India
  - Sensitization: Mild to highly allergenic.
- *Cocos nucifera*:
  - Local name: *Narikel*, *Nariyal*, and *Narikela*
  - Tall trunk (20–30 meters); smooth and gray bark, marked by ringed scars; pinnate leaves, 4–6 meter long, bright green leaflets

- Flowers: Bear lanceolate petals, 6 stamens and ovary contains 3 connate carpels
- Fruits: Large (30 cm long, 1–2 kg), thin smooth gray-brownish epicarp, contains one seed which is partially liquid (coconut milk), partly solid (flesh)
- Flowering season: Round the year
- Distribution: Maharashtra and West Bengal
- Sensitization: Highly allergenic.

- *Coriandrum sativum*:
  - Local name: *Dhunya*, *Dhania*, Coriander, and *Danga*
  - Strongly smelling herb; mature seeds aromatic (sweet–spicy fragrance); fern-like finely divided upper leaves
  - Flowers: Purplish to white in loose compound umbels
  - Flowering season: December to April
  - Distribution: Dehradun
  - Sensitization: Mild.

- *Cynodon dactylon*:
  - Local name: Bermuda grass, Doob ghas
  - Long rapid-growing (20 meters), creeping, perennial grass; leaves are 2.5–20 cm, flat or folded
  - Flowers: Inflorescence digitate, 2–12 spikes arranged star-like at apex of stem
  - Flowering season: Late summer (July to October)
  - Anemophilous
  - Distribution: Delhi, Dehradun, Kanpur, Bhopal, Aligarh, Lucknow, Jaipur, Bengaluru, and Tirupati
  - Sensitization: Highly allergenic.

- *Dodonaea viscosa*:
  - Local name: *Vilayati mehndi*
  - Evergreen shrub or small tree (2–8 meters); gray bark; branchlets are rusty red and sticky; shiny leaves (5–10 cm), round or pointed tip; black seeds
  - Flowers: Greenish yellow; brown stamens
  - Flowering season: June to December

- Distribution: Jammu & Kashmir, Himachal Pradesh, Delhi, and Lucknow
- Sensitization: Highly allergic.
- *Eucalyptus* spp.
  - Local name: Blue gum, *Safeda*
  - Evergreen tall grown trees up to 100 meters; leathery leaves, opposite, sessile, cordate-ovate and covered with a bluish white bloom; adult leaves are alternate, 6–12 inches long and 1–2 inches broad
  - Flowers: Cream colored flowers, petals are united to form a cap which drops during flowering, leaving numerous colored stamens free
  - Fruit: Surrounded by a woody, cup-shaped receptacle and contains numerous minute seeds
  - Flowering season: Round the year
  - Distribution: Hot, arid regions from different parts of India
  - Sensitization: Moderate.
- *Gynandropsis gynandra*:
  - Local name: *Hulhul*, *Kathal*, *Safed Bagro*, Spider flower, Cat's whiskers, African spider flower, and Bastard mustard
  - Erect, aromatic, annual herb, covered in glandular hairs; leaves palmate with 3–5 leaflets
  - Flowers: White to fading pinkish on a long stalk; stamens purple
  - Flowering season: August to October
  - Distribution: Delhi, Punjab, Rajasthan, UP, and Central India
  - Sensitization: Moderate.
- *Holoptelea integrifolia*:
  - Local name: Chilbil, *Papri*, Indian elm, and Kanju
  - Large deciduous tree (18 meters); gray bark, covered with blisters; leaves alternate, elliptic-ovate, 8–13 cm long and 3.2–6.3 cm wide; leaf base rounded or heart-shaped; unpleasant odor from crushed leaves. Found commonly along roadsides

- Flowers: Small greenish-yellow to brownish in numerous fascicles; velvety sepals
- Fruit: Circular, 2.5 cm diameter, membranous net-veined wings; flat seeds
- Flowering season: February to March
- Entomophilous
- Distribution: All over India
- Sensitization: Mild to highly allergenic.

- *Imperata* spp. *(Cylindrica)*:
  - Local name: *Bhurighas*, Cogon grass, cotton wool grass, silver spike, and sword grass
  - Erect, slender grass, 60 cm or less; leaves linear, flat (about 2 cm wide), narrow at apex, mid-rib white, upper surface hairy, underside hairless
  - Flowers: Silvery, spike like, cylindrical dense; orange anthers
  - Flowering season: June to October
  - Distribution: Delhi and other parts of North India
  - Sensitization: Moderate to high.

- *Lolium perenne*:
  - Local name: Ryegrass
  - Wiry, loosely tufted perennial grass up to 50 cm; smooth stem and leaves; culms light green, hairless; alternate leaves on lower-third of culm; leaf blades are 2–5 mm and 6 inches long, medium to dark green, hairless; leaf blades have ear-like basal lobes (whitened auricles) at their base
  - Flowers: Glumes of spikelets are usually alternate on two sides of a stalk, spikelets change color from light green to light tan on maturity
  - Flowering season: Most part of summer
  - Anemophilous
  - Distribution: Dehradun and Himachal Pradesh
  - Sensitization: Highly allergenic.

- *Mallotus philippensis*:
  - Local name: *Kamala* tree, Monkey face tree, *Rohan*, and *Kesari*
  - Shrub or small branched evergreen tree (up to 10 meters); ovate-rhombic, alternate, rusty-velvety leaves
  - Flowers: In spike with globose capsule, covered with a bright crimson layer of minute, easily detachable reddish powder
  - Flowering season: October and December
  - Distribution: All over India, predominant in Himachal Pradesh
  - Sensitization: Moderate.
- *Mangifera indica*:
  - Local name: *Aam*, Mango, *Amra*, and *Mamadichitoo*
  - Evergreen tree with a broad, rounded canopy (20–100 feet tall); grayish-brown bark, branchlets are brown; leaves are lanceolate to oblong, thin leathery, crowded, bronze-red initially, dark green later, alternately arranged
  - Flowers: Yellowish-green
  - Flowering season: March to April
  - Distribution: Almost all over India, mainly West Bengal and Bihar
  - Sensitization: Mild.
- *Melia azedarach*:
  - Local name: *Neem*, *Bewa*, *Dek*, *Nimba*, Persian lilac, and *Vepa*
  - Medium-sized tree (20 meters); long branches form loose open crown; bark gray-brown, smooth; bipinnate opposite leaves; leaflets in 3–7 pairs
  - Flowers: Lilac-blue to white, fragrant
  - Fruit: Yellowish-brown globular drupe
  - Flowering season: March to May
  - Distribution: Delhi, MP, North East, Punjab, and Karnataka
  - Sensitization: Moderate.

- *Morus alba*:
  - Local name: *Sehtoot*, Mulberry
  - Medium-sized tree (15 meters); short trunk, rounded crown; broad, leaves are alternate, ovate, 6–18 cm long, 5–13 cm wide, shiny green on upper side, paler and slightly hairy underneath; bark is light brown to gray
  - Flowers: Monoecious, male spikes catkin-like, elongated
  - Fruits: White or dark purple
  - Flowering season: January to March
  - Distribution: Delhi, Bangalore, Jaipur, Kolkata, Mumbai, Bhopal, and Aligarh
  - Sensitization: Mild to highly allergenic.
- *Parthenium hysterophorus*:
  - Local name: Congress grass, *Gajar ghas*
  - Erect, much branched, aromatic herb; 30–90 cm height; basal rosette of pale green, strongly dissected, deeply bilobed leaves, 8–20 cm in length and 4–8 cm in width
  - Flowers: Terminal, axillary, pedunculated and slightly hairy, many florets formed into small white capitula
  - Flowering season: June to July
  - Distribution: Bengaluru, Delhi, Aurangabad, Imphal, Mumbai, and Hyderabad
  - Sensitization: Highly allergenic.
- *Pennisetum typhoides*:
  - Local name: *Bajra*, Pearl millet, Horse millet, Dark millet, Candle millet, and Cattail millet
  - Perennial, creeping grass with hairy leaves, up to 3 meter height with a profuse root system; leaves are alternate, minutely serrated, up to 1.5 meter long and 8 cm wide
  - Flowers: Lower floret male or barren, upper hermaphrodite
  - Fruits: Grains
  - Flowering season: September to October
  - Distribution: All over India cultivated for its grain as crop and fodder
  - Sensitization: Highly allergenic.

- *Phoenix sylvestris*:
  - Local name: Wild date palm, date-sugar palm, Indian wild date, Indian wine palm, Silver date palm, Sugar date palm, Sugar palm, *Khajoor*, *Sendhi*, and *Khurjjooree*
  - Tall or stunted palm (4–15 meters) with a large thick crown; leaves are 3 meter long, grayish-green, emerge as a tuft from summit; seeds are pale brown
  - Flowers: White
  - Fruit: Single-seeded fruit ripens to purple-red color
  - Flowering season: January to April
  - Distribution: Orissa, Kerala, and Tamil Nadu
  - Sensitization: Highly allergenic.
- *Pinus strobus*:
  - Local name: White pine, Pin blanc
  - Tall coniferous tree (30–67 meters), conic crown; bark is blackish, thick, deeply furrowed; irregular rectangular purple-tinged scaly plates; branches whorled; dark green-blue green needles in fascicles of five
  - Flowers: Ovulate cones shedding seeds and falling soon after, clustered, pendent, symmetric, gray-brown to pale-brown; seeds compressed, obovoid, tapering at both ends, red-brown mottled with black
  - Flowering season: Early summer
  - Anemophilous
  - Distribution: Shillong, Almorah, and Dehradun
  - Sensitization: Moderately allergenic.
- *Poa annua*:
  - Local name: *Ghas*, *Champa*, annual winter grass, and goosegrass
  - Annual grass with characteristic "tramlines" on flat leaves; leaves abruptly contract at apices to give "boat-shaped tip", often transversely wrinkled, folded in a smooth and compressed sheath
  - Flowers: Yellow colored

- Flowering season: March to November
- Distribution: North and Central India
- Sensitization: Moderate to highly allergenic.
- *Prosopis juliflora*:
  - Local name: Mesquite, *Kabuli kikar*, Mexican thorn, *Belari jail*, *Vilayati kikar*, and *Vilayati babul*
  - Medium-sized (3-12 meters), deciduous tree or shrub; spreading branches, hard wood; green foliage; axillary spines; leaves are bipinnate with numerous pairs of leaflets (11-15 pairs), elliptic-oblong
  - Flowers: Very small fragrant, greenish-white turning to bright yellow, crowded cylindrical spikes; seeds are oval, brown, transverse
  - Flowering season: April to September
  - Anemophilous
  - Distribution: Delhi, Rajasthan, Aligarh, and Madhya Pradesh
  - Sensitization: Mild to highly allergenic.
- *Ricinus communis*:
  - Local name: *Bherenda*, *Haralu*, *Arundi*, *Citnavara*, Castor, Castor bean, and African coffee tree
  - Evergreen shrub or small tree (1-5 meters); shoots green-red; stem and branches with conspicuous nodes and ring-like scars of the bracts; leaves are spirally arranged, dark green when old; found in wastelands
  - Flowers: Female flowers occupy the upper portion of branching racemes, male flowers toward base with many stamens
  - Fruits: Ellipsoid to subglobose (15-25 mm long), brown, spiny or smooth; seeds ellipsoid (9-17 mm long)
  - Flowering season: Round the year
  - Anemophilous
  - Distribution: All over India
  - Sensitization: Mild to highly allergenic.

- *Salix caprea*:
  - Local name: *Bedmushk, Jalavetasa, Vajjula, Vanjula, Varnara, Vidula*, Goat willow, Pussy willow, and Great sallow
  - Deciduous shrub or small tree (4.5–7.5 meter tall); elliptic-oblong leaves (2–4 inches long and 1–3 inches wide), alternate arrangement, dark green above, grayish and hairy beneath, and faintly tooth on the margins
  - Flowers: Soft silky and silvery 3–7 cm long catkins; yellow anthers
  - Flowering season: Spring
  - Distribution: Himalayan regions, Himachal Pradesh, and Uttaranchal
  - Sensitization: Highly allergenic.
- *Suaeda fruticosa*:
  - Local name: *Lonia, Nankhuri, Lunaki*, and Shrubby seablight
  - Erect branched shrub (1 meter); stems pale or purplish; crowded leaves round the axis
  - Flowers: Greenish, bisexual, turns red at maturity
  - Flowering season: December to January
  - Distribution: Rajasthan, Delhi, UP, and Punjab
  - Sensitization: Moderate.
- *Sorghum vulgare*:
  - Local name: *Jawar, Jowar, Karbi, Jaundri*, Green millet, Indian millet, *Durra, Shallu, Cholam*, and *Jonna*
  - Tall annual grass (0.6–2.4 meters); broad linear leaves (76 cm long and 5 cm broad); white wax over stalk and leaves
  - Flowers: Incomplete sessile, each cluster 800–3,000 kernels
  - Flowering season: September to October
  - Distribution: All over India
  - Sensitization: Highly allergenic.
- *Syzygium cumini*:
  - Local name: *Jamun*, black plum, Indian blackberry, *Jambolan*, Malabar plum, and *Jambu*

- Medium-sized or large tree (up to 30 meters), broad crown; bark is rough, cracked, flaking, and discolored on the lower part of trunk; evergreen leaves with turpentine smell, 5–25 cm long, 2.5–10 cm wide, oblong-oval or elliptic, tapering to apex, pinkish when young, leathery glossy dark-green above, lighter beneath, yellowish midrib when mature
- Flowers: Greenish-white, fragrant; in clusters
- Fruits: Ovoid-oblong, dark purple, one-seeded, thin glossy skin; pulp purple-white, juicy
- Flowering season: April to June
- Distribution: Tamil Nadu, Kerala, Orissa, Himachal Pradesh, and UP
- Sensitization: Mild.

- *Xanthium strumarium*:
  - Local name: Cocklebur, *Adhisishi*, and *Chota dhatura*
  - Coarse erect, often branching herb; stems 30–150 cm tall, short dark spots, short hairs; alternate leaves, long stalked, deltoid ovate
  - Flowers: Many-flowered heads clustered at the tips of branches above the female flowers
  - Fruit: Hard brown, ovoid bur, 1.5–2.5 cm long; hooked spines; readily sticking to clothes
  - Flowering season: Most of summer to late fall
  - Anemophilous
  - Distribution: Delhi and Madhya Pradesh
  - Sensitization: Highly allergenic.

- *Zea mays*:
  - Local name: *Mokka*, *Bhutta*, *Makki*, and *Mokka-juna*
  - Erect, monoecious grass; overlapping sheaths; broad and flat leaves; whole structure enclosed in numerous large foliaceous bracts and a mass of long styles (silky threads) protrude from the tip
  - Anemophilous
  - Flowering season: Winter
  - Distribution: Dehradun
  - Sensitization: Mild.

CROSS-REACTIVE POLLEN ALLERGENS

Ability of an antigen to bind with an antibody in the serum, to which the patient was never exposed previously, is due to cross-reactivity phenomenon. Different species share similar epitopes, responsible for sensitization and cross-reactivity. Different pollens share similar epitopes, hence more cross-reactivity, if belongs to common genus or tribe and epitope sharing gradually reduces, while riding the classification ladder toward order and phylum. This phenomenon leads to false positivity of allergy tests with many nonrelevant allergens. This phenomenon should also be considered while selecting allergen test panel or immunotherapy for a particular patient. Tables 6 and 7 depict known cross-reactivity among various allergens.

Table 6: Cross-reactivity amongst pollens.

Family	Name of cross-reactive allergens
Grasses	
Pooideae	*Phleum pratense* (Timothy)*, *Anthoxanthum odoratum*, *Festuca*, *Lolium*, *Poa*, *Dactylis*, *Holcus*, *Phalaris*, Cereals (wheat, rye, barley)
Chloridoideae	*Cynodon dactylon* (Bermuda)*, *Eragrostis* (Lovegrass)
Panicoideae	*Sorghum halepense* (Johnson)*, *Paspalum notatum*, *Zea mays*, *Saccharum officinarum*
Weeds	
Asteraceae	*Artemisia vulgaris* (Mugwort)*, other species of *Artemisia*
	Ambrosia (Ragweed)*, *Parthenium hysterophorus*
Trees	
Cupressaceae	*Juniperus ashei* (Mountain cedar)*, cedar trees
Pinaceae	*Pinus strobus* (White pine)*, other pine trees
Betulaceae	*Betula**, *Alnus**, *Corylus* (Hazelnut)
Fagaceae	*Quercus alba* (White Oak)*, other oaks

*Designated as recommended representative allergen for allergen immunotherapy in case of cross-reactivity between many allergens.

Source: Weber RW. Patterns of pollen cross-allerengicity. J Allergy Clin Immunol. 2003;112(2):229-39.

Table 7: Cross-reactivity between inhalant and food allergens.

Inhalant allergen	Food allergen
Tree pollen	Apple, cherry, nectarine, peach, hazelnut, carrot, soybean, peanut, potato, kiwi fruit, Sharon fruit, and jackfruit
Mugwort pollen	Spice, carrot, lychee, mango, sunflower seeds, grapes, and peach
Ragweed and Mugwort pollen	Melon, zucchini, cucumber, and banana
Grass pollen and grain	Flour, bran, tomato, and legumes

A pollen allergic patient might experience symptoms during certain food administration, wrongly labeling food as the culprit for his problems.

Source: Worm M, Jappe U, Kleine-Tebbe J, et al. Food allergies resulting from immunological cross-reactivity with inhalant allergens. Allergo J Int. 2014;23(1):1-16.

AVOIDANCE MEASURES FOR AEROALLERGENS

- *Pollen*:
  - Allergenically significant trees should be replaced by nonallergenic trees
  - Avoid going outdoors on days of high pollen count in air
  - Close windows in evening time when pollens are settling down
  - Use air conditioners to reduce indoor pollen count
  - Eliminate weed and grasses in near vicinity
  - After coming home, take bath and wear fresh clothes
  - General awareness through media would be helpful.
- *Fungal*:
  - Identification of source and environmental conditions
  - Substances, predisposing fungus growth, should be removed
  - Kitchen or eating area and bathroom should be kept clean and dry
  - Work places should be well ventilated and hygienic
  - Dehumidifiers are recommended to help in moisture reduction
  - Improve air quality by periodic maintenance of air treatment plant, fumigation and application of antifungal agents
  - Personal filter masks of sufficient pore size should be used
  - Regular health check-up of patients.

3.1 COMMON AEROALLERGENS (WITH LOCAL NAME)

(For color version of the following figures, see Plates 1 to 16).
1. Acacia arabica (*Gursoonder, Babool, Kikar*)

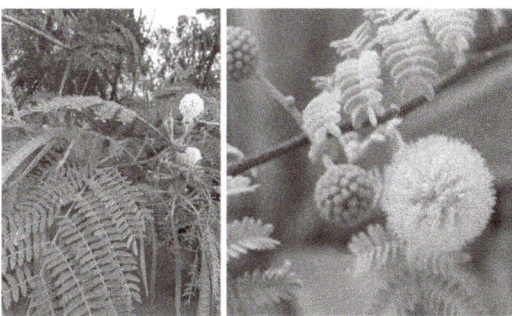

2. Ageratum conyzoides (*Nilam*, Billy goat weed)

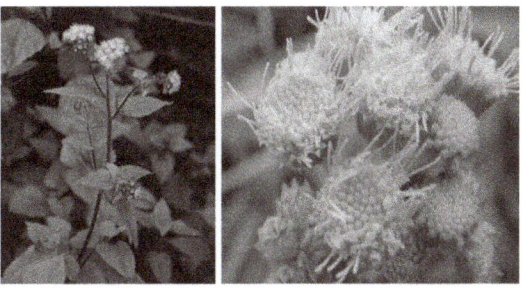

3. Ailanthus excelsa (*Urru, Aralu*, Indian tree of Heaven, *Neem*)

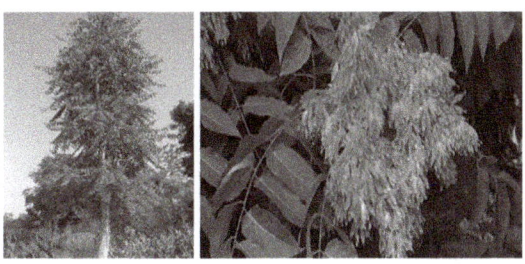

4. *Albizia lebbeck* (*Siras*, Woman's tongue tree)

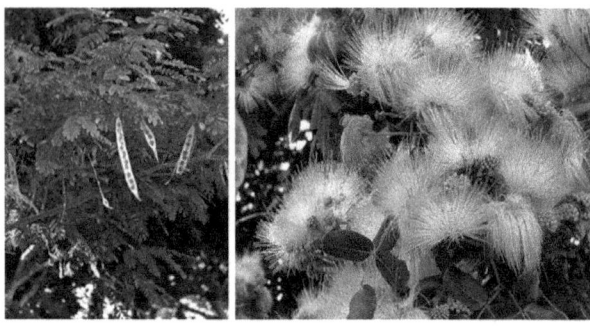

5. *Alnus nitida* (Gray alder)

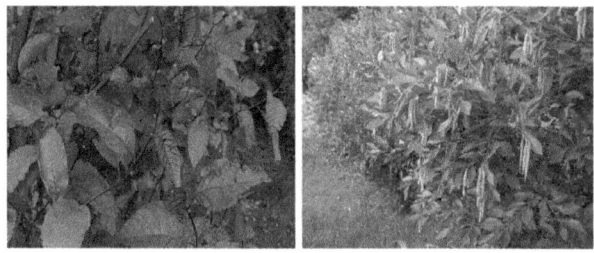

6. *Amaranthus spinosus* (*Kantewali chaulai*, Needle burr)

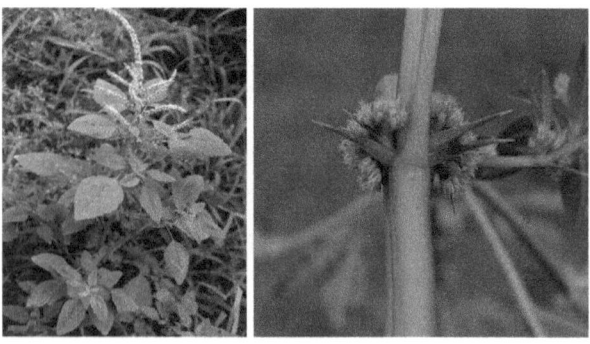

7. *Argemone mexicana* (*Siyal-kanta, Satyanashi*)

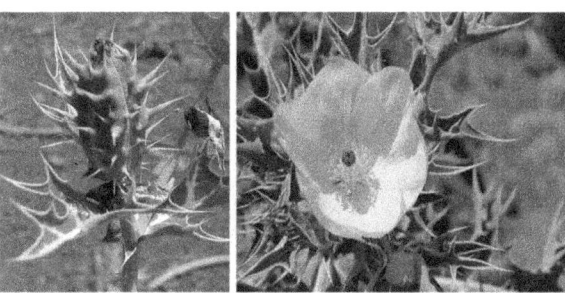

8. *Artemisia vulgaris* (Mugwort, Nagdona, Common wormwood)

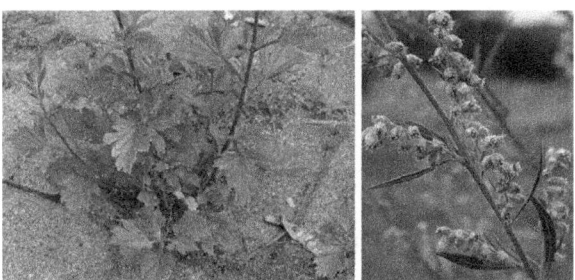

9. *Asphodelus tenuifolius* (*Jungle piyaz*)

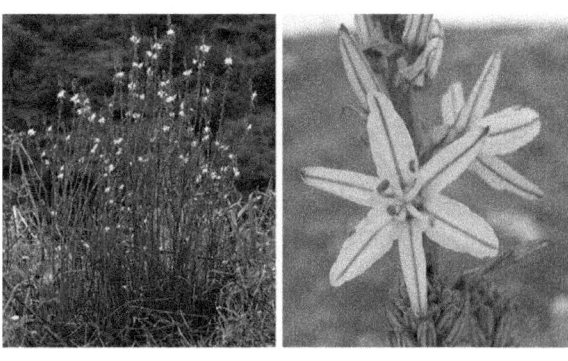

10. *Azadirachta indica* (*Neem*)

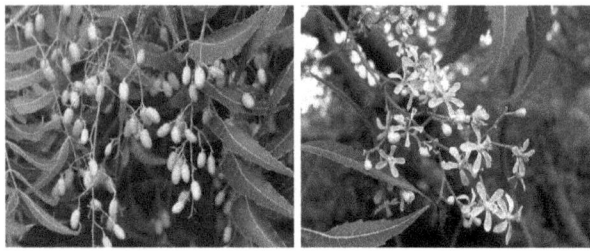

11. *Betula utilis* (Silver birch, *Bhojpatra*)

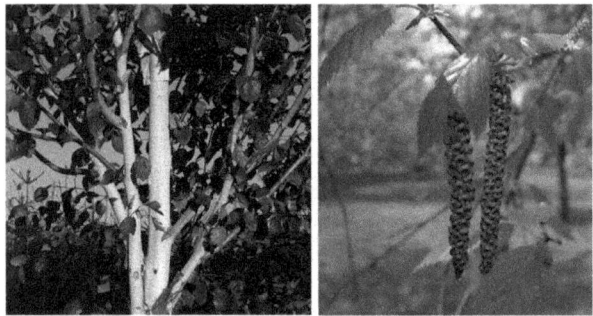

12. *Borassus flabellifer* (*Tal, Taad*)

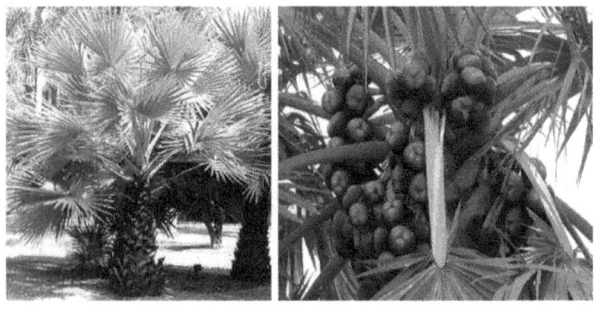

13. *Brassica campestris* (*Sarson*, Mustard)

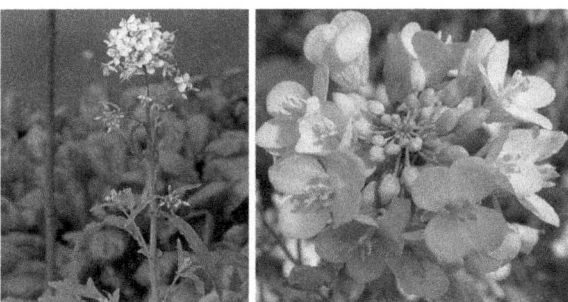

14. *Cannabis sativa* (*Ganja, Bhang*)

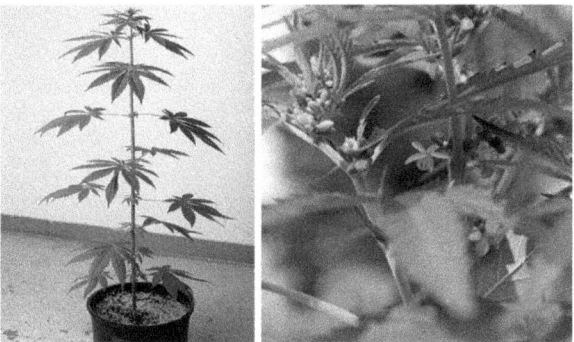

15. *Cassia fistula* (*Sonali, Ahilla,* Golden shower tree)

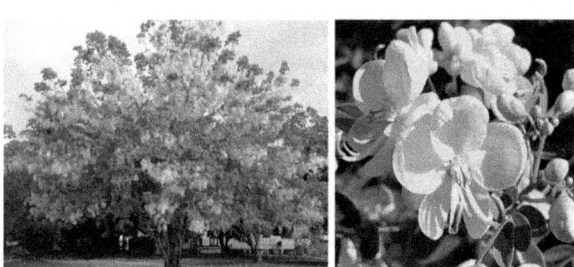

16. *Casuarina equisetifolia* (*Kasagaha*, Beefwood tree)

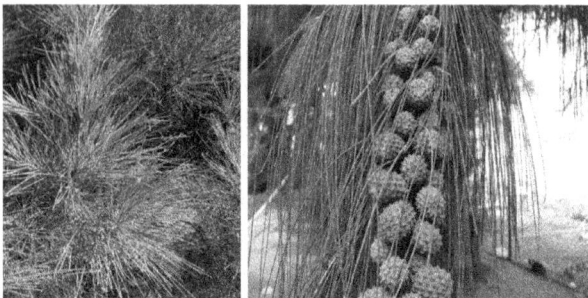

17. *Cenchrus ciliaris* (*Anjhan, Anjan*)

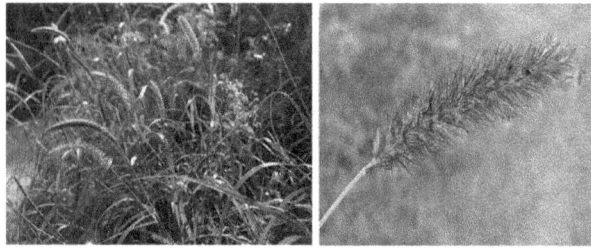

18. *Cedrus deodara* (*Devdar*)

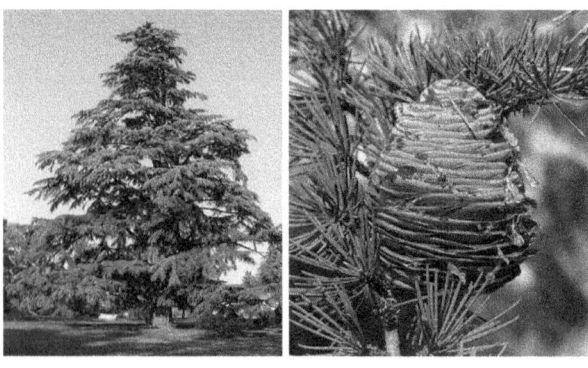

19. *Chenopodium album* (*Bathua*)

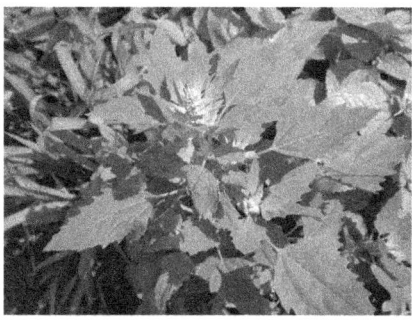
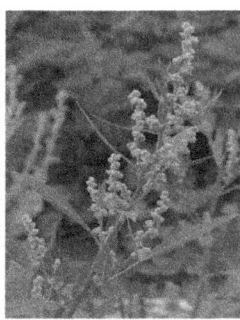

20. *Cocos nucifera* (*Narikel, Nariyal*)

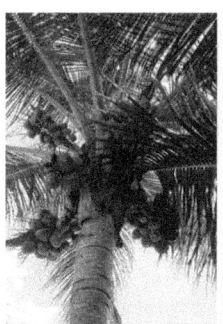
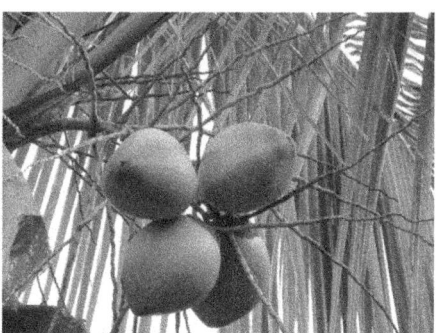

21. *Coriandrum sativum* (*Dhania*)

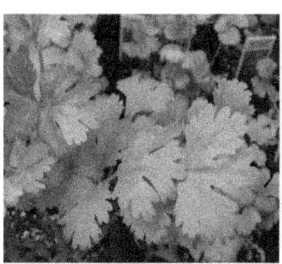
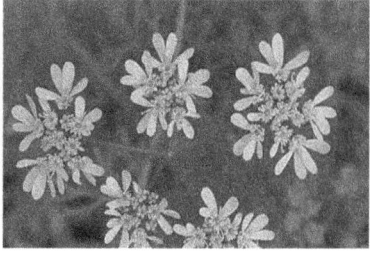

22. *Cynodon dactylon* (Bermuda grass, *Doob ghas*)

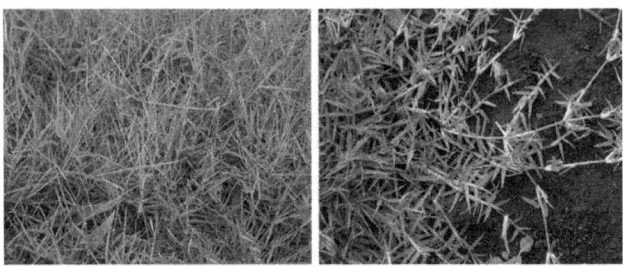

23. *Dodonaea viscosa* (*Vilayati mehndi*)

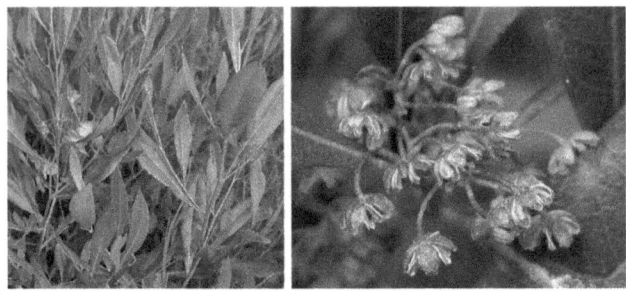

24. *Eucalyptus* spp. (Blue gum, *Safeda*)

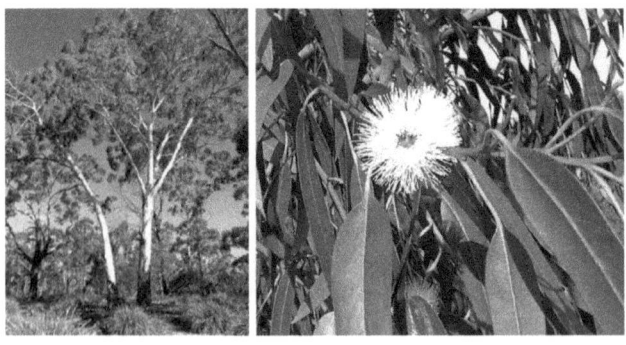

25. *Gynandropsis gynandra* (*Hulhul, Kathal*)

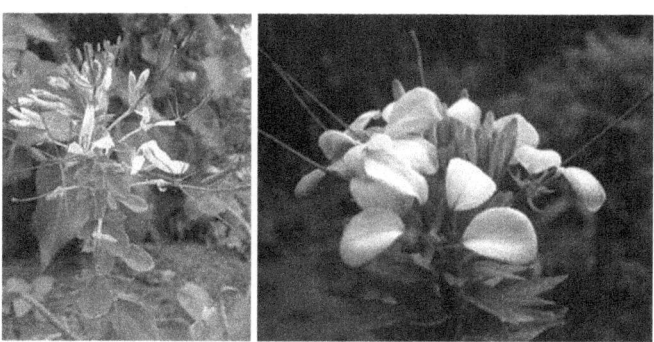

26. *Holoptelea integrifolia* (Chilbil, *Papri*, Indian elm)

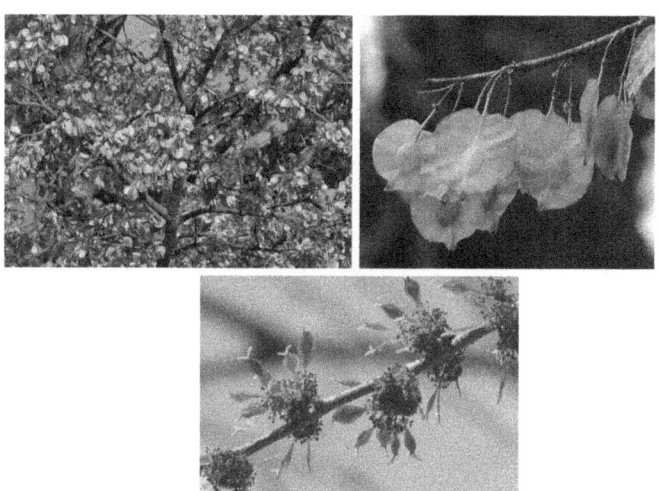

27. *Imperata cylindrica* (*Bhurighas*)

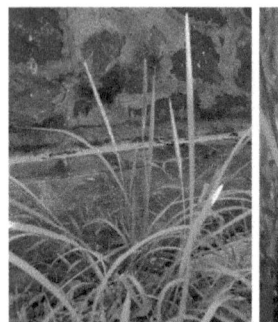
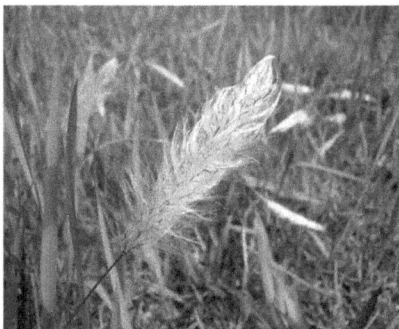

28. *Lolium perenne* (*Ryegrass*)

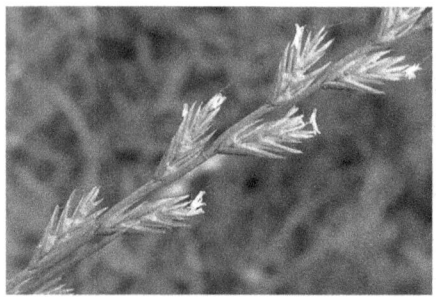
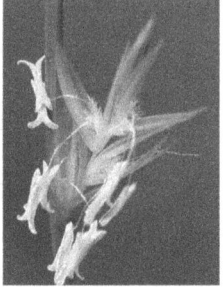

29. *Mallotus philippensis* (Kamala tree)

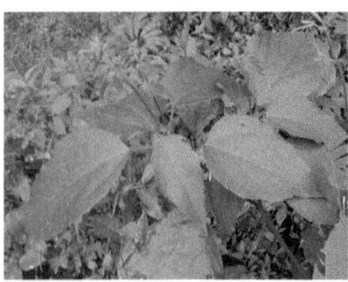
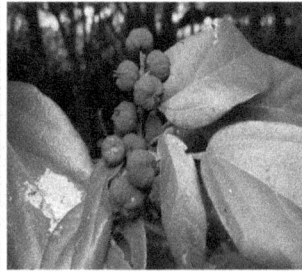

30. *Mangifera indica* (*Aam*, Mango)

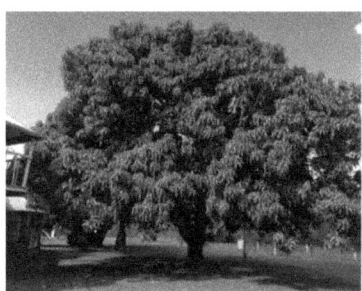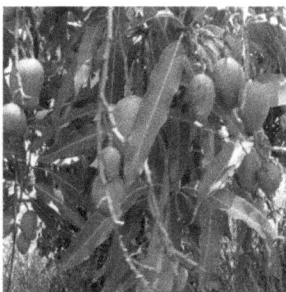

31. *Melia azedarach* (*Dek*, Nim)

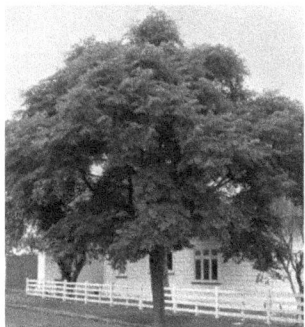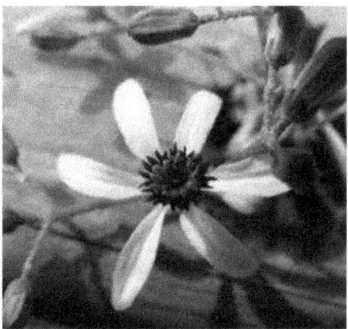

32. *Morus alba* (*Sehtoot*, Mulberry)

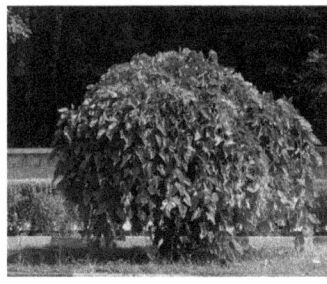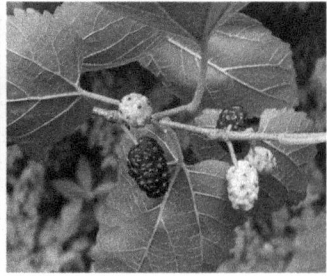

33. *Parthenium hysterophorus* (*Congress grass*)

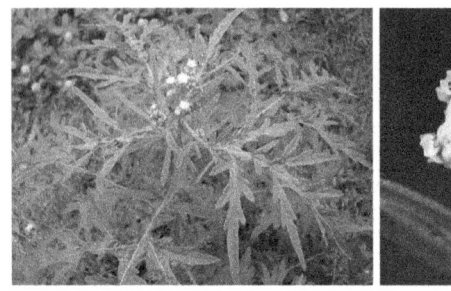
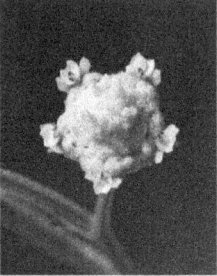

34. *Pennisetum typhoides* (*Bajra*)

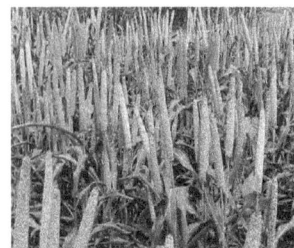
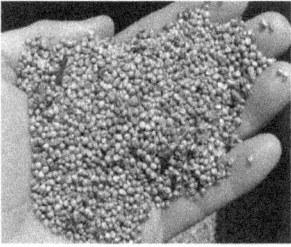

35. *Phoenix sylvestris* (Wild date palm, *Khajoor*)

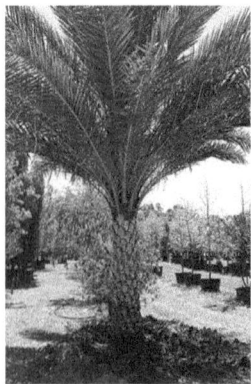
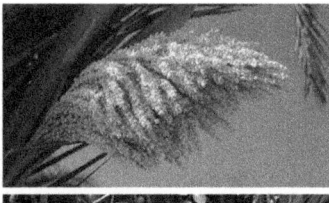
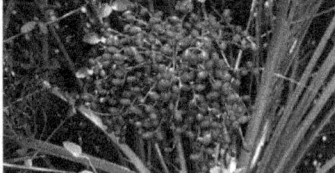

36. *Pinus strobus* (White pine)

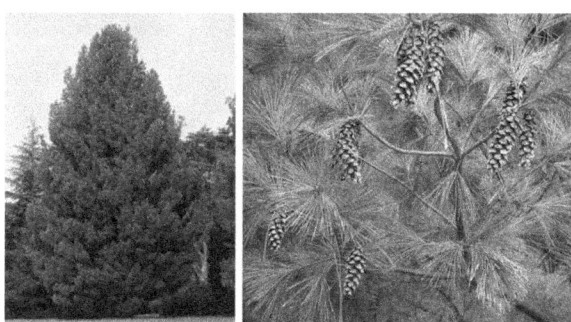

37. *Poa annua* (*Ghas*)

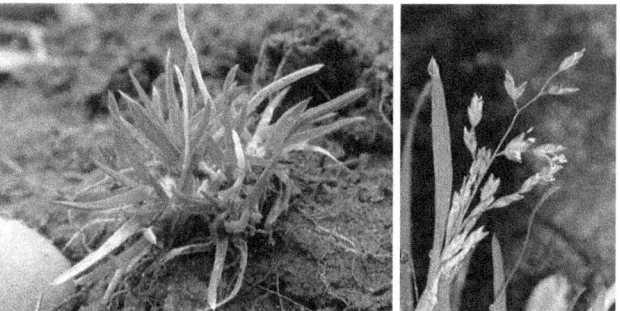

38. *Prosopis juliflora* (*Kabuli kikar*)

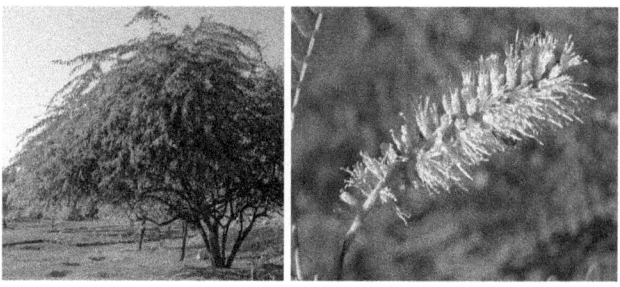

39. *Ricinus communis* (Castor, Castor bean, African coffee bean)

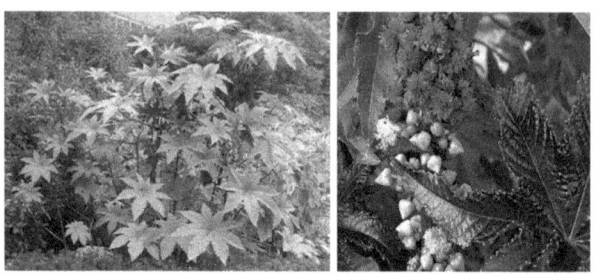

40. *Salix caprea* (Goat willow, Pussy willow)

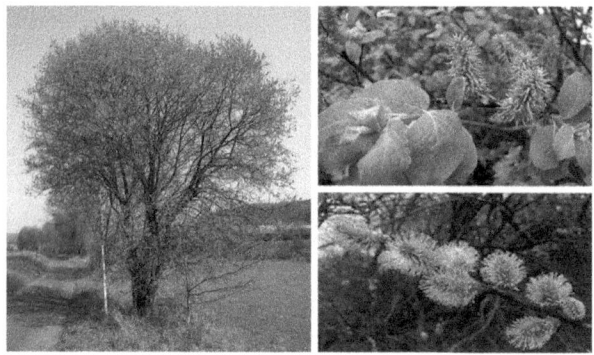

41. *Sorghum vulgare* (*Jowar, Karbi*)

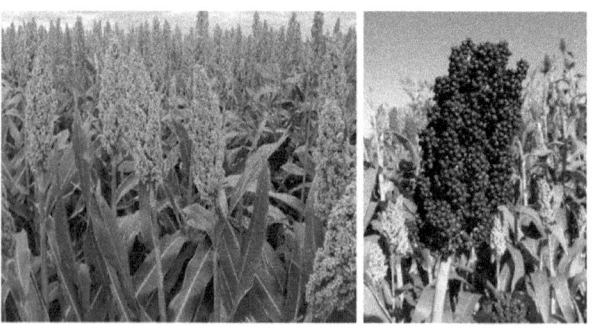

42. *Suaeda fruticosa* (Shrubby seablight, Lonia)

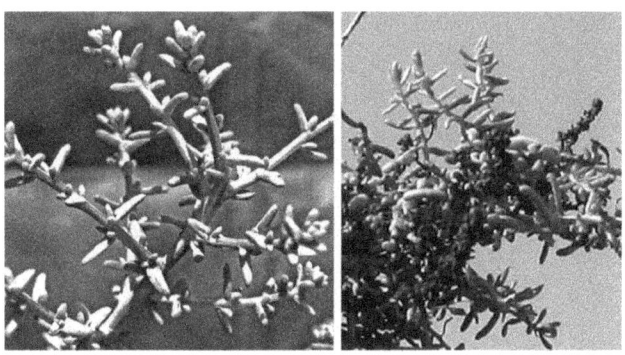

43. *Syzygium cumini* (Jamun, Black plum, Indian blackberry)

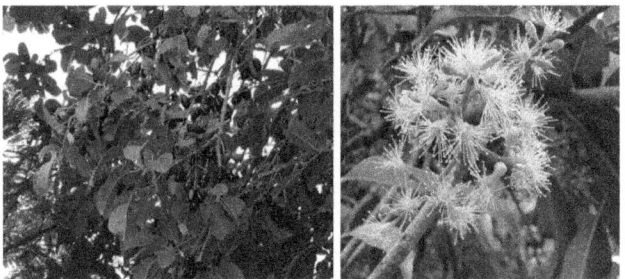

44. *Xanthium strumarium* (*Adhisishi, Chota dhatura*)

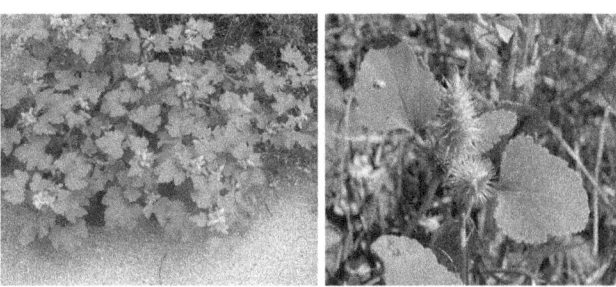

45. *Zea mays* (*Mokka, Bhutta, Makki*)

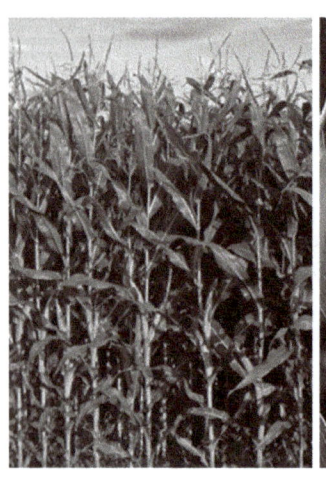
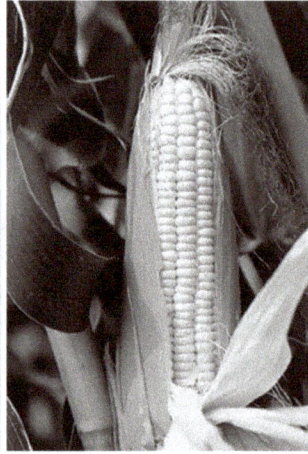

SUGGESTED READING

1. Gill NK, Kumar K, Rai NK. Risk assessment of outdoor airborne biological allergens in India: A review. J Entomol Zool Stud. 2017;5(4):1069-75.
2. Kumar R, Kumar M, Robinson K, et al. Atmospheric pollen count in North Delhi region. Indian J Allergy Asthma Immunol. 2015;29:32-9.
3. Levetin E. Methods for Aeroallergen Sampling. Current Allergy and Asthma Reports. 2004;4:376-83.
4. Singh AB. Glimpse of Clinical Aerobiology in India: An Overview. Glob J Otolaryngol. 2017;12(3):555-840.
5. Singh AB, Khandelwal A. An Atlas of Allergenically Significant Plants of India, 1st edition. 2016.

Respiratory Allergies

AN OVERVIEW

Allergic disorders can affect any of the organs with respiratory system bearing most of the burden. "United airway concept" signifies that an inflammatory allergic reaction involves entire respiratory tract (from nose to lungs) heterogeneously with predominant problems of rhinosinusitis in some patients and of asthma in others. Approximately 500 million people suffer from allergic rhinitis (AR) and 300 million from asthma worldwide. South Asia itself accounts for 100 million cases of AR.

Allergic disorders are often underdiagnosed and undertreated. These account for 1% of all disability-adjusted life years lost worldwide. As per the recent International Study of Asthma and Allergy in Childhood (ISAAC) data, AR affects 10–30% of all adults and 40% of all children. In India, it is still considered a trivial disease, though 75% of children and 80% of all asthmatic adults suffer from AR. AR has been reported from 11.3%–61.9% in some Asian studies, whereas asthma accounted for 25–30%.

The direct estimated cost for diagnosing and managing allergic disorders is approximately 7.3 billion USD and an additional 4.3 billion USD, due to loss of productivity, makes it 11.6 billion USD in USA, which is double of India's total health budget of 5.9 billion USD and 30 times more of expenditure on medications of AR and asthma in India.

Among the major allergens, responsible for respiratory allergies, house dust mites were responsible in 89.7%, followed by pollens as 10–20% and animal dander as 2.8%. Environmental pollutants [oxides of nitrogen and sulfur, particulate matter (PM)] were the major contributor in outdoor surroundings. The main sources were fuel combustion from vehicles, construction and agricultural operations, power plants, and industries. PM is a mixture of organic and inorganic solid and liquid particles of different origins, size, and composition. Particles up till 10 μm (PM_{10}) can invade nose and upper airway, whereas smaller particles up till 2.5 μm ($PM_{2.5}$) reach the lower airways and are responsible for most of the clinical problems like asthma.

It is the felt need of community to recognize and treat respiratory allergies at the earliest, especially in children, so that clinical, economical, and psychological aspects of allergic diseases can be minimized.

4.1 ALLERGIC RHINITIS

INTRODUCTION

Allergic rhinitis is a very common entity, affecting 10–30% adults and nearly 40% children at some parts of their life. Approximately 60 million people are currently affected in United States alone with AR, as per the latest national survey. Along with the clinical burden, it significantly affects the quality of life of an individual, directly reflecting on work or school performance and sleep quality. Effects of AR are not just limited to patients, rather it creates a huge economic burden on the family due to medications, lifestyle changes, and many associated comorbidities. The ill effects of AR, both clinical and economical, can be prevented if the disease is managed appropriately in early phase. Correct diagnosis and effective management, at the root level, are the keys to success.

DEFINITION

Allergic rhinitis is a symptomatic disorder, there is no set definition. It is an immunoglobulin E (IgE)-mediated reaction, in an already sensitized individual, to certain trigger factor or allergen. It can be characterized by four cardinal symptoms:
- Watery rhinorrhea
- Nasal obstruction

- Nasal itching
- Sneezing.

These symptoms can present either alone or in various combinations in an affected patient. Itching of the palate, postnasal drip, and cough are commonly associated complaints.

NONALLERGIC RHINITIS

- Atrophic rhinitis
- Chemical or irritant-induced rhinitis
- Drug-induced rhinitis: Antihypertensive medications, aspirin and other nonsteroidal anti-inflammatory drugs (NSAIDs), oral contraceptives, and rhinitis medicamentosa
- Emotional rhinitis
- Exercise-induced rhinitis
- Gustatory rhinitis
- Hormone-induced rhinitis: Hypothyroidism, menstrual cycle, oral contraceptives, and pregnancy
- Infectious rhinitis: Acute (mostly viral) and chronic (rhinosinusitis)
- Nonallergic rhinitis with eosinophilia syndrome
- Occupational rhinitis (irritant)
- Perennial nonallergic rhinitis: Vasomotor rhinitis
- Postural reflexes
- Primary ciliary dyskinesia
- Reflux-induced rhinitis or gastroesophageal reflux disease.

CONDITIONS THAT MAY MIMIC SYMPTOMS OF RHINITIS

- Cerebrospinal fluid rhinorrhea
- Inflammatory or immunologic conditions:
    - Midline granuloma
    - Nasal polyposis
    - Sarcoidosis
    - Sjogren's syndrome

- Systemic lupus erythematosus
- Wegener's granulomatosis.
- Relapsing polychondritis
- Structural or mechanical conditions:
  - Choanal atresia
  - Deviated septum
  - Enlarged adenoids
  - Foreign bodies
  - Hypertrophic turbinates
  - Nasal tumors.

TRIGGERS OF ALLERGIC RHINITIS

- *Allergens*:
  - Aeroallergens—outdoor and indoor pollens
  - Dust, animal and insect allergens—house dust, house dust mites, cockroaches, and pet dander
  - Occupational
  - Latex—important in healthcare professionals.
- *Pollutants*:
  - Indoor—biomass fuel, tobacco, and gas pollutants
  - Outdoor—ozone, oxides of nitrogen and sulfur from diesel exhaust.
- *Drugs*:
  - Aspirin and other NSAIDs.

PATHOPHYSIOLOGY

When an allergen presents to the dendritic cells (one of the many types of antigen presenting cells), $CD4^+$ T cells are stimulated via major histocompatibility complex (MHC) class II involvement. $CD4^+$ T cells differentiates into T helper 2 (Th2) cells in an atopic individual, triggering the type I hypersensitivity, reaction which induces IgE production, through B cells, and proliferation of eosinophils, mast cells, and basophils (Fig. 1). This free IgE binds to mast cells and basophils and wait for the re-exposure of allergenic

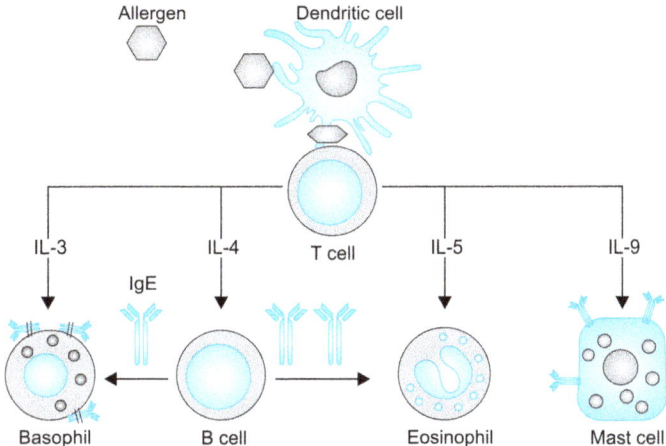

Fig. 1: Sensitization and shift toward Th2 pathway in an atopic individual.
(IL: interleukin; Ig: immunoglobulin)
Source: Min YG. The pathophysiology, diagnosis and treatment of allergic rhinitis. Allergy Asthma Immunol Res. 2010;2:65-76.

stimulus. On second hit, allergens bind to bound IgE (on mast cells) and produces allergic reaction in an already sensitized individual.

Early versus Late Reaction

Stimulated mast cells releases the already formed chemical mediators (histamine, prostaglandins, and leukotrienes) immediately in the near vicinity. Symptoms like repeated sneezing and watery nasal discharge appears within few minutes to 2 hours. Few hours later, eosinophils, more mast cells, and T cells migrate to the affected area, nasal mucosa, under the influence of released mediators and remodeling of tissue occurs resulting in nasal obstruction. Newly formed mediators are responsible for persistence of nasal symptoms for hours to days. Apart from type I hypersensitivity, there are certain other mechanisms involved in the pathogenesis of AR:

- *Neurogenic inflammation*: During the tissue remodeling phase, nerve endings, in nasal mucosa, are denuded and become hyperresponsive to nonspecific stimuli or even in absence of any external stimuli. This will create a "retrograde axonal reflex" dictating the secretion of substance P and neurokinin A from sensory nerve fibers. These newly formed mediators are responsible for smooth muscle contraction, mucus production, and exudative leakage, resulting in neurogenic inflammation.
- *Nonspecific hyperresponsiveness*: Exposed nerve ending and breached nasal mucosa become hypersensitive to external nonallergenic stimuli like tobacco, cold or dry air, sudden change in temperature, smoke, fragrant substances or extreme emotional states.
- *Minimal persistent inflammation*: Recent concept in AR is persistence of minimal inflammation in atopic patients during asymptomatic period. This requires a minimal trigger by an allergen to produce intermittent exacerbations.

CLASSIFICATION

The initial classification of AR was based on timing of symptomatology. Regular symptoms caused by indoor allergens like house dust mites, cockroaches, animal dander or fungi were classified under "perennial" group, whereas periodic symptoms caused by outdoor allergens like pollens were labelled as "seasonal" (Table 1).

This classification was unable to delineate causative allergens clearly, as on the one hand, multiple pollens may cause symptoms round the year and on the other hand, perennial allergen concentration may vary causing periodic exacerbations. In 2001, AR and its Impact on Asthma (ARIA) group reclassified AR in "Intermittent" (<4 days per week OR <4 weeks per year) and "Persistent" (>4 days per week AND >4 weeks per year) category. Severity of symptoms, depending on work or school performance, daily activities and sleep quality, demanded further categorization as "mild" and "moderate-severe" (Fig. 2).

Table 1: Pattern of rhinitis.

Feature	Seasonal allergic	Perennial allergic	Nonallergic
Symptoms	Rhinorrhea, sneezing, itchy nose, watery and itchy eyes	Rhinorrhea, sneezing, itchy nose, watery and itchy eyes	Nasal blockage and postnasal drainage prominent
Other atopic diseases	Common	Common	Less common
Age of onset	Most before 20 years	Most before 20 years	Over 20 years
Timings	During affected seasons only	Throughout the year	Perennial, can coexist with allergic rhinitis
Triggers	Grass cutting, windy weather, walking out of house, walking through parks, gardening	Vacuuming, dry dusting, pet exposure, opening old cupboards	No readily identifiable aeroallergens. Respiratory irritants: Cigarette smoking, strong scents, fragrances Weather changes: temperature, humidity Others: Spicy foods, medications, infections
Likely allergens	Grass, weed, tree, pollens	House dust mite, cats, dogs, fungus	None

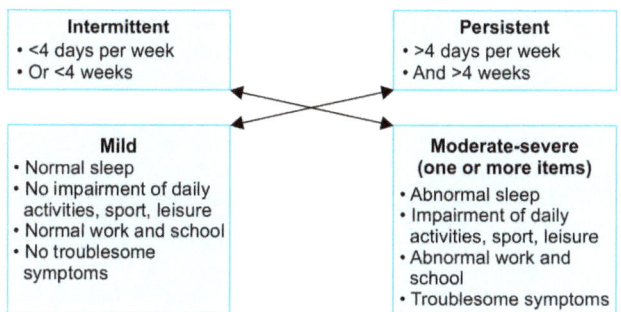

Fig. 2: Classification of allergic rhinitis.
Source: Min YG. The pathophysiology, diagnosis and treatment of allergic rhinitis. Allergy Asthma Immunol Res. 2010;2:65-76.

DIAGNOSIS

Allergic rhinitis is suspected on clinical, when two or more symptoms out of watery rhinorrhea, sneezing, nasal obstruction, and nasal pruritus last for 1 hour or more on most days. There are limited findings on clinical examination. One may find clear rhinorrhea, bluish or pale swelling of nasal mucosa, ocular findings (watery discharge, swollen conjunctivae, scleral injection), allergic shiners, and nasal crease. Disease severity should be classified as per ARIA guidelines (*see* Fig. 2) and diagnosis should be confirmed with either laboratory tests or nasal provocation. Presence of unilateral nasal stuffiness, mucopurulent discharge, mucoid postnasal drip, local pain, recurrent epistaxis, and anosmia warrant search for alternate diagnosis.

Laboratory Diagnosis

The ideal test for AR diagnosis is nasal provocation test but it requires hospital settings and facilities for emergency care due to risk of severe reaction or anaphylaxis. Its utility is also limited due to nonavailability of standard allergen extract for all the possible allergens. It is routinely not recommended. There are various in vitro and in vivo tests available.

- *In vitro test*:
  - *Total IgE*: It is the most commonly used serum test but has got many false-positives and negatives. Serum free IgE production may be increased in many conditions apart from allergic reactions especially parasitic infestations, more prevalent in developing countries. It could be low if a type I hypersensitivity reaction is unable to produce significant amount of IgE. It is no more considered as diagnostic marker for type I hypersensitivity reaction.
  - *Specific IgE (sIgE)*: This is a better marker than total IgE estimation. It detects free IgE levels in response to a specific allergen. This could also be falsely elevated, in

presence of increased total IgE, due to nonspecific binding to other allergens in the laboratory estimation techniques. Specificity and negative predictive value of sIgE is higher than sensitivity and positive predictive value, which means that normal sIgE values to a particular allergen virtually rule out type I hypersensitivity to that allergen while positive value should be supported with suggestive clinical history and other laboratory markers.

- *In vivo test*:
  - *Skin test*: It detects the presence of bound IgE on the mast cells and simulates the exact clinical reaction, in controlled manner, in the affected individual. Skin test is considered gold standard, for all the practical purposes, to identify sensitization. Its sensitivity, specificity, positive and negative predictive values are excellent for aeroallergens, however, it lacks sensitivity for food allergens. Patient's clinical symptoms and local flora should be considered, while selecting an allergen panel for testing. It is widely available, simple, economical, and requires only 15–20 minutes. Non availability of standardized allergen extracts might be the limiting factor in certain situations. Antihistamine intake, extremes of age, diffuse dermatologic diseases, long-term immunosuppressant (including steroids), and different test sites (forearm, back) might influence the test results.
  - *Nasal provocation test*: Though an extremely helpful test, it is rarely done in clinical settings due to many logistic reasons.
- *Supportive tests*:
  - *Radiology*: Might suggest comorbid conditions like sinusitis and adenoid hypertrophy.
  - *Nasal endoscopy*: Pale boggy nasal mucosa or nasal polyp may be identified.
  - *Nasal eosinophilia*: Moderately high sensitivity and high specificity for diagnosis of AR.

TREATMENT

Allergen Avoidance

An effort should be made for identification of specific allergen/s, based on careful history and supportive tests, so that targeted avoidance measures may be instituted. Patients should be advised to avoid areas with high pollen/fungal/dusty environment. Daily pollen counters are helpful to predict and prevent pollen exposure. Pest control measures should be rigorously implemented. House dust mite is the most common culprit, responsible for aeroallergies. Frequent changing and washing of carpets, mattresses, bed sheets, and sun drying are desirable measures, but far from practical. There are special bed covers available, with very small pore size to prevent mite intrusion, at very high cost. Reduction in relative humidity below 50% is an alternative measure for reducing house dust mite concentration in the environment. Avoidance measures work best for occupational allergies.

Nasal Clearance

Normal saline irrigation is commonly used as an adjunctive therapy to other pharmacological measures. Nasal sprays, drops, nebulizers, and irrigations are among the many modes of delivery. Saline delivered by high pressure and more volume is more effective. Available saline solutions could be hypotonic (<0.9% NaCl), isotonic (0.9% NaCl) or hypertonic (>0.9% NaCl). The proposed mechanism of normal saline in AR is through mechanical clearance of mucus and inflammatory mediators like histamine. Mucociliary function also improves due to better ciliary beat function. Some individuals may experience ear fullness, stinging of the nasal mucosa, and epistaxis.

Pharmacological Treatment

Pharmacologic agents help in symptomatic management of patients with AR. Commonly used agents are antihistamines, steroids, and leukotriene receptor antagonists (LTRAs).

- *Oral antihistamines*: These are effective for rhinorrhea, sneezing, nasal itching, and eye symptoms but can worsen nasal stuffiness. First-generation antihistamines cause sedation, memory impairment, and psychomotor disturbances. Dry mouth, dry eyes, urinary retention, constipation, and tachycardia are reported due to nonspecific cross binding of first-generation antihistamines with cholinergic, α-adrenergic, and serotonergic receptors. Second-generation antihistamines do not cross blood–brain barrier, so provide better neurosafety profile than its predecessor. However, terfenadine and astemizole (both are second-generation antihistamines) can cause QT prolongation and increased risk for arrhythmia. Ebastine affects liver and kidney functions along with QT prolongation. Table 2 depicts different antihistamines, their therapeutic doses, and selective action on various receptors.
- *Intranasal antihistamines*: These agents are helpful in nasal pruritus, sneezing, and rhinorrhea. Azelastine and olopatadine nasal sprays are the commonly available preparation.
- *Intranasal corticosteroids*: They inhibit both early- and late-phase reactions. Local steroids penetrate cell membrane, bind to cytoplasmic receptors, reach to nuclear DNA, and directly affect the protein synthesis. IgE and eosinophil production reduce via downregulation of interleukin (IL)-4, IL-5, and IL-13 within a week time. The therapeutic effect of nasal steroids starts by 6–7 hours of administration and peaks by 2 weeks. It is effective for all clinical manifestations of AR (Table 3) and is considered to be the best therapeutic agent. Systemic absorption is limited (20–50% for flunisolide, triamcinolone acetonide, and beclomethasone dipropionate; <0.1% for mometasone furoate and <2% for fluticasone propionate).
- *Anticholinergic agents*: These have limited role for controlling nasal discharge.
- *Local chromones*: These are known to benefit in allergic conjunctivitis with lesser effect on nasal symptoms.

Table 2: Antihistamines—pharmacological properties.

Antihistamine	Dose (mg)	Dosing Interval (hrs)	Sedative effects	Anti-H_1 activity	Anti-M activity	Antiemetic
First generation: Propylamines						
Brompheniramine	4	4–6	+	+++	++	-
Chlorpheniramine	4	4–6	+	++	++	-
Dexchlorpheniramine	2	4–6	+	+++	++	-
Triprolidine	2.5	4–6	+	+++	++	-
Phenindamine	25	4–6	±	++	+++	-
First generation: Ethanolamines (Aminoalkyl ethers)						
Clemastine	1	12	++	++	+++	+++
Carbinoxamine	4–8	6–8	++	++	+++	+++
Diphenhydramine	25–50	6–8	+++	+	+++	+++
First generation: Ethylenediamines						
Pyrilamine	25–50	6–8	+	++	±	-
Tripelennamine	25–50	4–6	++	++	±	-
First generation: Phenothiazines						
Promethazine	12.5–25	6–24	+++	+++	+++	++++
Trimeprazine	2.5	6	++	+++	+++	++++
Methdilazine	8	6–12	+	+++	+++	++++
First generation: Piperazines (Cyclizines)						
Hydroxyzine	25–100	4–8	+++	+++	++	+++
First generation: Dibenzocycloheptenes/heptanes						
Azatadine	1–2	12	++	++	++	-
Cyproheptadine	4	8	+	++	++	-
First generation: Phthalazinone						
Azelastine	0.5	12	±	+++	±	-
Second generation: Piperazine						
Cetirizine	5–10	24	±	+++	±	-
Second generation: Piperidines						
Astemizole	10	24	±	+++	±	-
Fexofenadine	60	12	±	-	±	-
Loratadine	10	24	±	+++	±	-

Source: Modified from DeRuiter J. Histamine H1-Receptor antagonists: Antihistaminics agents. Principles of Drug Action 2, Fall 2001.

Table 3: Therapeutic drug categories in allergic rhinitis and their effect on various symptoms.

Drug class	Sneezing	Itching	Congestion	Rhinorrhea	Ocular
Oral H_1 antihistamines	+++	+++	?	++	++
Intranasal antihistamines	+++	+++	+	++	–
Oral decongestants	–	–	+	–	–
Intranasal steroids	+++	+++	+++	+++	++
Anticholinergics	–	–	–	++	–
Leukotriene receptor antagonist	+	+	+	+	+

- *Leukotriene receptor antagonists (LTRA)*: These can be used as an adjunctive therapy along with intranasal corticosteroids. LTRAs block cysteinyl leukotriene 1 (CysLT1) receptor, thus inhibiting leukotrienes, inflammatory mediators of mast cells, eosinophils, basophils, macrophages, and monocytes, which are important contributor for allergic manifestations in AR and asthma. Some response in nasal and eye symptoms has been witnessed by researchers in patients with isolated AR or AR with asthma. The widely used combination regimens of LTRAs and antihistamines requires more investigations before it can be advocated for generalized use.
- *Anti-IgE antibody*: Recombinant humanized monoclonal antibody, binds with free IgE, reducing its availability for attachment to mast cells and basophils and reduces the allergic reaction. It has potential use in severe asthma, though use in AR still debated. Safety profile of this costly therapy needs to be kept in mind before implementing as anaphylaxis has been reported apart from headache, upper respiratory infection, and sinusitis.

Immunotherapy

Immunotherapy (IT) is the only disease modifying therapeutic measure to cure allergic phenomenon. IT shifts the T_{reg} cells response toward nonallergic Th1 cells rather than allergic Th2 cells, with the help of downregulating IL-4 and IL-13 and upregulating IL-10. Standardized allergen extracts are used in therapeutic doses to desensitize the patients by various routes. Subcutaneous immunotherapy (SCIT) and sublingual immunotherapy (SLIT) are used for various allergens across the world. SCIT is more efficacious with some risk factors as compared to SLIT, whose safety profile is better. IT is beneficial in patients with AR, AR with asthma, and allergic asthma in descending order. It prevents onset of asthma and neosensitization in patients with AR. Long-term IT, 3–5 years, is effective in preventing late onset allergic symptoms. Flowchart 1 enumerates management steps for patients with AR.

COMPLICATIONS AND COMORBID DISEASES

Poorly controlled AR can be commonly associated with comorbid conditions, thus leading to many avoidable complications, so appropriate management at early stage is warranted.

- *Allergic conjunctivitis*: It is more common with outdoor allergens such as pollens and is the most common entity associated with AR.
- *Rhinosinusitis*: Sinusitis has been found in certain patients along with AR, requiring attention for better disease control. Chronic use of nasal decongestants may cause ciliary dysfunction predisposing for hypertrophic sinusitis.
- *Nasal polyposis*: Nasal mucosal edema and recurrent sneezing potentiate protrusion of nasal mucosa predisposing for polyposis.
- *Adenoid hypertrophy*: It is commonly associated with IL-4, IL-5, and increase eosinophil production.
- *Eustachian tube dysfunction and otitis media with effusion.*
- *Changes in cognitive abilities*: Symptomatic AR increases school or work absenteeism, reduces quality of life and poor

Flowchart 1: Stepwise approach to a patient with allergic rhinitis.
(Ig: immunoglobulin)

```
┌─────────────────────────────────────────────────────────────┐
│  Diagnosis on basis of history ± skin prick test or specific IgE │
└─────────────────────────────────────────────────────────────┘
                              │
                   ┌──────────────────────┐
                   │  Allergen avoidance  │
                   └──────────────────────┘
                     │                  │
        ┌────────────────────┐   ┌────────────────────┐
        │ Intermittent symptoms │   │ Persistent symptoms │
        └────────────────────┘   └────────────────────┘
```

Intermittent symptoms

Mild
- Oral H₁ antihistaminic
- Intranasal H₁ blocker
- And/or decongestant

Moderate-severe
- Oral H₁ antihistaminic
- Intranasal H₁ blocker
- And/or decongestant
- Intranasal steroids
- Chromone

In persistent rhinitis, review the patient after 2–4 weeks

- If failure: Step-up
- If improved: Continue for 1 month

Persistent symptoms

Mild

Moderate-severe
Intranasal steroids

Review after 2–4 weeks

Improved
Step-down and continue × 1 month

Failure
Review diagnosis
Review compliance
Query infections or other causes

- Increase intranasal steroid dose
- Itch/sneeze-add H₁ blocker
- Rhinorrhea-add decongestant or oral steroid (short-term)
- If still fails—surgical referral

If conjunctivitis add:
- Oral H₁-blocker or intraocular H₁ blocker or intraocular chromon or saline

Consider specific immunotherapy

Source: Min YG. The pathophysiology, diagnosis and treatment of allergic rhinitis. Allergy Asthma Immunol Res. 2010;2:65-76.

work performance. Irritability, daytime somnolence, fatigue, depression, attention deficit, learning and memory deficit, sexual dysfunction, and sleep-disordered breathing are commonly reported comorbidities with AR.

CONCLUSION

Allergic rhinitis is a common entity, mostly diagnosed on clinical suspicion, supported by certain diagnostic tests. Allergen avoidance, pharmacotherapy, and IT seem promising tools for appropriate management, if instituted timely.

4.2 SINUSITIS

INTRODUCTION

Sinusitis is an under recognized entity, affecting approximately 16% of adults in United States. As per a recent survey, 134 million Indians (more than population of Japan) suffer from chronic sinusitis. It is more common than diabetes, asthma and coronary heart disease. The rising pollution levels, congested living conditions and diverse flora are some of the predisposing factors. A clear understanding and early suspicion are warranted for its proper management.

ANATOMY

Sinuses, situated around nasal area, are pneumatized spaces with pseudostratified and ciliated columnar epithelial lining interspersed with goblet cells. Figures 3 and 4 depict anatomical aspects of paranasal sinuses and internal nose. Ciliary movement sweeps mucus toward the ostial opening. Ventilation for anterior ethmoid, frontal and maxillary sinuses is provided by ostiomeatal complex (OMC), a narrow drainage pathway in the middle meatus.

DEFINITION

Sinusitis is defined as inflammation of one or more of the sinuses. Based on clinical manifestations, sinusitis may be classified as:

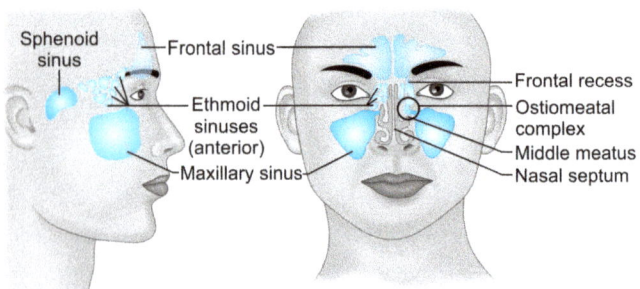

Fig. 3: Anatomical location of paranasal sinuses.

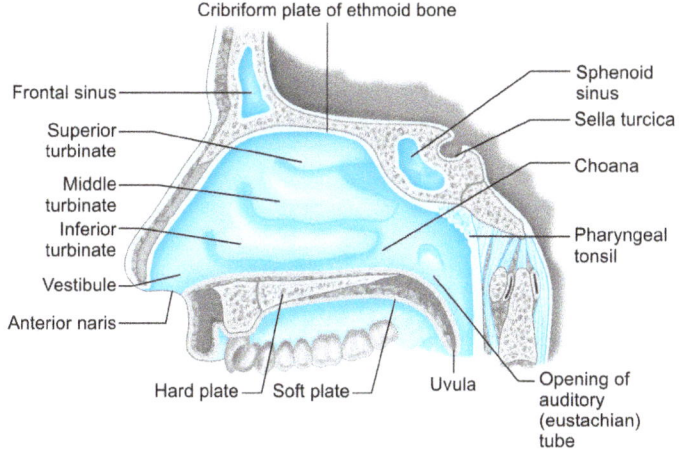

Fig. 4: Anatomy of internal nose.

- Acute—symptoms lasting less than 4 weeks (usually more than 10 days)
- Subacute—symptoms between 4 weeks and 8 weeks
- Chronic—symptoms which persists more than 8 weeks
- Recurrent—three or more acute episodes in a year.

Classifying sinusitis as per different time limits, may help in delineating etiological agents, and thus better management, in individual patients. Chronic sinusitis may further be categorized as infectious, allergic or vasomotor as per the proposed etiology.

PATHOPHYSIOLOGY

Acute Sinusitis

It is usually infective in origin. Viral upper respiratory infections cause inflammation of sinuses and blockage of OMC, resulting in reduced drainage and ventilation. Functional loss of cilia and mucosal damage, due to reduced pH and oxygen content, predisposes to secondary infections. Rhinovirus is the most common virus and *Streptococcus pneumoniae*, *Haemophilus influenza* and *Moraxella catarrhalis* are among the most common bacterial pathogens. Researchers suggest that forceful nose blowing creates negative intranasal pressure, sucking nasal fluid from middle meatus into the sinus cavity, thus causes sinus inflammation and predispose to infections.

Chronic Sinusitis

Etiology for chronic sinusitis is usually multifactorial viz. anatomic, infectious, allergic and inflammatory. Chronicity of the inflammatory process is contributed by mucociliary dysfunction, mucostasis, hypoxia, and release of microbial products. Among the infectious causes, anaerobes, *Staphylococcus aureus* and coagulase-negative *Staphylococci* are the predominantly cultured microbes from sinus aspirate especially in patients with immunodeficiency states and mucociliary dysfunction (cystic fibrosis, immotile cilia syndrome, Kartagener syndrome). Immune hyperresponsiveness to an inciting agent (bacterial or fungal protein) may trigger chronic inflammation and formation of polyps. It is closely associated with other allergic diseases like rhinitis, asthma and aspirin sensitivity. Gastroesophageal reflux can contribute to sinusitis by causing ostium inflammation. Vasomotor sinusitis includes physical hypersensitivity to temperature change, barometric pressure, irritants and changing emotional states.

CONDITIONS PREDISPOSING TO SINUSITIS

- Allergic and nonallergic rhinitis
- Anatomic abnormality of the OMC
- Nasal anatomic variants:
  - Septal deviation
  - Septal spur
  - Concha bullosa
  - Paradoxical curvature of the middle turbinate
  - Haller cells

- Cystic fibrosis
- Common variable immunoglobulin (Ig) deficiency
- Specific antibody deficiency
- IgG subclass deficiency
- IgA deficiency
- Ciliary dyskinesia, Kartagener syndrome, Young syndrome
- Aspirin sensitivity
- Acquired immunodeficiency syndrome
- Churg—Strauss syndrome
- Rhinitis medicamentosa
- Environmental irritants
- Foreign bodies
- Adenoid hypertrophy
- Nasal polyp
- Smoking
- Cocaine abuse
- Swimming and diving.

DIAGNOSIS

Sinusitis is mostly diagnosed on clinical suspicion and confirmed with supportive labs. A careful history about classical symptoms and local examination is usually sufficient for initiating therapy.

History

- Nasal congestion, purulent rhinorrhea, postnasal drainage, facial or dental pain, headache (worse in morning hours), cough (worsening at night time) and sensation of pressure in paranasal area (worse on leaning forward), pressure or pain in ear.
- Less frequent symptoms are fever, nausea, malaise, fatigue, halitosis, hyposmia and sore throat.
- Additional symptoms in children are increased irritability and vomiting.

Physical Examination

- Nasal mucosa should be examined for color, swelling and character of secretions, polyps, and structure of nasal septum
- Palpate for tenderness in maxillary and frontal sinus area
- Transillumination of frontal and maxillary sinuses
- Dark circles beneath the eyes, periorbital edema
- Pharyngeal edema, lymphoid hyperplasia, purulent material in posterior pharynx
- Ear examination—middle ear effusion, eustachian tube dysfunction
- Complicating factors—presence of facial swelling-erythema over the sinus, visual changes, abnormal extraocular movements, proptosis, periorbital inflammation-edema-erythema, any sign of intracranial involvement as abnormal neurological signs.

Diagnostic Criteria

At least 2 major or 1 major and atleast 2 minor symptoms among the following:
- Major:
    - Purulent anterior nasal discharge
    - Purulent or discolored posterior nasal discharge
    - Nasal congestion or obstruction
    - Facial congestion or fullness
    - Facial pain or pressure
    - Hyposmia or anosmia
    - Fever (for acute sinusitis only).
- Minor:
    - Headache
    - Ear pain, pressure, or fullness
    - Halitosis
    - Dental pain
    - Cough
    - Fever (for subacute or chronic sinusitis)
    - Fatigue.

Imaging

- X-ray paranasal sinuses—opacification or mucosal thickening and air-fluid level in frontal, maxillary and sphenoid sinuses:
    - Mucosal thickening of more than 6 mm in adults or more than 4 mm in children for maxillary sinus
    - More than 33% loss of air space volume within the maxillary sinuses
    - Opacification or air-fluid levels in any of the paranasal sinuses.
- Computed tomography (CT) scan—it is the investigation of choice, ethmoid sinuses can be studied in better manner
- Ultrasonography—alternative tool for frontal and maxillary sinus especially in pregnancy, due to radiation free technique
- Magnetic resonance imaging (MRI)—helps in evaluation of soft tissues, differentiation between inflammatory or malignant disease and to evaluate intracranial or orbital complications.

Indications

- Computed tomography without contrast—images bone, sinus anatomy, ostiomeatal complex, better soft-air-bone contrast:
    - Recurrent acute sinusitis
    - Chronic sinusitis
    - Preoperative for sinus surgery
    - Nasal polyposis
    - Persistent nasal congestion—obstruction
    - Immunocompromised patient with fever
    - Dentomaxillary pain
    - Facial pressure-headache unresponsive to medical therapy
    - Anosmia after appropriate workup.
- Computed tomography with contrast—differentiates soft tissue opacification:
    - Complications of sinusitis (periorbital edema, subperiosteal abscess).

- Magnetic resonance imaging with contrast—excellent soft tissue differentiation:
    - Skull base dehiscence with opacification
    - Unilateral sinonasal opacification (on CT scan)
    - Sinonasal process with cranial extension
    - Expansible sinonasal mass with bony erosion (? Remodeling)
    - Sinonasal mass with orbital extension
    - Biopsy—proved tumor
    - Fungal sinusitis.

Microbiology

- Responsible pathogen may be cultured through maxillary sinus aspiration.

Differential Diagnosis

- Infectious rhinitis:
    - Viral upper respiratory tract infections.
- Allergic rhinitis:
    - Seasonal
    - Perennial.
- Nonallergic rhinitis:
    - Vasomotor rhinitis
    - Aspirin intolerance
    - Eosinophilic nonallergic rhinitis.
- Rhinitis medicamentosa:
    - Decongestants
    - β-blockers
    - Birth control pills
    - Antihypertensives.
- Rhinitis secondary to:
    - Pregnancy
    - Hypothyroidism
    - Horner syndrome
    - Wegener granulomatosis—midline granuloma.

- Anatomic abnormalities causing rhinitis:
  - Foreign body
  - Nasal polyps
  - Nasal septal deviation
  - Enlarged tonsils and adenoids.
- Concha bullosa and other middle turbinate abnormalities
- Tumors
- Cerebral spinal fluid rhinorrhea
- Vascular headache (migraine).

TREATMENT

Acute Sinusitis

Antibiotics (Table 4) for at least 2 weeks are the mainstay of therapy as infectious etiology is more likely in acute sinusitis. Amoxicillin-clavulanate is commonly used as initial empirical therapy. Anti-inflammatory agents like intranasal steroids may act as adjunctive therapy. Surgical interventions might be required, in case of any complications or nonresponsiveness.

Chronic Sinusitis

Anti-inflammatory agents like inhaled nasal corticosteroids are the mainstay of treatment with antibiotics as an adjunct in some of the patients. Aspirin desensitization should be done in case of aspirin sensitivity. Leukotriene modifiers might be useful with nasal polyposis and aspirin exacerbated respiratory disease (AERD).

Adjunctive Therapies
- Saline: Saline nasal sprays or lavage liquefies secretions
- Steam inhalation (with or without added astringents)—membrane warming effect usually works as decongestant
- Mucolytics: No evidence
- Antihistamines: Occasionally helpful
- α-adrenergic decongestants: Topical (oxymetazoline, xylometazoline and phenylephrine) and oral decongestants

Table 4: Antibiotics (with dosage) for sinusitis.

Antibiotic	Pediatric dose	Adult dose
Amoxicillin	45 mg/kg BID	500 mg BID
Amoxicillin/potassium Clavulanate	22.5–45 mg/kg (of amoxicillin) BID	500–875 mg BID
Erythromycin/sulfisoxazole	12.5/37.5 mg/kg QID	—
Sulfamethoxazole/trimethoprim	200/40 mg/kg BID	800/160 mg/kg BID
Cefuroxime	7.5 mg/kg BID	250–500 mg BID
Cefpodoxime	5 mg/kg BID	200–400 mg BID
Cefixime	8 mg/kg QD	400 mg QD
Azithromycin	Day 1–10 mg/kg Day 2 to 5–5 mg/kg QD	Day 1–500 mg Day 2 to 5–250 mg QD
Clarithromycin	7.5 mg/kg BID	500 mg BID
Ciprofloxacin	—	500–700 mg BID
Levofloxacin	—	500 mg QD
Clindamycin	15 mg/kg TID	150–450 mg TID, QID
Metronidazole	7.5 mg/kg TID	250–500 mg TID, QID

(BID: twice daily; QID: 4 times daily; QD: every day; TID: 3 times a day)

Source: Slavin RG, Spector SL, Bernstein IL. The diagnosis and management of sinusitis: a practice parameter update. J Allergy Clin Immunol. 2005;116:S13-47.

(pseudoephedrine) reduce tissue edema by vasoconstriction, enhance secretion drainage; 3–5 days course is usually sufficient
- Surgery—reserved for partial or nonresponders or advanced disease with complications (removal of disease tissue, polyps and/or drainage of sinuses)
- Environmental control:
  - Changing workplace (if symptoms are in a particular place like office building)
  - Increasing fresh air ventilation
  - Using high-efficiency particulate air and electrostatic filters.

- Changing habits:
  - No more than usual time in reclining position in bed, as recumbent position increases nasal congestion
  - Quit smoking or drug abuse.
- Education:
  - Advise comfort measures—adequate rest, hydration, analgesics, warm facial packs, steamy showers, head end of bed elevated during sleep
  - Avoid adverse factors—relevant allergens, pollution, barotrauma, aspirin or other nonsteroidal anti-inflammatory diseases (NSAIDs)
  - Early and appropriate treatment—allergies, viral upper respiratory infections.

Indications for Referral to a Specialist

- Severe infection—high persistent fever with temperature more than 39°C (>102°F); orbital edema, severe headache, visual disturbance, altered mental status, meningeal signs
- Recalcitrant infection with failure to respond to extended courses of antimicrobial therapy
- Immunocompromised host
- Multiple medical problems along with sinusitis (e.g. hepatic or renal impairment, hypersensitivity to antimicrobial agents, organ transplant)
- Unusual or resistant pathogens
- Fungal sinusitis or granulomatous disease
- Nosocomial infection
- Anatomic defects causing obstruction and requiring surgical intervention
- Multiple recurrent episodes of acute bacterial rhinosinusitis (3-4 episodes per year) suggesting chronic sinusitis
- Chronic rhinosinusitis (with or without polyps or asthma) with recurrent exacerbations
- Evaluation of immunotherapy for allergic rhinitis.

Allergic Fungal Rhinosinusitis (AFRS)

The characteristic features of AFRS are nasal polyposis, type I and possibly type III hypersensitivity reaction, production of allergic mucin with abundant eosinophils and noninvading fungal hyphae. Fungal allergens create hypersensitivity reactions in the atopic individual. There are various factors, which have a role in pathogenesis of AFRS (Fig. 5).

AFRS is commonly seen in young immunocompetent males from rural background, which work in warm climates, and are colonized with fungus frequently. People from African-American origin, structural anomalies and low socioeconomic status are more prone to develop this disease. AFRS should be suspected

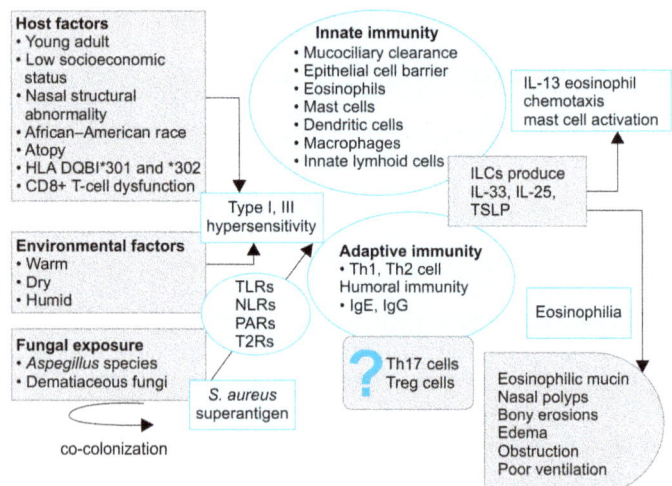

(HLA: human leukocyte antigen; ILC: innate lymphoid cell; IL: interleukin; TLRs: toll like receptors; NLRs: NOD like receptors; PARs: protease activated receptors; TSLP: thymic stromal lymphopoitin; Th: T-helper)

Fig. 5: Interplay of various factors in pathophysiology of allergic fungal rhinosinusitis.

Source: Chakrabarti A, Kaur H. Allergic aspergillus rhinosinusitis. J Fungi. 2016;2:32.

in immunocompetent hosts showing symptoms of chronic rhinosinusitis with nasal polyposis and viscid, dark mucoid discharge with greenish black nasal casts and who are not responding to conventional medical and surgical interventions, and targeted bacterial etiology. Visual disturbances, proptosis, telecanthus, facial deformity, neuropathies or intracranial abscess are known complications.

Among the several diagnostic criteria, Bent and Kuhn criteria (1994) are widely used for AFRS diagnosis, which includes:

- Major criteria:
    - Type I hypersensitivity
    - Nasal polyposis
    - Typical CT findings—multiple sinus opacifications with central hyperattenuation, sinus mucocele, skull base erosions, central low T1 and T2 void in sinuses, due to eosinophilic mucin, surrounded by low T1 and high T2 signal intensity of inflamed mucosa enhanced by intravenous gadolinium contrast
    - Eosinophilic mucin containing fungus (without evidence of invasion).
- Minor criteria:
    - Asthma
    - Charcot-Leyden crystals
    - Eosinophilia
    - Unilateral disease
    - Culture positive for fungus
    - Bony erosion.

Type I hypersensitivity to fungi can be demonstrated by either specific IgE (ImmunoCAP) or skin prick test. Total IgE, though nonspecific test, value is usually more than 1,000 IU/mL. Eosinophilic mucin is viscid, tenacious and peanut butter-like and has a dark-greenish to brown color. On staining, onion laminations of eosinophils surrounded by Charcot-Leyden crystals and mucin are visible.

MANAGEMENT

The management of AFRS includes combined surgical and medical therapy. Fungal load (antigenic stimulus) is reduced, mucus and debris are removed with functional endoscopic sinus surgery (FESS), which helps in improving ventilation and restoring mucociliary function. Saline irrigations and oral steroids (12 weeks postoperatively) are recommended for medical treatment. Antifungal therapy might be helpful in reducing fungal load, steroid dependence and tendency of recurrence. There is no consensus on role of specific immunotherapy and leukotriene modulators. Anti-IL-5 antibody (mepolizumab) has been shown of potential benefit in reducing polyp size and sinus opacification.

CONCLUSION

Sinusitis is an important entity with significant effect on physical, mental and social wellbeing of an individual. It has got diverse etiology. Allergic factors play significant role in pathogenesis of chronic sinusitis. An early suspicion, especially in children, followed by relevant investigations and appropriate management is the key to prevent many complications. Flowchart 2 depicts a comprehensive approach to a patient with sinusitis.

4.3 OTITIS MEDIA

INTRODUCTION

Otitis media (OM) is very common inflammatory disorder of middle ear in children. Almost 80% of children get at least one episode of OM by their 3rd birthday and up to three episodes in half of them. Infants are most vulnerable for OM. It is rare after 6 years of life. Children are at higher risk due to partially developed immune system, shorter and horizontal eustachian tube, presence of lymphoid follicles and adenoids in the nasopharyngeal area. OM imposes a huge burden on economic status, costing approximately 3.8 billion US dollar (USD) in United States alone, mainly contributed to cost of antimicrobials use.

Flowchart 2: Approach to a patient with sinusitis.

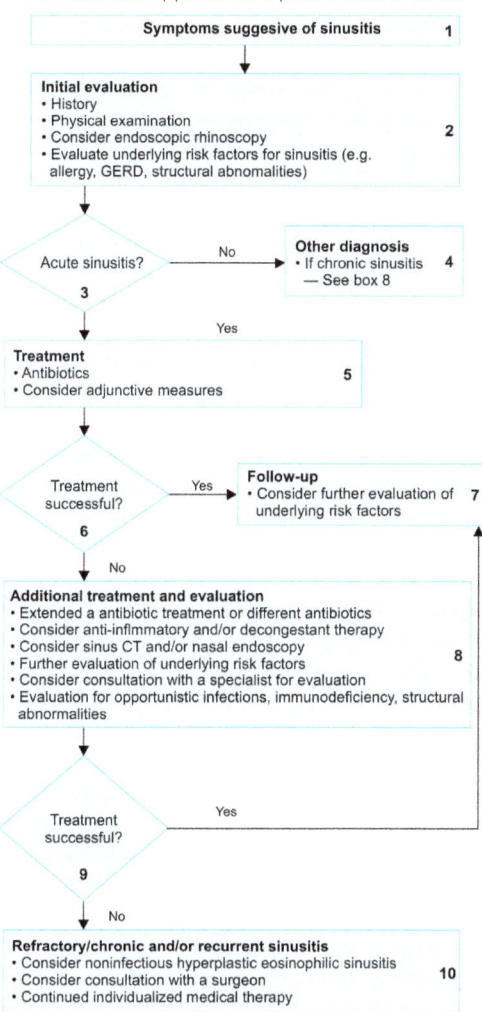

(GERD: gastroesophageal reflux disease; CT: computed tomography)
Source: Slavin RG, Spector SL, Bernstein IL. The diagnosis and management of sinusitis: a practice parameter update. J Allergy Clin Immunol. 2005;116:S13-47.

DEFINITIONS

Acute OM may be characterized by rapid onset inflammation of the middle ear cleft, which is usually infective and frequently associated with middle ear effusion. Acute OM may be further categorized as:
- Sporadic episodes—infrequent isolated events, mostly with upper respiratory tract infections
- Resistant—persistent symptom and signs beyond 3-5 days of antibiotic treatment
- Persistent—persistent or recurrent symptoms and signs within 6 days of completion of an antibiotic course
- Recurrent—more than or equal to three episodes of acute OM within 6 months, or more than or equal to four episodes within 12 months period.

PREDISPOSING FACTORS

- Age—maximum incidence between 3 months and 3 years
- Ethnicity—native American, Alaskan and Canadian children are more predisposed
- Male sex
- More than one sibling at home
- Parental smoking and exposure to wood smoke—major risk factor
- Upper respiratory tract infections (rhinitis, nasopharyngitis)—direct spread of infectious agent from nasopharynx to middle ear
- Day care attendance
- Familial tendency—history of allergic rhinitis, asthma, milk protein allergy, parental atopy and OM predisposes for acute OM due to eustachian tube blockage and malfunction, by lymphoid hyperplasia
- Short duration of breastfeeding—breastfeeding increases IgA concentration in baby and also reduces aspiration of contaminated secretions in middle ear space
- Use of pacifiers, presence of digit sucking and bottle feeding

- Gastroesophageal reflux
- Overcrowding and poor socioeconomic status—easy transmission depending on room space and adequacy of ventilation
- Infections (measles, pertussis, diphtheria, tuberculosis) and immunosuppression (defects of chemotaxis, phagocytosis and killing)
- Cleft palate, Down syndrome and other craniofacial defects—predisposition to chronic OM (with effusion) due to eustachian tube dysfunction
- Genetic factors—certain human leukocyte antigen (HLA) classes have been shown to be associated with recurrent acute OM. Maternal blood group A is known to be an independent risk factor for OM in children.

PATHOGENESIS

The common viral pathological agents are respiratory syncytial virus (RSV), rhinovirus, parainfluenza and coronavirus whereas *Streptococcus pneumoniae* is the most common bacteria involved followed by *Moraxella catarrhalis*, and nontypeable *Haemophilus influenza*. Organism may infect middle ear mucosa via eustachian tube (most common route), tympanic membrane perforation (pathological or grommet insertion) and hematogenous spread. The culprit organism initially affects the eustachian tube followed by inflammation, tube blockage and ultimately its dysfunction. The normal functions of eustachian tube are:
- Primary defense mechanism of middle ear
- Equilibration of middle ear pressure with atmospheric pressure
- Protection of middle ear from reflux of nasopharyngeal secretions
- Drains middle ear secretions into the nasopharynx.

As the eustachian tube is smaller, wider and more horizontal in younger children, they are more prone to OM than adolescents and adults.

CLINICAL FEATURES

- Acute OM—earache, fever, purulent foul smelling discharge, hearing impairment, irritability, restlessness
- Otitis media with effusion—mostly asymptomatic with some times "plugged ear" feeling, hearing impairment
- Chronic suppurative OM (CSOM)—purulent ear discharge for more than 6 weeks, perforation of tympanic membrane, hearing impairment.

STAGES

Four stages can be differentiated in clinical course of otitis media:
- Tubotympanitis—nonspecific discomfort, loss of mobility of tympanic membrane
- Hyperemia—otalgia, hyperpyrexia, opaque tympanic membrane with reduced mobility
- Exudative—severe otalgia with loss of anatomical features
- Suppurative—severe pulsatile otalgia, yellow tympanic membrane, purulent or bloody otorrhea.

INVESTIGATIONS

- Otoscopy—conventional and pneumatic—pneumatic is preferred, as mobility of tympanic membrane can be assessed
- Tympanometry—to detect middle ear effusion with sensitivity of 70% and specificity of 90%
- Respiratory assays—may be utilized to identify the common viral etiology
- Microbiological culture—bacterial swab of ear discharge
- Complete blood count—anemia and white blood cell disorders are known to be associated with acute OM
- Immunoglobulin profile—may be appropriate in children with recurrent infections
- Work-up for primary ciliary dyskinesia—if nasal and pulmonary symptoms coexist.

DIAGNOSIS

- Acute OM—yellowish-pink bulging tympanic membrane, eardrum perforation, discharge, reduced eardrum mobility
- Otitis media with effusion—air-fluid levels in middle ear, clear or amber color middle ear fluid, negative middle ear pressure (prominent lateral process and shortening of long arm of malleus with horizontal orientation), tympanometry may be used to determine mobility of eardrum in children over 6 months of age
- Chronic suppurative OM (CSOM)—perforated tympanic membrane, polyp and discharge from middle ear might be visualized.

TREATMENT (TABLE 5)

- Acute OM:
    - First-line antibiotic—amoxicillin
    - Second-line antibiotic—amoxicillin-clavulanate combination
    - Antihistamine or decongestant role—controversial
    - Analgesics
    - Antipyretics
    - Local heat
    - Myringotomy.
- Recurrent OM:
    - Chemoprophylaxis
    - Tympanostomy tubes
    - Immunization *(Pneumococcus)*
    - Adenoidectomy—short-term benefit as prophylaxis.
- Otitis media with residual and persistent effusion:
    - Wait and watch (for spontaneous resolution of effusion)
    - Antibiotics ±
    - Corticosteroids may be used
    - Ventilation tubes.

Table 5: Pharmacotherapy in otitis media.

Agent	Dose	Comments
Antimicrobials (course of 10 days is recommended, unless specified)		
Amoxicillin	80–90 mg/kg/day in two divided doses	First-line drug
Amoxicillin/clavulanate	90 mg/kg of amoxicillin in two divided doses	Second-line drug
Azithromycin	30 mg/kg single dose 20 mg/kg/day for 3 days	In penicillin allergy, recurrent infection
Cefdinir	14 mg/kg/day in one or two divided doses	In penicillin allergy
Cefpodoxime	30 mg/kg once daily	In penicillin allergy
Ceftriaxone	50 mg/kg once daily	In penicillin allergy, recurrent or persistent infection
Cefuroxime	30 mg/kg/day in two divided doses	In penicillin allergy
Clarithromycin	15 mg/kg/day in three divided doses	In penicillin allergy
Clindamycin	30–40 mg/kg/day in four divided doses	In penicillin allergy
Topical agents (for 7–10 days in chronic suppurative otitis media)		
Ciprofloxacin	3 drops twice daily	
Hydrocortisone/neomycin/polymyxin B	4 drops 3–4 times daily	
Ofloxacin	5 drops twice daily	
Analgesics		
Acetaminophen	15 mg/kg every 6 hours	
Ibuprofen	10 mg/kg every 6 hours	

Source: Ramakrishnan K, Sparks RA, Berryhill WE. Diagnosis and treatment of otitis media. Am Fam Physician. 2007;76(11):1650-8.

- Chronic suppurative OM:
  - Systemic antibiotics (for *Pseudomonas* and anaerobes)
  - Topical quinolones

- Regular cleaning of ear canals
- Repair procedures—paper patch, fat myringoplasty, tympanoplasty.

STRATEGIES FOR PREVENTING RECURRENT OTITIS MEDIA

- Check for undiagnosed allergies leading to chronic rhinorrhea
- Eliminate bottle propping and pacifiers
- Eliminate exposure to passive smoke
- Routinely immunize with the pneumococcal conjugate and influenza vaccines.

COMPLICATION

- Intracranial:
    - Meningitis
    - Extradural abscess
    - Subdural empyema
    - Sigmoid sinus thrombosis
    - Focal otitic encephalitis (cerebritis)
    - Brain abscess
    - Otitic hydrocephalus.
- Extracranial:
    - Tympanic membrane perforation—being the most common complication, it can heal spontaneously or persists with or without otorrhea
    - Acute mastoiditis
    - Petrositis—infection extends to apex of petrous bone. The classical Gradenigo's triad (VI nerve palsy, severe pain in trigeminal nerve distribution and middle ear infection) need not to be present always
    - Facial nerve palsy
    - Labyrinthitis.

CONCLUSION

Otitis media is common among small children. It can cause significant acute symptoms and long-term sequelae, if left undetected. Most of the patients recover spontaneously still antibiotics are used to eradicate the causative pathogens from middle ear cavity. Careful selection of antibiotics is very important, to tackle emerging resistance. Surgical interventions might be required, as an adjunct, in some of the cases. Flowchart 3 enumerates the steps of management for a patient with otitis media. Universal immunization including pneumococcal conjugate and Influenza A vaccines should be implemented for primary protection.

4.4 ASTHMA

DEFINITION

Asthma is a heterogeneous disease, characterized by chronic airway inflammation. The typical features are wheezing, shortness of breath, chest tightness, and cough along with variable expiratory airflow limitation.

PHENOTYPES

As many disease processes result in airflow limitation, asthma is usually defined by phenotypic expression based on demographic, clinical, and/or pathophysiological characteristics in a particular patient (Fig. 6). This might help in guiding management, with variable treatment responses (Table 6). The most common phenotypes are:

- *Allergic asthma*: Symptoms often start in early childhood. There is personal or familial history of atopy/allergic diseases like dermatitis, rhinitis, and food or drug allergy. It is usually characterized by eosinophilic airway inflammation and has a good response to inhaled corticosteroids (ICS).
- *Nonallergic asthma*: Often starts in adults, with neutrophilic or eosinophilic inflammation, without any atopic history. These patients do not respond to ICS well.

Flowchart 3: Approach to a patient with otitis media.

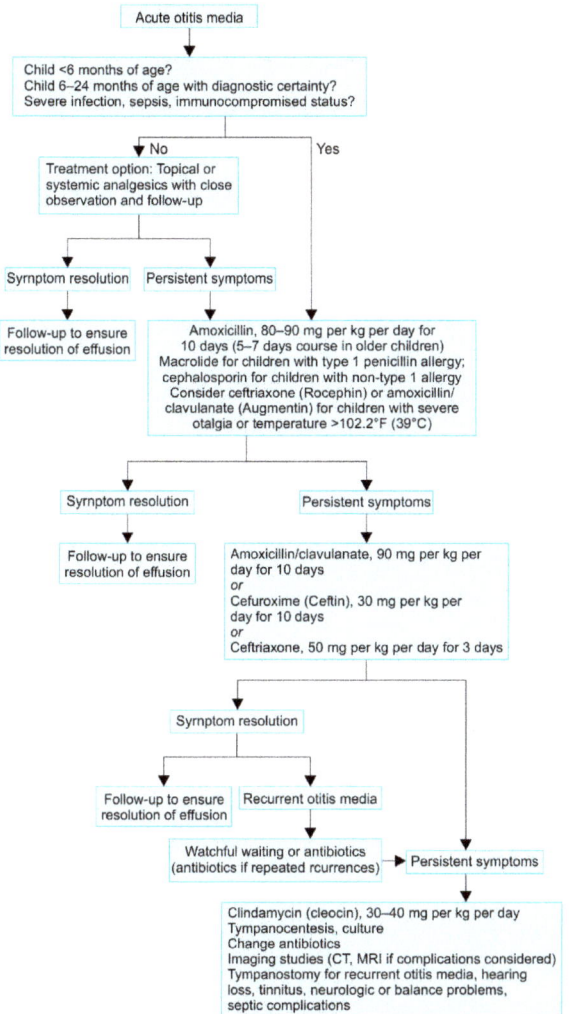

Source: Ramakrishnan K, Sparks RA, Berryhill WE. Diagnosis and treatment of otitis media. Am Fam Physician. 2007;76(11):1650-8.

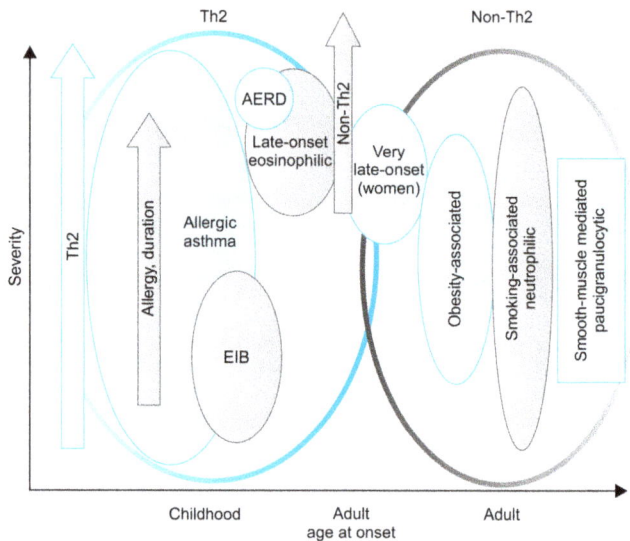

Fig. 6: Asthma phenotypes for difficult to control asthma.
(AERD: aspirin-exacerbated respiratory disease; EIB: exercise-induced bronchoconstriction; Th: T-helper)
Source: Wenzel SE. Asthma phenotypes: the evolution from clinical to molecular approaches. Nat Med. 2012;18:716-25.

- *Late-onset asthma*: Nonatopic adult women with first-time onset, poor responders to ICS.
- *Asthma with fixed airflow limitation*: Airway wall remodeling in long-standing asthma.
- *Asthma with obesity*: Prominent asthmatic symptoms in obese patients with little eosinophilic inflammation.
- *Biomarker based*: Eosinophilic and neutrophilic.

PARAMETERS FOR EOSINOPHILIC INFLAMMATION IN ASTHMA

- Fractional exhaled nitric oxide (FENO): More than or equal to 35 (children) ppb and more than or equal to 50 (adults) ppb as cutoff for positive value

Table 6: Asthma phenotypes characteristics.

Phenotype	Natural history	Clinical and physiological features	Pathobiology and biomarkers	Genetics	Response to therapy
Early-onset allergic	Early onset; mild to severe	Allergic symptoms and other diseases	Specific IgE; Th$_2$ cytokines	17q12; Th$_2$-related genes	Corticosteroid responsive
Late-onset eosinophilic	Adult onset, often severe	Sinusitis; less allergic	Eosinophilia; IL-5		Responsive to antibody to IL-5 and cysteinyl leukotriene modifiers; corticosteroid refractory
Exercise-induced		Mild; intermittent with exercise	Mast cell activation; Th$_2$ cytokines; cysteinyl leukotrienes		Responsive to cysteinyl leukotriene modifiers, beta agonists and antibody to IL-9
Obesity-related	Adult onset	More common in females; very symptomatic	Lack of Th$_2$ biomarkers; oxidative stress		Responsive to weight loss, antioxidants and possibly to hormonal therapy
Neutrophilic		Low FEV$_1$; more air trapping	Sputum neutrophilia; Th$_{17}$ pathways; IL-8		Possibly responsive to macrolide antibiotics

(FEV: forced expiratory volume; IL: interleukin; Th: T-helper; Ig: Immunoglobulin)

- *Eosinophils in the blood differential count*: More than or equal to 4% or more than or equal to 400/mm^3
- *Eosinophils in induced sputum or bronchoalveolar lavage (BAL)*: More than or equal to 3%
- *Eosinophilic cationic protein (ECP) in serum*: More than or equal to 20 μg/L
- Eosinophilia is indirectly supported by:
  - Clinically relevant allergies
  - Reversible bronchial hyperreactivity
  - Good response to inhaled corticosteroids
  - Presence of nasal polyps and aspirin sensitivity.

MAKING A DIAGNOSIS (IN >6 YEARS, ADOLESCENTS, AND ADULTS)

- *History of variable respiratory symptoms*: Wheeze, shortness of breath, chest tightness, and cough:
  - Multiple respiratory symptoms
  - Variable over time and intensity
  - Worse at night or early morning
  - Exercise, laughter, allergens, and cold air being common triggers
  - Worsen during viral infections.
- *Confirmed variable expiratory airflow limitation*: Forced expiratory volume (FEV_1)/forced vital capacity (FVC) reduced (normally >0.75–0.80 in adults, >0.90 in children)
  - Positive bronchodilator reversibility test (withhold SABA ≥4 hours, LABA ≥15 hours):
    - Adults—increase in FEV_1 of more than 12% and more than 200 mL from baseline, 10–15 minutes after 200–400 μg of inhaled salbutamol
    - Children—increase in FEV_1 of more than 12% predicted
  - Excessive variability in twice daily peak expiratory flow (PEF) over 2 weeks [(day's highest minus day's lowest/mean of day's highest and lowest) averaged over 2 weeks]

- Adults: More than 10%
 - Children: More than 13%
- Significant increase in lung function after 4 weeks of anti-inflammatory treatment:
 - Adults: Increase in FEV_1 by more than 12% and more than 200 mL (or PEF >20%) from baseline after 4 weeks of treatment
- Positive exercise challenge test:
 - Adults: Fall in FEV_1 of more than 10% and more than 200 mL from baseline
 - Children: Fall in FEV_1 of more than 12% predicted, or PEF more than 15%
- Positive bronchial challenge test—performed in adults:
 - Fall in FEV_1 of more than or equal to 20% with standard doses of methacholine or histamine, or more than or equal to 15% with hyperventilation, hypertonic saline, or mannitol challenge
- Excessive variation in lung function between subsequent visits:
 - Adults: Variation in FEV_1 of more than 12% and more than 200 mL
 - Children: Variation in FEV_1 of more than 12% or more than 15% in PEF.

*Table 7 represents differentials of asthma in children and adults.

Supportive Tests

- *Allergy tests*: Skin prick test (in-vivo) or specific IgE (in-vitro), to carefully selected relevant allergens, can be used to identify atopic status of an individual. Skin prick test is simple, rapid, economical, and has better sensitivity and specificity than blood tests, with limitations in extensive skin diseases, immediate postanaphylaxis period and in a patient on antihistaminics.
- *Fractional concentration of exhaled nitric oxide (FENO)*: Higher concentration of FENO is directly proportional to type-2 airway inflammation like allergic asthma, though the levels can rise in non-asthmatic conditions (eosinophilic bronchitis,

atopy, allergic rhinitis, eczema) and levels will be normal in neutrophilic asthma. FENO levels are falsely low in smokers, during bronchoconstriction and in early phase of allergic response or the levels may be variable in viral respiratory infections. FENO levels are widely used for monitoring asthma control but, till date, there is no consensus for its utility in asthma management.

ASTHMA ASSESSMENT (IN >6 YEARS, ADOLESCENTS, AND ADULTS)

- *Assess asthma control*: Symptom control and future risk of adverse outcomes:
  - *Assess symptom control* (over last 4 weeks)—based on day symptoms, night symptoms, reliever use, and level of activity; level of asthma control is classified as well controlled (none of four symptoms), partly controlled (one to two of four symptoms) and uncontrolled (three or more symptoms).
    - Day symptoms—cough, wheeze, dyspnea, symptom trigger, and way of achieving control
    - Night symptoms—cough, awakenings, tiredness during day
    - Reliever use—frequency of use
    - Level of activity—as compared to peers or siblings
  - Various asthma symptom control tools are:
    - For adults and adolescents:
      - Asthma Control Questionnaire (ACQ): Score 0–6 (higher score is worse)
      - Asthma Control Test (ACT): Score 5–25 (higher score is better)
    - For children 6–11 years:
      - Childhood Asthma Control Test (c-ACT)
      - Asthma Control Questionnaire (ACQ)

- *Assess asthma severity*:
    - Mild: Well controlled on as-needed reliever medication alone or with low-intensity controller treatment such as low dose ICS, leukotriene receptors, or chromones (Step 1 or Step 2 in Fig. 7)
    - Moderate: Well controlled on low dose ICS/LABA combination or moderate dose ICS (Step 3)
    - Severe: Asthma that requires higher treatment like high-dose ICS/LABA combination (Step 4 or Step 5)
- *Identify risk factors for exacerbations*:
    - High SABA use (>1 × 200-dose canister/month)
    - Inadequate ICS, poor adherence, incorrect inhaler technique
    - Low FEV_1 (<60% of predicted)
    - High bronchodilator reversibility
    - Major psychological or socioeconomic problems
    - Smoking, allergen exposure
    - Comorbidities—obesity, chronic rhinosinusitis, confirmed food allergy
    - Sputum or blood eosinophilia
    - Elevated FENO
    - Pregnancy
    - Past history of intubation on admission in intensive care unit for asthma (independent risk factor)
    - More than or equal to 1 severe exacerbation in last 12 months
- *Identify risk factors for fixed airflow limitations*:
    - Preterm birth, low-birth weight
    - Lack of ICS treatment
    - Exposure to tobacco smoke, noxious chemicals, occupational exposures
    - Low initial FEV_1, chronic mucus hypersecretion, sputum or blood eosinophilia

Table 7: Differential diagnosis of asthma (in >6 years, adolescents, and adults).

Age	Condition	Symptoms
6–11 years	Chronic upper airway cough syndrome (postnasal drip)	Sneezing, itching, blocked nose, throat-clearing
	Inhaled foreign body	Sudden onset of symptoms, unilateral wheeze
	Bronchiectasis	Recurrent infections, productive cough
	Primary ciliary dyskinesia	Recurrent infections, productive cough, sinusitis
	Congenital heart disease	Cardiac murmurs, ±cyanosis
	Bronchopulmonary dysplasia	History of premature birth, symptoms since birth
	Cystic fibrosis	Excessive cough and mucus production, gastrointestinal symptoms
12–39 years	Chronic upper airway cough syndrome (postnasal drip)	Sneezing, itching, blocked nose, throat-clearing
	Vocal cord dysfunction	Dyspnea, inspiratory stridor
	Hyperventilation, dysfunctional breathing	Dizziness, paresthesia, sighing
	Bronchiectasis	Recurrent infections, productive cough
	Cystic fibrosis	Excessive cough and mucus production
	Congenital heart disease	Cardiac murmurs, ±cyanosis
	Alpha$_1$-antitrypsin deficiency	Shortness of breath, family history of early emphysema
	Inhaled foreign body	Sudden onset of symptoms
40+ years	Vocal cord dysfunction	Dyspnea, inspiratory stridor
	Hyperventilation, dysfunctional breathing	Dizziness, paresthesia, sighing
	Chronic obstructive pulmonary disease (COPD)	Cough, sputum, dyspnea on exertion, smoking or noxious exposure
	Bronchiectasis	Productive cough, recurrent infections
	Cardiac failure	Dyspnea with exertion, nocturnal symptoms
	Medication-related cough	Treatment with angiotensin converting enzyme (ACE) inhibitor
	Parenchymal lung disease	Dyspnea with exertion, non-productive cough, finger clubbing
	Pulmonary embolism	Sudden onset of dyspnea, chest pain
	Central airway obstruction	Shortness of breath, no response to bronchodilators

- *Identify risk factors for medication side effects* (easy bruising, osteoporosis, cataracts, glaucoma, adrenal suppression, oral thrush and dysphonia)
  - Systemic—frequent oral corticosteroids (OCS), long-term high dose and/or potent OCS, taking P450 inhibitors
  - Local—high dose or potent ICS, poor inhaler technique
- *Measure lung function* at diagnosis/start of treatment, 3-6 months after starting controller treatment, then periodically
- *Assess treatment issues*:
  - Document the patient's current treatment step
  - Watch inhaler technique, assess adherence and side effects
  - Check for availability of written asthma action plan with patient
  - Ask about the patient's attitudes and goals for their asthma symptoms and medications
- *Assess comorbidities* (contributes to poor quality of life and poor asthma control)
  - Rhinitis
  - Rhinosinusitis
  - Gastroesophageal reflux
  - Obesity
  - Obstructive sleep apnea
  - Depression and anxiety
- *Other investigations* (if needed):
  - 2-week diary—document symptoms, reliever use, PEF readings
  - Exercise challenge—document airway hyperresponsiveness.

MANAGEMENT (>6 YEARS, ADOLESCENTS, AND ADULTS)

Controlling the acute symptoms and minimizing the future risk of exacerbations with minimal or no side effects are the key in management of asthma. Figure 7 depicts various steps of asthma management. Doses of inhaled steroids are enumerated in Table 8.

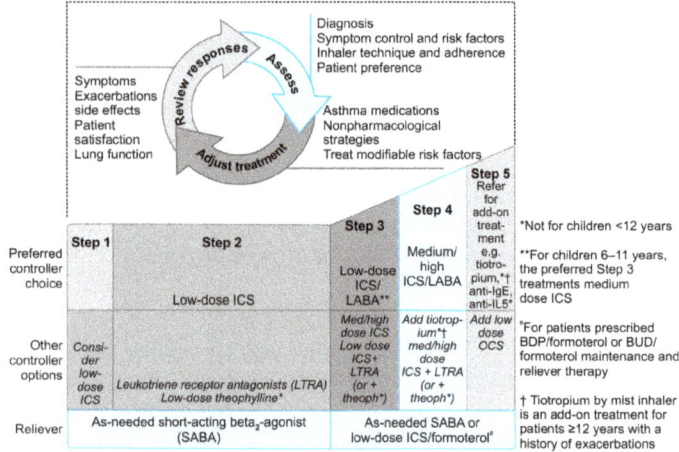

Fig. 7: Steps of asthma management in children more than 6 years, adolescents, and adults.
(ICS: inhaled corticosteroids; IgE: immunoglobulin E; LABA: long-acting beta agonists)
Source: Global Initiative for Asthma (2018). Global strategy for Asthma management and prevention.

Step 1: *As-needed reliever medication*:
- SABA (as quick reliever) should be used for occasional day time symptoms (less than twice a month), lasting for only few hours, no night waking and normal lung functions.
- Low dose ICS may be started to decrease exacerbation risk.

Step 2: *Low dose controller medication plus as-needed reliever medication*:
- Regular low-dose ICS should be started as it effectively reduces symptoms, risk of exacerbations, asthma-related hospitalizations and death, improves lung functions, and quality of life.
- Leukotriene receptor antagonist (LTRA), though less effective, may be used as an alternate to ICS, if ICS cannot be used and in patients with associated allergic rhinitis.

Table 8: Various doses of inhaled corticosteroids (ICS) for adolescents and adults.

Drug	Daily dose (mcg)		
	Low	Medium	High
Adults and adolescents (12 years and older)			
Beclomethasone dipropionate (CFC)	200–500	>500–1,000	>1,000
Beclomethasone dipropionate (HFA)	100–200	>200–400	>400
Budesonide (DPI)	200–400	>400–800	>800
Ciclesonide (HFA)	80–160	>160–320	>320
Fluticasone furoate (DPI)	100	NA	200
Fluticasone propionate (DPI)	100–250	>250–500	>500
Fluticasone propionate (HFA)	100–250	>250–500	>500
Mometasone furoate	110–220	>220–440	>440
Triamcinolone acetonide	400–1,000	>1,000–2,000	>2,000
Children 6–11 years			
Beclomethasone dipropionate (CFC)	100–200	>200–400	>400
Beclomethasone dipropionate (HFA)	50–100	>100–200	>200
Budesonide (DPI)	100–200	>200–400	>400
Budesonide (nebules)	250–500	>500–1,000	>1,000
Ciclesonide	80	>80–160	>160
Fluticasone furoate (DPI)	NA	NA	NA
Fluticasone propionate (DPI)	100–200	>200–400	>400
Fluticasone propionate (HFA)	100–200	>200–500	>500
Mometasone furoate	110	≥220–<440	≥440
Triamcinolone acetonide	400–800	>800–1,200	>1,200

(CFC: chlorofluorocarbon propellant; DPI: dry powder inhaler; HFA: hydrofluoroalkane propellant; NA: not applicable)

- Weak efficacy of sustained-release theophylline with many side effects
- Favorable safety profile of chromones (nedocromil sodium and sodium cromoglycate) but low efficacy; inhalers require daily washing.

Step 3: *One or two controllers plus as-needed reliever medication*:
- Combination of low-dose ICS/LABA combination as maintenance plus as-needed SABA (in adults or adolescents), Or
- Combination of low-dose ICS (budesonide or beclomethasone)/formoterol as both maintenance and reliever treatment (in adults and adolescents), Or
- Moderate-dose ICS plus as-needed SABA (in children)
- Low-dose ICS plus either LTRA or low dose, sustained-release theophylline—less effective
- Sublingual immunotherapy (SLIT) should be considered when culprit allergen is identified and pulmonary functions are adequately controlled (FEV_1 is >70% predicted).

Step 4: *Two or more controllers plus as-needed reliever medication*:
- Combination of low-dose ICS/formoterol as maintenance and reliever (in adults and adolescents), Or
- Combination medium-/high-dose ICS/LABA plus as-needed SABA
- Tiotropium (long-acting muscarinic antagonist) by mist inhaler may be used as an add-on therapy (in adults or adolescents)
- Sublingual immunotherapy should be considered when culprit allergen is identified and $F2EV_1$ is more than 70% predicted.

Step 5: *Higher level care and/or add-on treatment*:
- Add-on tiotropium (in adults and adolescents) with uncontrolled symptoms on ICS/LABA combination
- *Add-on anti-IgE (omalizumab) treatment*: More than or equal to 6 years with moderate or severe allergic asthma uncontrolled on Step 4
- Add-on anti-interleukin-5 (subcutaneous mepolizumab or benralizumab for ≥12 years; intravenous reslizumab for ≥18 years) for patients uncontrolled on Step 4 treatment
- *Sputum-guided treatment*: Target eosinophils less than 3% in induced sputum

- Bronchial thermoplasty—may be used in adult patients with severe uncontrolled asthma
- Add-on low-dose OCS (≤7.5 mg/day prednisone equivalent)—for adults in severe uncontrolled asthma.

Red flag signs in a patient with asthma—which suggest threat to life:
- Altered sensorium (drowsy or very agitated)
- Bradycardia
- Poor pulse volume
- Cyanosis
- Excessive use of accessory muscles or a state of exhaustion
- Vocalization limited to 1-2 words
- Silent chest on auscultation
- Peripheral capillary oxygen saturation (SpO_2) on room air less than 92%.

Management of an Acute Asthma Flare-up (Flowchart 4 and Table 9)

Management plan for acute asthma is discussed in Flowchart 4.

Table 9: Pulmonary score (PS) to determine severity of asthma exacerbation.

Score	RR (<6 years)	RR (>6 years)	Wheezing	Accessory muscle usage
0	<30	<20	None	No apparent activity
1	31–45	21–35	Terminal expiration with stethoscope	Questionable increase
2	46–60	36–50	Entire expiration with stethoscope	Increase apparent
3	>60	>50	During inspiration and expiration without stethoscope or wheezing absent due to absent airflow	Maximum activity
Total		0–3: Mild, 4–6: Moderate, >6: Severe		

(RR: respiratory rate)

Flowchart 4: Management plan for acute asthma.

Mild (PS 0–3)	Moderate (PS 4–6)	Severe (PS >6)	**Red flag signs**
Home plan	Emergency room plan	Ward plan	**ICU plan**

Mild (Home plan):
- SABA (2–4 puf q 20 min. × 3)
  - Sustained effect → Yes → Home or discharge plan
  - No → First dose rescue steroid @ 1 mg/kg/day

Moderate (Emergency room plan):
- Oxygen
- SABA nebulizer or puff q 20 min. × 3
- Rescue steroid (if not given earlier)
- SABA q 1 hourly/prn
- Obsrve hourly for 3–4 hours
- Sustained effect for 4–6 hours → Yes → Home or discharge plan; No → Ward plan

Severe (Ward plan):
- Oxygen
- IV fluids
- IV steroids
- SABA nebulizer q 20 min × 3, the 1 hour/continuous
- Ipratropium nebulizer q 30 min × 3, then q 6 hrs × 24 hours
- Monitor vital signs, SpO₂, pulmonary score q 15–30 mins
- IV Magsulf infusion over 30 min
- IV Aminophylline infusion
- Monitor K⁺
- CBC, CXR to identify complications
- Continuous monitoring
- Blood gas if SpO₂ <92%

Sustained effect for 4–6 hours → Yes → Meet discharge criteria; No → ICU plan

Red flag signs (ICU plan):
- Continue intensified ward plan
- Blood gas
- Trial of non-invasive ventilation
- Possible invasive ventiblation ketamine and Midazolam/fentanyl infusion
- Vecuronium (if required)

Improvement present → No → back to ICU / Yes → discharge criteria

Home or discharge plan
- Continue SABA prn till asymptomatic
- Rescue steroid (3–7 days)
- Trigger elimination
- Preventer adherence
- Follow-up within 7–14 days

Home or discharge plan
- Pneumothorax
- Pneu momediastinum
- Subcutaneous emphysema
- Atelectasis
- Bacterial/viral penumonia

Meet discharge criteria:
- Pulmonary score <3
- Comfortable
- Slept well at the night
- Eating well

Do not routinely use:
- Antibiotics, mucolytics, cough suppressants, chest physiotherapy

(CBC: complete blood count; CXR: chest X-ray; IV: intravenous; SpO₂: peripheral capillary oxygen saturation)

Source: Modified from Global Initiative for Asthma (2018). Global strategy for Asthma management and prevention.

Indications for Short Course of Oral Corticosteroids

For children (6–11 years): 1–2 mg/kg/day, maximum of 40 mg/day for 3–5 days; for adolescents and adults 40–50 mg/day for 5–7 days.

- Failure to respond to an increase in reliever and controller medication for 2–3 days
- Deteriorate rapidly or who have a PEF or FEV_1 less than 60% of their personal best or predicted value
- Have a history of sudden severe exacerbation.

Review for Response

- 1–3 months after starting treatment and 3–12 months thereafter.

Stepping up Asthma Treatment

- Sustained step-up for 2–3 months—if uncontrolled symptoms after correcting inhaler technique and adherence, removing modifiable risk factors
- Short-term step-up for 1–2 weeks—if exacerbations during viral infections or seasonal allergen exposure
- Day-to-day adjustment—if patient is on ICS (budesonide or beclomethasone)/formoterol combination.

Stepping down Asthma Treatment

- Once good control is achieved and maintained for 3 months
- Reduce ICS by 25–50% of the highest dose at 3-month interval
- Combination low-dose ICS/LABA may be stepped down to low-dose ICS alone (with or without addition of LTRA)
- After minimal dose of ICS—consider stopping controller after 6–12 months of asymptomatic period.

Nonpharmacological Interventions

- Cessation of smoking and environmental tobacco smoke (ETS) exposure
- Engage in regular physical activities
- Avoidance of occupational exposures

- Avoidance of medications that make asthma worse—aspirin, nonsteroidal anti-inflammatory drugs (NSAIDs)
- Encourage healthy diet
- Avoidance of indoor allergens (house dust mite, molds, cockroaches, etc.)
- Weight reduction for obese patients
- Specific allergen immunotherapy (provided FEV_1 is >70%)
- Breathing exercises
- Avoidance of indoor air pollution (use nonpolluting heat and cooking sources)
- Vaccination—routine pneumococcal and influenza vaccination
- Bronchial thermoplasty—in adults with severe uncontrolled disease
- Avoidance of outdoor allergens—pollens and molds, close windows and doors, remain indoors, use air conditioners
- Dealing with emotional stress—relaxation strategies and breathing exercises, mental health assessment
- Avoidance of outdoor air pollutants/weather conditions—very cold weather, low humidity, or high-air pollution
- Avoidance of sensitive food and food chemicals.

Indications for Referral or Expert Opinion

- Difficulty in confirming the diagnosis:
    - Symptoms of chronic infection
    - Features suggestive of cardiac or other nonpulmonary cause
    - No or partial response to ICS trial
    - Features of both chronic obstructive pulmonary disease (COPD) and asthma.
- Suspected occupational asthma:
    - For confirmatory testing and identification of sensitizing or irritant agent
    - For specific advice about eliminating exposure
    - For pharmacological treatment.

- Persistent uncontrolled asthma or frequent exacerbations:
  - Despite adequate controller and checking inhaler technique.
- Any risk factors for asthma-related death:
  - Near-fatal asthma attack (ICU admission, or mechanical ventilation for asthma) in past
  - Anaphylaxis or confirmed food allergy in asthmatic patient.
- Evidence or risk of significant treatment side effects:
  - Significant medication side effects
  - Long-term OCS treatment
  - Frequent need for OCS (two or more courses per year).
- Symptoms suggesting complications or subtypes of asthma:
  - Aspirin-exacerbated respiratory disease
  - Allergic bronchopulmonary aspergillosis.
- Additional reasons in children 6–11 years of age:
  - Doubt about diagnosis—partial/no response in a child who was born prematurely
  - Uncontrolled symptoms or frequent exacerbations on moderate-dose ICS
  - Suspected medication side effects
  - Confirmed food allergy.

Risk Factors for Asthma-related Death

- History of near-fatal asthma requiring intubation and mechanical ventilation
- Hospitalization or emergency care visit for asthma in the past year
- Currently using or having recently stopped using OCS
- Not currently using ICS
- Over-use of SABA (>1 canister/month)
- History of psychiatric disease or psychosocial problems
- Poor adherence with asthma medications and/or poor adherence with (or lack of) a written asthma action plan
- Food allergy in a patient with asthma.

Managing Comorbidities

- Obesity:
    - Problems could be due to different type of airway inflammation, obstructive sleep apnea, gastroesophageal reflux disease (GERD), mechanical factors, or certain undefined factors
    - ICS are mainstay of treatment
    - Weight loss program with aerobic and strength exercises
    - Bariatric surgery may be warranted in extreme cases.
- Gastroesophageal reflux disease:
    - Beta-2 agonists and theophylline can relax lower esophageal sphincter and worsen the asthmatic situation
    - Trial of antireflux medications—proton pump inhibitors or motility agents
    - Lifestyle changes, fundoplication.
- Anxiety and depression:
    - Psychiatric disorders have been associated with increased asthma-related exacerbations
    - Drug treatment and cognitive behavior therapy are helpful.
- Food allergy and anaphylaxis:
    - Food-induced anaphylaxis can present as life-threatening event
    - Food avoidance
    - Epinephrine autoinjector.
- Rhinitis, sinusitis, and nasal polyps:
    - Chronic rhinosinusitis with nasal polyp is associated with severe asthma
    - Intranasal corticosteroids along with asthma management is usually helpful.

ASTHMA IN SPECIAL SITUATIONS

- Exercise-induced bronchoconstriction (EIB):
    - As-needed SABA before exercise should be used
    - Stepping up of regular controller treatment, if more frequent exacerbations.

- Athletes:
  - Prevent air pollutants, allergens and chlorine levels in pool
  - Avoid training in extreme cold weather or pollution
  - Minimize use of beta-2 agonists to avoid tolerance development.
- Pregnancy:
  - Exacerbations in second trimester due to mechanical or hormonal changes, cessation of asthma medications by mother/healthcare provider
  - Poor symptom control leads to worse outcome for mother (preeclampsia) and for baby (preterm delivery, low-birth weight, increased perinatal mortality)
  - Adequate control of asthma is warranted
  - Aggressive treatment, of exacerbation, with SABA, oxygen, and systemic corticosteroids
  - Respiratory infections should be monitored and managed appropriately
  - If SABA is used during labor and delivery, monitor blood glucose in the baby.
- Women—perimenstrual asthma (catamenial asthma):
  - Worse asthmatic symptoms in premenstrual phase, particularly in older women with severe asthma, higher body mass index, long duration of asthma, and aspirin-exacerbated respiratory disease
  - Oral contraceptives and LTRA are useful adjuncts to regular therapy.
- Occupational asthma:
  - Work history and symptom relationship are very important
  - For latex allergy—using nonpowered low-allergen gloves may be helpful.
- The elderly:
  - Reduced lung function in elderly due to stiff chest wall, reduced respiratory muscle function, loss of elastic recoil, and airway wall remodeling

- Comorbid arthritis may contribute to reduced exercise capacity and lack of fitness and difficult inhaler use
- Side effects of beta-2 agonists (cardiotoxicity) and corticosteroids (skin bruising, osteoporosis, cataracts) are more common
- Careful selection of inhaler device
- Large print versions of written information.
- Surgery:
  - As far as possible, good asthma control should be achieved before any surgical procedure.
- Aspirin-exacerbated respiratory disease (AERD):
  - Aspirin challenge (oral, bronchial, or nasal) is the gold standard for diagnosis
  - COX-2 inhibitor (celecoxib or etoricoxib) or paracetamol should be used instead of NSAIDs
  - ICS is the mainstay of therapy
  - OCS and LTRA may be helpful
  - Desensitization may be conducted at specialist centers.

ASTHMA VERSUS COPD VERSUS ASTHMA—COPD OVERLAP (ACO) SYNDROME

The features of asthma versus COPD versus asthma–COPD overlap (ACO) syndrome are discussed in Table 10.

Asthma versus COPD Investigations

Investigations for asthma and COPD are listed in Table 11.

WHEEZING IN UNDER-FIVE

Wheezing phenotypes have been classified based on symptom- or time trend-based:
- Symptom-based classification:
  - Episodic wheeze—during discrete time periods, mostly in association with upper respiratory infections

Table 10: Features of asthma, chronic obstructive pulmonary disease (COPD), and asthma–COPD overlap (ACO) syndrome.

Feature	Asthma	COPD	ACO
Age of onset	Usually childhood, but can commence at any age	>40 years	Usually >40 years, but may had symptoms in earlier age
Pattern of respiratory symptoms	Vary over time (day-to-day, or over longer periods), often limiting activity. Often triggered by exercise, emotions, dust or allergen exposure	Chronic usually continuous symptoms, particularly during exercise, with "better" and "worse" days	Symptoms on exertion with variability
Lung function during symptoms	Current and/or historical variable airflow limitation with BD reversibility	FEV_1 may be improved by therapy, but no BD reversibility	Airflow limitation not fully reversible
Lung function in-between symptoms	May be normal	Persistent airflow limitation	Persistent airflow limitation
Past or family history	History of allergies or asthma may be present	Exposure to noxious particles and gases (tobacco, biomass fuels)	History of allergies or asthma and noxious particles may be present
Time course	Often improves spontaneously or with treatment, may result in fixed airflow limitation	Slow progressive over years despite treatment	Intermittent symptomatic improvement, progressive and requires higher treatment
Chest X-ray	Usually normal or hyperinflated	Severe hyperinflation and other changes of COPD	Severe hyperinflation and other changes of COPD
Exacerbations	Can occur, risk can be reduced by appropriate treatment and avoidance measures	Can occur, risk can be reduced. Comorbidities contribute to impairment	More than COPD. Comorbidities contribute to impairment

Contd...

Contd...

Feature	Asthma	COPD	ACO
Airway inflammation	Eosinophils and/or neutrophils	Neutrophils ± eosinophils in sputum, lymphocytes in airways, may have systemic inflammation	Eosinophils and/or neutrophils in sputum
Spirometric variables			
Normal FEV_1/FVC pre- or post-BD	Compatible with diagnosis	Not compatible with diagnosis	Not compatible with diagnosis
Post-BD FEV_1/FVC < 0.7	Indicates airflow limitation but may improve spontaneously or on treatment	Required for diagnosis as per GOLD criteria	Usually present
Post-BD $FEV_1 \geq$ 80% predicted	Compatible with diagnosis	Compatible with GOLD classification of mild airflow limitation if post-BD FEV_1/FVC <0.7	Compatible with diagnosis of mild ACO
Post-BD FEV_1 <80% predicted	Compatible with diagnosis, risk factor for early exacerbation	Indicator of severity of airflow limitation and risk of future events (e.g. mortality and exacerbations)	Indicator of severity of airflow limitation and risk of future events (e.g. mortality and exacerbations)
Post-BD increase in $FEV_1 \geq 12\%$ and 200 mL from baseline (reversible airflow limitation)	Usual at some time in course of asthma, but may not be present when well-controlled or on controllers	Common and more likely when FEV_1 is low	Common and more likely when FEV_1 is low
Post-BD increase in $FEV_1 > 12\%$ and 400 mL from baseline (marked reversibility)	High probability of asthma	Unusual	Compatible with diagnosis of ACO

(ACO: asthma–COPD overlap; BD: bronchodilator; FEV_1: forced expiratory volume in 1 second; FVC: forced vital capacity; GOLD: global initiative for obstructive lung disease)

Table 11: Asthma versus chronic obstructive pulmonary disease (COPD)—investigations.

Investigations	Asthma	COPD
Lung function tests:		
DLCO	Normal or slightly elevated	Often reduced
Arterial blood gas	Normal between exacerbations	May be chronically abnormal
Airway hyperresponsiveness	Higher levels favor asthma	
Imaging:		
High-resolution CT scan	Usually normal, air trapping and increased bronchial wall thickness may be observed	Low-attenuation areas denoting air trapping or emphysematous change, bronchial wall thickening and features of pulmonary hypertension may be seen
Inflammatory biomarkers:		
Test for atopy (skin prick or specific IgE tests)	Modestly increases probability of asthma	Conforms background prevalence, does not rule out COPD
FENO	>50 ppb in nonsmokers is associated with eosinophilic airway inflammation	Usually normal, low in current smokers
Blood eosinophilia	Supports eosinophilic airway inflammation	May be present in COPD during exacerbations
Sputum inflammatory cell analysis	Role in differential diagnosis is not established	

- Multi-trigger wheeze—wheeze present in-between the episodes also.
- Time trend-based classification:
  - Transient wheeze—symptom began and ended before the age of 3 years
  - Persistent wheeze—symptom began before the age of 3 years and continued beyond the age of 6 years
  - Late-onset wheeze—symptom began after the age of 3 years.

However, the management based on these phenotypes is unreliable in real life. Following features are utilized (in under-five children) for asthma diagnosis:

- Cough—recurrent or persistent cough, worse at night
- Wheezing—recurrent wheezing during sleep or with triggers like activity, laughing, crying, or exposure to tobacco smoke or air pollution
- Shortness of breath—occurring with exercise, laughing, or crying
- Reduced activity—as compared to peers
- Past or family history—other allergic diseases (atopic dermatitis, allergic rhinitis, asthma in first-degree relatives)
- Therapeutic trial with low-dose inhaled corticosteroids—improvement during 2–3 months of controllers and worsening when treatment is stopped.

Lung function testing requires expiratory maneuvers, which is difficult in children. Similarly, bronchial provocation tests also have limited role in children. Elevated FENO value in preschool children with recurrent coughing and wheezing can assist in asthma diagnosis.

Indications for Referral to a Specialist (in Under-five Wheeze)

- Failure to thrive
- Neonatal or very early onset of symptoms
- Vomiting associated with respiratory symptoms
- Continuous wheezing
- Failure to respond to asthma controller medications
- No association of symptoms with typical triggers, such as viral upper respiratory infections
- Focal lung or cardiovascular signs, or finger clubbing
- Hypoxemia out of proportion to viral illness.

Differential Diagnosis of Asthma (in Under-five Children)

- Recurrent viral respiratory tract infections—cough is predominant feature sometimes associated with runny congested nose, asymptomatic in-between episodes
- Gastroesophageal reflux—cough when feeding, recurrent chest infections
- Foreign body aspiration—abrupt onset severe cough and/or stridor during eating or playing, recurrent chest infections, focal lung signs may be present
- Tracheomalacia—noisy breathing during crying, eating, or upper airway infections, harsh cough, symptoms since birth, poor response to bronchodilators or steroids
- Tuberculosis—persistent cough and/or noisy breathing, prolonged fever, history of recent contact with a patient suffering from tuberculosis is highly suggestive
- Congenital heart disease—cardiac murmur, cyanosis, failure to thrive, tachycardia, tachypnea, hepatomegaly, poor response to bronchodilators
- Cystic fibrosis—recurrent chest infections, persistent cough, failure to thrive (malabsorption), loose greasy bulky stools
- Primary ciliary dyskinesia—cough and recurrent chest infections, chronic ear infections and purulent nasal discharge, poor response to asthma medications, situs inversus in 50% of children
- Vascular ring—persistent noisy breathing, poor response to asthma medications
- Bronchopulmonary dysplasia—preterm low-birth weight babies who require prolonged ventilation or supplemental oxygen in early neonatal period
- Immunodeficiency—recurrent fever and infections, failure to thrive.

Indications for Immediate Transfer to Hospital in Under-five Children with Asthma

- At initial or subsequent assessment:
  - Unable to speak or drink
  - Cyanosis
  - Subcostal retractions
  - Oxygen saturation less than 92% on room air
  - Silent chest on auscultation.
- Lack of response to initial bronchodilator treatment:
  - Lack of response to initial 6 puffs (3 aliquots of 2 puffs each) of SABA over 1–2 hours
  - Persistent tachypnea despite three aliquots of inhaled SABA.
- Adverse social environment impairing acute treatment, or parent/caregiver unable to manage acute asthma at home.

Approach to an Under-five Child with Wheeze

Procedure to approach an under-five child with wheeze is discussed in Flowchart 5.

Management of Asthma (in Under-five Children)

Management of asthma in under-five children is discussed in Figure 8 and Table 12.

Factors affecting Asthma Development in Children

- Maternal diet—introduction of allergenic foods (peanut and milk) in pregnant mother's diet is associated with decrease in allergies and asthma in children
- Maternal obesity and excessive weight gain during pregnancy—increased risk of asthma in children
- Breastfeeding—decreases wheezing episodes in early life
- Delayed introduction of solids—initially delayed introduction of allergenic foods was recommended as an effective strategy for allergy prevention in children, this has been recently challenged in "LEAP" study, which suggests early introduction helps in tolerance development to allergenic food items.

Respiratory Allergies **139**

Flowchart 5: Approach to an under-five child with wheeze.

```
Child (<5 years) with wheezing in clinic:
• Good history and clinical examination
• Classify phenotypes and the severity
```

- **Episodic viral wheezers**
  - **Infrequent**
    - No regular prophylaxis
    - Treat episodes symptomatically
  - **Frequent**
    - Consider regular LTRA or ICS
    - **No or partial improvement**
      - Re-affirm the diagnosis
      - Try alternative drugs

- **Multiple trigger wheezers** (Symptom pattern consistent with asthma) **AND** not well controlled **OR** >3 exacerbations/year
  - Trial of ICS/LTRA for 12 weeks
  - **Response**
    - **Good**
      - Stop medications
      - Watch for reappearance of symptoms
      - If symptoms reccur and respond to a second drug of same therapy → Manage as asthma in under-five
    - **Poor**
      - Refer for specialist opinion

- **Unclear phenotypes**
  - Keep under follow-up

Table 12: Inhaled corticosteroid doses in under-five children.

Drug	Low daily dose
Beclomethasone dipropionate (HFA)	100 (ages ≥5 years)
Budesonide nebulized	500 (ages ≥1 year)
Fluticasone propionate (HFA)	100 (ages ≥4 years)
Mometasone furoate	110 (ages ≥4 years)
Budesonide pMDI + spacer	Insufficient evidence
Ciclesonide	Insufficient evidence
Triamcinolone acetonide	Insufficient evidence

(HFA: hydrofluoroalkane propellant; pMDI: pressurized metered dose inhaler)

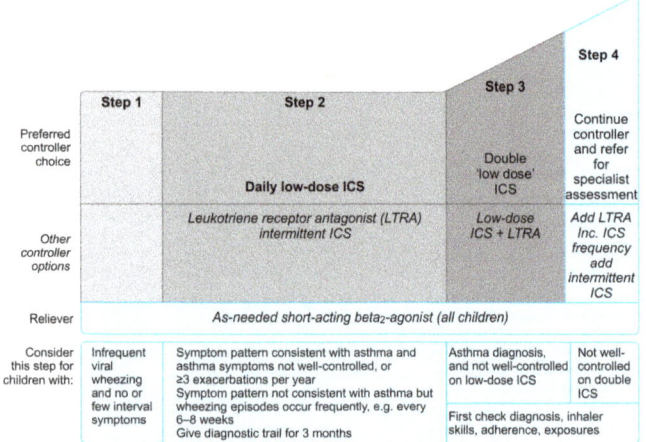

Fig. 8: Management of asthma in under-five children.
(ICS: inhaled corticosteroids)
Source: Global Initiative for Asthma (2018). Global strategy for Asthma management and prevention.

- Vitamin D—vitamin D and E supplementation during pregnancy is associated with lower risk of wheezing in infants
- Probiotics—insufficient evidence till date for any preventive effect on allergies
- Inhalant allergens—exposure to mold allergen in early childhood increases the risk of asthma
- Pollutants—maternal tobacco smoke and exposure to high levels of pollution during pregnancy are associated with greater likelihood of allergic disorders in children
- Microbial effects—vaginal delivery and exposure to pets in early life reduce the risk for allergies
- Medications and other factors—antibiotic use during pregnancy is associated with increased risk of asthma in childhood
- Psychosocial factors—maternal stress (during pregnancy and early years of child's life) is associated with childhood asthma in offspring.

PRIMARY PREVENTION OF ASTHMA

- Prevent environmental tobacco smoke during pregnancy and after birth
- Vaginal delivery should be encouraged as much as possible
- Exclusive breastfeeding for at least 4-6 months is recommended
- Prolonged breastfeeding is advised
- Use of broad-spectrum antibiotics should be avoided during 1st year of life
- Solid foods should be started at 4-6 months of age.

SUGGESTED READING

1. Allergic Rhinitis and its Impact on Asthma (ARIA) Guidelines—2016. J Allergy Clin Immunol. 2017;140(4):950-8.
2. Chakrabarti A, Kaur H. Allergic Aspergillus Rhinosinusitis. J Fungi (Basel). 2016;2(4):32.
3. Chester AC. Chronic sinusitis. Am Fam Physician. 1996;53(3):877-997.
4. Chow AW, Benninger MS, Brook I, et al. IDSA Clinical Practice Guideline for Acute Bacterial Rhinosinusitis in Children and Adults. Clin Infect Dis. 2012;54(8):e72-e112.
5. Desai M, Oppenheimer J. Elucidating asthma phenotypes and endotypes: progress towards personalized medicine. Ann Allergy Asthma Immunol. 2016;116:394-401.
6. Dykewicz MS, Wallace DV, Baroody F, et al. Treatment of seasonal allergic rhinitis: An evidence-based focused 2017 guideline update. Ann Allergy Asthma Immunol. 2017;119(6):489-511.
7. Global Initiative for Asthma (2018). Global strategy for Asthma management and prevention. [online] Available from https://ginasthma.org/2018-gina-report-global-strategy-for-asthma-management-and-prevention/. [Accessed December, 2018].
8. Harmes KM, Blackwood A, Burrows HL, et al. Otitis Media: Diagnosis and Treatment. Am Fam Physician. 2013;88(7):435-40.
9. Hernandez-Vaquero GE, Soto-Galindo GA, Gonzalez JL. Update in Pediatric Acute Otitis Media: A Review. Ann Otolaryngol Rhinol. 2017;4(4):1173.
10. Ilechukwu GC, Ilechkwu CG, Ubesie AC, et al. Otitis Media in Children: Review Article. Open J Pediatrics. 2014;4:47-53.
11. Leibovitz E, Greenberg D. Acute Otitis Media in Children: Current Epidemiology, Microbiology, Clinical Manifestations and Treatment. Chang Gung Med J. 2004;27(7):475-88.

12. Leung RS, Katial R. The Diagnosis and Management of Acute and Chronic Sinusitis. Prim Care Clin Office Pract. 2008;35(1):11-24.
13. Lockey RF. Asthma Phenotypes: An Approach to the Diagnosis and Treatment of Asthma. J Allergy Clin Immunol Pract. 2014;2:682-3.
14. Min YG. The Pathophysiology, Diagnosis and Treatment of Allergic Rhinitis. Allergy Asthma Immunol Res. 2010;2(2):65-76.
15. Quillen DM, Feller DB. Diagnosing Rhinitis: Allergic vs. Nonallergic. Am Fam Physician. 2006;73(9):1583-90.
16. Ramakrishnan K, Sparks RA, Berryhill WE. Diagnosis and Treatment of Otitis Media. Am Fam Physician. 2007;76(11):1650-8.
17. Rea P, Graham J. Chapter 73, Acute otitis media in children. Pediatr Otorhinolaryngol. pp. 912-27.
18. Ruiter JD. Histamine H1-Receptor Antagonists: Antihistaminic Agents. Principles of Drug Action. 2001;2.
19. Seidman MD, Gurgel RK, Lin SY, et al. Clinical Practice Guideline: Allergic Rhinitis. Otolaryngol Head Neck Surg. 2015;152:S1-S43.
20. Slavin RG, Spector SL, Bernstein IL. The diagnosis and management of sinusitis: A practice parameter update. J Allergy Clin Immunol. 2005;116(6 Suppl):S13-47.
21. Sood A. Diagnostic significance of nasal eosinophilia in allergic rhinitis. Indian J Otolaryngol Head Neck Surg. 2005;57(1):13-6.
22. Wenzel SE. Asthma phenotypes: the evolution from clinical to molecular approaches. Nature Med. 2012;5:716-25.

Anaphylaxis

CHAPTER 5

INTRODUCTION

Anaphylaxis is the most severe form of hypersensitivity reaction with rapid onset, compromising airway, breathing and/or circulation. It may be associated with skin, mucosal or gastrointestinal symptoms. If proper treatment is not instituted in time, it can be life-threatening. There is plenty of scientific literature available for anaphylaxis management, still it is one of the most commonly mismanaged entities, mostly due to lack of awareness and confusion among the healthcare providers.

CAUSES OF ANAPHYLAXIS

Common

- Insect stings—most commonly honeybee, Australian native ants, and wasps. Honeybee stings are more common in bee keepers
- Foods—peanuts, tree nuts, egg, seafood, cow's milk, dairy products, seeds
- Medications—antibiotics, nonsteroidal anti-inflammatory drugs are the most common culprit
- Unidentified—despite a careful history and thorough investigations, the anaphylaxis cause remains elusive in some situations.

Less Common

- Physical triggers—exercise, cold
- Biological fluids—transfusions, immunoglobulin, anti-venoms, and semen

- Latex
- Tick bites
- Hormonal changes—breastfeeding, menstrual factors
- Dialysis membranes—hemodialysis associated anaphylaxis
- Hydatid cyst rupture
- Aeroallergens—domestic/laboratory animals, and pollen
- Food additives—monosodium glutamate, metabisulfite, preservatives, colors, natural food chemicals
- Topical medications—antiseptics.

IMMUNOLOGICAL MECHANISMS OF ANAPHYLAXIS

Immunoglobulin E-dependent Anaphylaxis

Immunoglobulin (Ig) E is the least abundant immunoglobulin in the circulation (normal value—50–200 ng/mL in healthy adults), however, it has been notoriously attributed to most cases of anaphylaxis. IgE binds to FcεRI receptors on the surface of mast cells and basophils after initial contact with a suspected allergen. On re-exposure to a bi-/multivalent allergen (Figs. 1A and B), cross-linking of FcεRI-bound IgE induces activation of mast cells and basophils, which releases preformed mediators (histamine and various proteases) and also stimulates de novo synthesis of many inflammatory mediators (certain leukotrienes, prostaglandins and cytokines). IgE is considered to be the most important mediator for diagnostic and therapeutic target, explaining the utility of anti-IgE molecules (omalizumab) for prevention of anaphylaxis in systemic mastocytosis patients.

Immunoglobulin E-independent Anaphylaxis

Despite, the proven role of IgE in many allergic reactions, high levels of IgE do not predispose for anaphylaxis and near-fatal anaphylaxis has been reported in patients with undetectable levels of circulating allergen-specific IgE also. This could be due to parallel pathways involving other molecules apart from IgE, like IgG (Fig. 1B) and complement activation. IgG-induced systemic

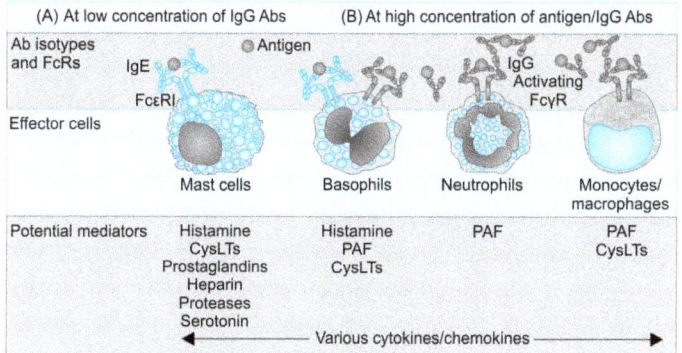

Figs. 1A and B: (A) IgE-mediated anaphylaxis, common in human; (B) Mouse models of anaphylaxis involving IgG molecules. Some examples of anaphylaxis involve both IgE and IgG pathways. Mediators: Histamine (strong evidence for involvement in human anaphylaxis); CysLTs, Prostaglandins, Heparin, PAF (importance in mice documented, but in human yet to be documented); Proteases, Serotonin (elements with potential to influence anaphylaxis, but importance in human or mouse anaphylaxis is not clear till date).
Source: Reber LL, Hernandez JD, Galli SJ. The pathophysiology of anaphylaxis. J Allergy Clin Immunol. 2017;140:335-48.

anaphylaxis has been demonstrated in mice, causing hypothermia, vasodilatation and cardiopulmonary changes. IgG-mediated anaphylaxis requires much higher dose of antigen/allergen than IgE. Activation of complement cascade causes generation of potent inflammatory mediators, called anaphylatoxins like C3a, C4a and C5a. Blood levels of these anaphylatoxins correlates with severity of anaphylaxis in humans. Table 1 shows role of various immune mechanisms in anaphylaxis.

GENE-HOST INFLUENCES

Gene-environment interaction plays crucial role in predisposition for allergy and anaphylaxis. Allergic reactions to drugs and latex have been linked with genetic polymorphisms, viz. IL-4 receptor-α, IL-10, and IL-13. Angiotensin-converting enzyme (ACE) levels have

Table 1: Potential roles of various mechanisms in causing anaphylaxis.

Mechanisms	Effects
Antibody isotypes	
IgE	• Levels are often raised in patients with allergies • Skin reactivity can be transferred via purified IgE from a sensitized subject to a naive host • Anti-IgE antibody (omalizumab) can significantly reduce anaphylaxis risk
IgG	• No definite evidence in human but it has documented anaphylaxis in mice • Anaphylaxis has been reported after treatment with monoclonal antibodies (with normal IgE levels)
Complement	
Anaphylatoxins (C3a, C4a, C5a)	• Wheal and flare reactions have been documented with low dose injections in healthy subjects • Higher blood levels correlate with increased chances of anaphylaxis
Effector cells	
Mast cells	• Raised tryptase levels have been demonstrated during acute anaphylaxis • Systemic mastocytosis is associated with high chances of anaphylaxis
Basophils	• Activation tests have been used to diagnose or confirm allergen sensitization • No definite evidence till date
Neutrophils	• Myeloperoxidase (MPO) levels are raised in anaphylaxis
Monocytes/macrophages	• Role not yet determined
Platelets	• Anaphylaxis in human has been documented with platelet activation • No definite evidence till date
Mediators	
Histamine	• Nebulized histamine induces bronchoconstriction • Intravenous administration can produce anaphylaxis • H1-antihistaminics are successfully used as adjunctive therapy for acute anaphylaxis and anaphylactoid reactions
CysLTs	• Levels increases in initial phase of anaphylaxis • Wheal and flare reaction have been observed after intradermal injection of LTB4, LTC4 and LTD4 • Aerosol administration of LT4 and LTD4 induces bronchoconstriction
Platelet-activating factor (PAF)	• Intradermal injection induces wheal-and-flare reactions • Circulating PAF levels increase and circulating PAF-acetyl hydrolase (PAF-AH) activity decreases in proportion to the activity of anaphylaxis
Others	• During anaphylaxis, quantity of many positive or negative mediators varies, e.g. certain cytokines, chemokines, prostaglandins, tryptase, bradykinin and serotonin.

been shown in inverse correlation with severe pharyngeal edema, secondary to decreased bradykinin metabolism. An activating mutation in *c-KIT D816V* promotes mast cell proliferation in patients with clonal mast cell disorders, including mastocytosis. Patients with autosomal-dominant hyper-IgE syndrome, due to loss-of-function mutation in signal transducer and activator of transcription 3, have less chances of anaphylaxis. Observation of increased disease severity in male versus female patients of 13–56 years of age and no sex difference in prepubescent and those older than 56 years, suggest potential role of hormones in anaphylaxis.

CLINICAL ANAPHYLAXIS

Anaphylaxis can be defined as "a serious allergic reaction that is rapid in onset and may cause death". There are several diagnostic criteria given by different societies, multiorgan involvement is the most common finding among all (Fig. 2).

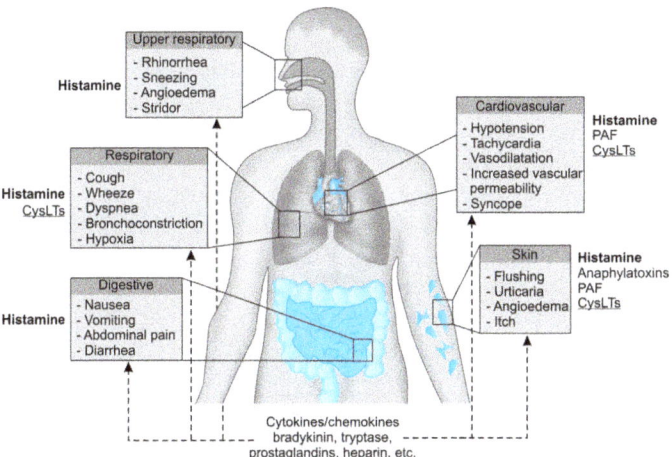

Fig. 2: Anaphylaxis—a multisystem disorder.

Source: Reber LL, Hernandez JD, Galli SJ. The pathophysiology of anaphylaxis. J Allergy Clin Immunol. 2017;140:335-48.

Majority of the anaphylactic reactions occur within few minutes to a maximum of few hours since the exposure of triggering agent. Biphasic reaction might be observed in minority of patients, in which signs and symptoms reoccur hours after the initial reaction. Occasionally late-phase reaction alone may occur without initial airway or hemodynamic compromise.

Early suspicion is the key in the presence of suspected allergen as delay in instituting injectable epinephrine in a probable case of anaphylaxis increases the morbidity and mortality by several folds.

DIAGNOSTIC CRITERIA

Anaphylaxis is usually suspected and diagnosed on clinical grounds. It is highly likely when any one of the following three criteria is fulfilled.

1. Acute onset of an illness (minutes to several hours) with involvement of the skin, mucosal tissue, or both (e.g. generalized hives, pruritus or flushing, swollen lips-tongue-uvula) and at least one of the following:
   - Respiratory compromise (e.g. dyspnea, wheeze-bronchospasm, stridor, reduced PEF, and hypoxemia)
   - Reduced BP or associated symptoms of end-organ dysfunction [e.g. hypotonia (collapse), syncope, and incontinence].
2. Two or more of the following that occur rapidly after exposure to a likely allergen for that patient (minutes to several hours):
   - Involvement of the skin-mucosal tissue (e.g. generalized hives, itch-flush, swollen lips-tongue-uvula)
   - Respiratory compromise (e.g. dyspnea, wheeze-bronchospasm, stridor, reduced PEF, and hypoxemia)
   - Reduced BP or associated symptoms [e.g. hypotonia (collapse), syncope, incontinence]
   - Persistent gastrointestinal symptoms (e.g. crampy abdominal pain, and vomiting).
3. Reduced BP after exposure to known allergen for that patient (minutes to several hours):

- *Infants and children*: Low systolic BP (age-specific) or greater than 30% decrease in systolic BP
- *Adults*: Systolic BP of less than 90 mm Hg or greater than 30% decrease from that person's baseline.

DIFFERENTIAL DIAGNOSIS

Tissue Swelling
- Idiopathic urticaria
- Isolated angioedema
- Idiopathic
- Angiotensin-converting enzyme inhibitor-induced
- Acquired or hereditary C1 esterase inhibitor deficiency.

Conditions Mimicking Upper Airway Edema
- Dystonic reactions mimicking symptoms of a swollen tongue after taking metoclopramide, prochlorperazine or antihistamines
- Acute esophageal reflux.

Flushing Syndromes
- Peptide-secreting tumors (e.g. carcinoid syndrome, VIPomas)
- Alcohol-related
- Medullary carcinoma of thyroid
- Red man syndrome.

Neurological Syndromes
- Epileptic seizure
- Stroke.

Other Causes of Collapse
- Vasovagal episodes
- Systemic inflammatory response syndrome
- Shock (septic, cardiogenic, and hemorrhagic).

Acute Respiratory Distress

- Asthma
- Panic disorders
- Globus hystericus
- Laryngospasm
- Vocal cord dysfunction.

Miscellaneous

- Scombroid fish poisoning
- Serum sickness
- Pheochromocytoma
- Systemic mastocytosis.

LABORATORY MARKERS

- *Histamine*: High histamine levels soon after IgE-mediated anaphylaxis are quite common but it is very difficult to document as half-life of histamine is only 2–3 minutes.
- *Tryptase*: It is a serine peptidase enzyme and exist in two forms as α and β:
  - α-tryptase is constantly being released in smaller concentration, along with pro-β-tryptase, hence tryptase is normally detectable in plasma. High concentration of α-tryptase are seen in systemic mastocytosis.
  - Mature β-tryptase is catalytically active, heparin-stabilized tetramer that is stored in mast cell secretory granules and is released during IgE-mediated anaphylactic reaction. It is the major isomer responsible for chemical diagnosis of anaphylaxis.

The serum tryptase concentration peaks between 15 to 20 minutes after encountering relevant allergen, with both timing and peak value dependent on route and dose of stimulus. Tryptase is catabolized in liver, with in vivo half-life of 2.5 hours. As tryptase levels can be affected by large volumes of fluid resuscitation, cardiac massage, defibrillation and baseline characteristics of an individual (systemic mastocytosis, myelodysplastic syndromes, mast cell leukemia and end-stage renal failure), both peak followed by trough levels should be documented to attribute high serum tryptase levels to anaphylaxis.

Blood should be collected into EDTA/heparin tubes or without anticoagulant. Sample should be transferred to laboratory with/without ice and analyzed at the earliest, preferably within 5–7 days. It may be frozen if there is an expected delay in analysis. Blood samples should be collected at approximately 1, 2, 3, 6, 12 and 24 hours post-reaction to measure peak and fall in tryptase levels. Facilities for tryptase estimation are scarce, making its utility doubtful in diagnosing anaphylaxis.

The reference range for serum tryptase is 2–14 µg/L. A peak concentration of more than 50 µg/L with corresponding symptoms and documented fall during convalescence is consistent with IgE-mediated anaphylaxis.

MANAGEMENT

Epinephrine virtually acts at every possible level and counteracts the pathophysiological changes, which happen during anaphylaxis. Various actions of epinephrine at different receptors are:
- *α_1-adrenergic receptors*: These induce vasoconstriction leading to diminished tissue and/or airway edema, hypotension and distributive shock.
- *β_1-adrenergic receptors*: These improve cardiac output by increasing heart rate and cardiac contractility.
- *β_2-adrenergic receptors*: Dilatation of airways and blockage of further release of mediators (histamine and eicosanoids) by mast cells and other effector cells.

H_1- and H_2-antihistamines resolve early cutaneous and upper respiratory signs and symptoms whereas corticosteroids might benefit in biphasic reaction but neither prevent nor treat airway obstruction or circulatory collapse and therefore cannot be considered alternatives to epinephrine.

Acute Management

The steps should be as under:
- *Immediate measures*:
  - *Allergen*: Remove the inciting allergen at the earliest, if possible
  - *Airway*: Assess airway, breathing, and circulation. If needed, support the airway (noninvasive/invasive)
  - *Cardiopulmonary resuscitation*: Start chest compression, in case of cardiac arrest or HR < 60 beats/min
  - *Epinephrine (intramuscular)*: It should be administered as soon as possible. Doses (Table 2) and technique (Fig. 3) need to be followed
  - Call for help
  - Position of comfort:
    - Adults and adolescents—recombinant
    - Children—supine
    - Pregnant women—left lateral
  - *Epinephrine (intramuscular)*: Repeat every 5–15 minutes up to 3 doses, if no or suboptimal response

Table 2: Doses of undiluted epinephrine (intramuscular) in case of anaphylaxis.

Adrenaline (epinephrine) dosages chart			
Age (years)	Weight (kg)	Vo. Adrenaline in mL (1:1000)	Adrenaline auto injector
<1	5–10	0.05–0.1	
1–2	10	0.1	10–20 kg (1–5 years) 0.15 mg (green labeled device)
2–3	15	0.15	
4–6	20	0.2	
7–10	30	0.3	>20 kg (>5 years) 0.3 mg (yellow labeled device)
10–12	40	0.4	
>12 and adults*	>50	0.5	

*For pregnant women, a dose of 0.3 mg should be used.

Anaphylaxis

- *Activate emergency medical system (EMS)*: If no response to first dose of epinephrine or if compromised mentation, airway or hemodynamics
- *Intravenous (IV) fluids*: 5-10 mL/kg of normal saline—up to 30 mL/kg in case of hypotension.
- *Additional measures*:
  - *Salbutamol*: 2.5-5 mg of nebulized salbutamol in 3 mL of normal saline if evidence of bronchoconstriction (dyspnea, wheeze, and desaturation), repeat in 15 minutes, if required.

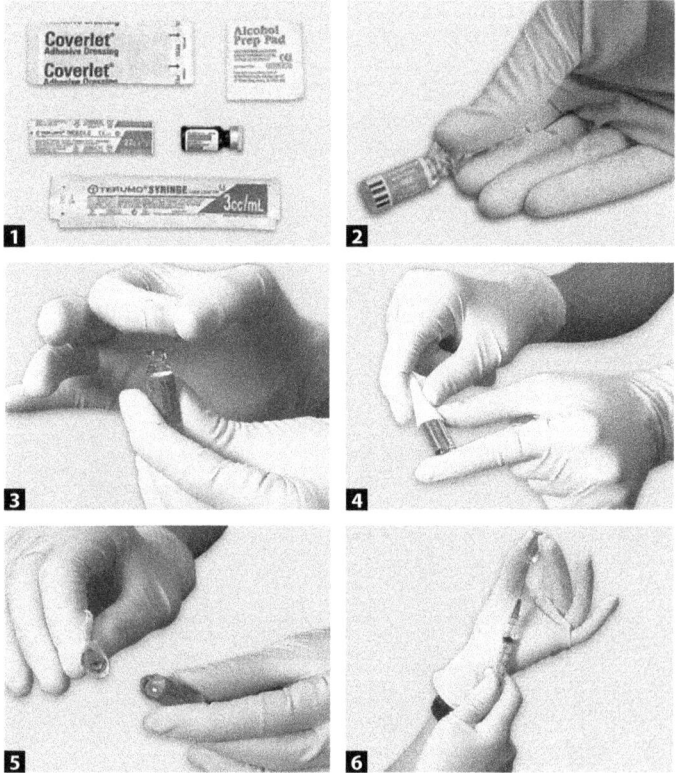

Contd...

Contd...

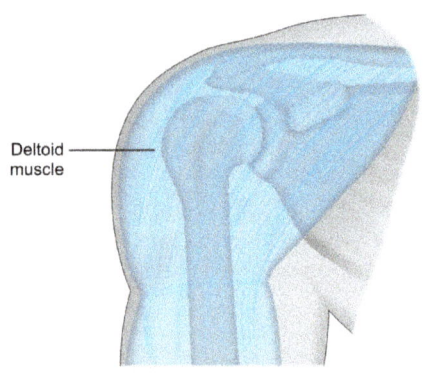

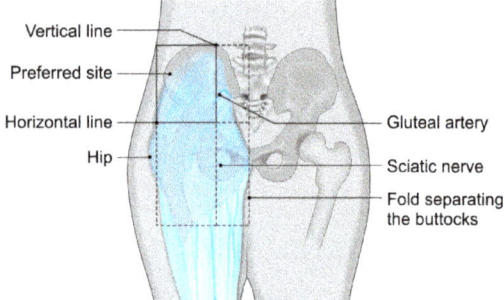

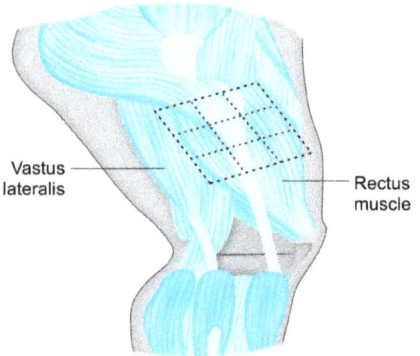

Contd...

Contd...

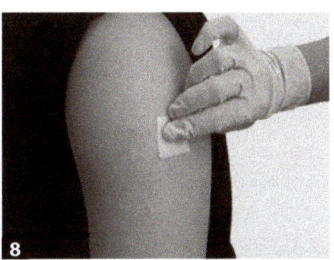

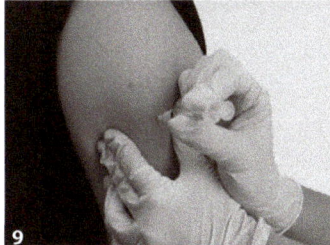
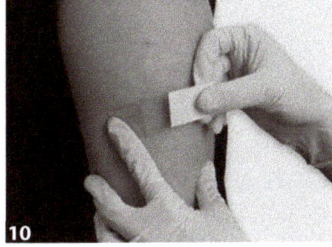

Fig. 3: Technique of administering intramuscular epinephrine. 1. Prepare the equipments; 2. Check the medication for expiry date; 3. Wear the gloves, hold the ampule upright and tap its top to dislodge any trapped solution; 4. Place gauze around the thin neck; 5. Snap it off with your thumb; 6. Draw up the medications, holding syringe with needle up, expel any air from the syringe; 7. Common intramuscular sites for injection; 8. Prepare the site with alcohol swab; 9. Insert the needle at 90° angle, aspirate for blood, if none, then inject the required dose; 10. Remove the needle and cover the site *(For color version, see Plate 17).*

- *Glucagon*: 1–5 mg of glucagon intravenously slowly over 15 minutes if patient is on β-blockers and not responding to epinephrine.
- *Epinephrine infusion*: If inappropriate response to previous epinephrine and IV fluids.
- *Intraosseous access*: If no IV access obtained with 3 attempts of IV canulation or 90 seconds, whichever is earlier and patient is in refractory anaphylaxis.

- Refractory anaphylaxis:
    - Advanced airway management
    - Vasopressors—Consider adding dopamine after epinephrine infusion.
- Optional treatment:
    - H_1-antihistaminic: 1 mg/kg in children (maximum 50 mg)
    - Corticosteroids: 1-2 mg/kg up to 125 mg/dose of methylprednisolone, for prevention of delayed reactions.
- Discharge checklist:
    - Education—about home recognition and treatment of anaphylaxis
    - Auto-injectable epinephrine (Epipen): Prescribe two doses to patients who experienced anaphylactic reaction or those who are at risk of severe anaphylaxis. If Epipen is not available, teach the patient and caregivers for treating anaphylaxis with regular epinephrine
    - Anaphylaxis action plan.

Disposition from Emergency Department

- Children requiring treatment with adrenaline should be observed for at least 6-8 hours as life-threatening manifestations can appear after apparent remission. They should be discharged on oral antihistamine and instructed to return immediately if there are any recurrent symptoms.
- All children who require more than a single dose of adrenaline should be admitted because of the possibility of recurrent symptoms over next 24 hours.

Long-term Management

For patients at risk of anaphylaxis:
- Individualized written management plan (in simple, nonmedical language) for an emergency situation; it should include:
    - *Personal identification data*: Name and address, contact details of the parents/guardian or next of kin, allergist,

family doctor and local ambulance service; and preferably a photograph and identity proof
- Clear identification of the source of the allergens to be avoided and allergen avoidance advice
- Clear identification of any non-allergen triggers or co-factors, such as exercise, and avoidance advice
- Anaphylaxis emergency action plan.

Copy of plan should be kept by the patient, any caregivers, school staff and family doctor.
- Provision of emergency kit with copy of anaphylaxis emergency action plan and medications for self-treatment, e.g.:
  - Adrenaline auto-injector for treating anaphylaxis, where appropriate
  - Fast acting, nonsedating, antihistamine for treating cutaneous allergic reactions, where appropriate.
- Venom immunotherapy and desensitization in drug allergy as appropriate
- Training of patients and caregivers, this should include:
  - Instructions on appropriate allergen avoidance measures, including consultation with an allergy dietitian, where appropriate
  - Instructions on prompt recognition of symptoms of anaphylaxis
  - Training on when and how to use an adrenaline auto-injector, where appropriate
  - Reinforcement with revision at regular yearly intervals.
- Psychological support as required
- Implementation of the patient's management plan in the community (e.g. nursery, school).

RECOVERY FROM ANAPHYLAXIS

Anaphylaxis is not always fatal. Many patients, who suffered from milder variety, survived without any medical intervention. In animal models of anaphylaxis and in human subjects undergoing insect sting challenge, substances with endogenous vasopressor activity like epinephrine, norepinephrine and angiotensin II are increased within minutes after anaphylaxis, which compensates for the vasodilation and fluid extravasation. Chymase released by mast cell degranulation converts angiotensin I to II, thus potentiating the compensatory phenomenon. Certain anti-anaphylactic mediators are released by mast cell activation, which helps to limit anaphylactic responses. Sphingosine-1-phosphate, on one hand, can enhance anaphylaxis via its effect on mast cells, and on the other hand, contributes to recovery by enhancing histamine clearance. Genetic differences in effector cell activation and mediator release might also contribute to varied presentation and recovery from anaphylaxis.

Is anaphylaxis always harmful?

Researchers have noticed that type 2 immune response to honeybee venom phospholipase A_2 (major allergen) could diminish the reduction in body temperature induced by challenge with "near-lethal" dose of venom. Snake or arthropod envenomation can result in systemic IgE dependent mast cell activation, which may produce clinical picture of anaphylaxis with systemic release of mast cell proteases that can degrade toxic component of venom itself. Thus, anaphylaxis can be beneficial if an individual survives the episode with both envenomation and anaphylaxis.

CONCLUSION

Anaphylaxis, a true medical emergency, in human is predominantly mediated by IgE mechanisms though other mediators are also known. Certain gene-environment interactions have potential effect on presentation and severity of anaphylaxis. It should be suspected and diagnosed early at the primary care level and injectable epinephrine should not be delayed at any cost followed by adequate supportive care.

SUGGESTED READING

1. ASCIA. (2016). Acute management of anaphylaxis. ASCIA guidelines 2016. [online] Available from https://www.allergy.org.au/images/stories/pospapers/ASCIA_Guidelines_Acute_Management_Anaphylaxis_Dec2016.pdf [Accessed Jan., 2019].
2. Brown SGA, Mullins RJ, Gold MS. Anaphylaxis: diagnosis and management. MJA practice essentials—Allergy. 2006;185(5):283-9.
3. European Academy of Allergy and Clinical Immunology (EAACI). (2018). Food allergy and anaphylaxis guidelines. EAACI. [online] Available from https://www.eaaci.org/resources/guidelines/faa-guidelines.html [Accessed Jan., 2019].
4. Lieberman P, Nicklas RA, Randolph C, et al. Anaphylaxis—a practice parameter update 2015. Ann Allergy, Asthma Immunol. 2015.
5. Mariana CC. (2011). Anaphylaxis and Hypersensitivity Reactions. [online] Available from https://www.google.com/search?client=firefox-b-ab&q=8.%09Anaphylaxis+and+Hypersensitivity+Reactions.+2011 [Accessed Jan., 2019].
6. Muraro A, Roberts G, Worm M, et al. Anaphylaxis: Guidelines from the European Academy of Allergy and Clinical Immunology. Allergy. 2014;69(8):1026-45.
7. Reber LL, Hernandez JD, Galli SJ. The pathophysiology of anaphylaxis. J Allergy Clin Immunol. 2017;140:335-48.
8. Sheldon J, Philips B. Laboratory investigation of anaphylaxis: not as easy as it seems. Anesthesia. 2015;70:1-17.

Gastrointestinal Allergies

6.1 MILK ALLERGY

INTRODUCTION

Among the common food items responsible for adverse health effects or allergic symptoms, milk and egg play most important role. Though cow's milk protein is the leading cause of allergy in children younger than 3 years, it can present with predominant gastrointestinal symptoms at any age. Perceived food allergy prevalence is much higher due to attribution of various nonspecific symptoms to many food items. This is due to lack of allergy knowledge and prevalence of various social taboos among both healthcare providers and receivers. The actual estimated prevalence of cow's milk protein allergy (CMPA) is 2–3% in infants, which reduces to less than 1% in children beyond 6 years of age. These numbers refer to immunoglobulin E (IgE)-mediated CMPA whereas non-IgE-mediated group is still underestimated. Early suspicion and timely intervention are the keys to manage CMPA.

PATHOPHYSIOLOGY

Milk allergy can be mediated via various IgE, non-IgE or combined mechanisms in an individual. Table 1 demonstrates salient features between two types of immune reactions. The major allergens belong to casein fraction (αs1-, αs2-, β-, and κ-casein) and to whey proteins (α-lactalbumin and β-lactoglobulin). Acute urticaria and angioedema are common IgE-mediated manifestations, whereas gastrointestinal symptoms like enterocolitis, enteropathy, colitis, and pulmonary hemosiderosis (Heiner syndrome) may be non-IgE mediated. Low serum vitamin D level is a risk factor for development of asthma, atopic dermatitis, and food allergy.

Table 1: Characteristics of IgE and non-IgE-mediated immune reactions.

Characteristic	IgE-mediated	Non-IgE-mediated
Time of exposure to reaction	Minutes to 2 hours	Several hours to days
Severity	Mild to anaphylaxis	Mild to moderate
Duration	May persist beyond 1 year of age	Usually resolved by 1 year
Diagnosis	Specific IgE, skin prick test	Oral challenge

(Ig: immunoglobulin)

Source: Lifschitz C, Szajewska H. Cow's milk allergy: evidence-based diagnosis and management for the practitioner. Eur J Pediatr. 2015;174:141-50.

CLINICAL PRESENTATION

There will be heterogeneous presentation with varying intensities in individual patients. The adverse reactions can happen within 2 hours (immediate) or up to 1 week (delayed) after milk exposure. Milk or dairy products may be exposed after ingestion or more commonly via skin contact. Immediate reactions are usually mediated by IgE pathway with increased chances of anaphylaxis whereas various non-IgE mechanisms operate during late reactions. The symptoms might involve any of the body systems; gastrointestinal and respiratory being the common one. Nonspecific extraintestinal manifestations may include fatigue, allergic shiners, mouth ulcers, joint pain or hypermobility, poor sleep, night sweats, headache, and bed wetting. Table 2 depicts common signs and symptoms of CMPA.

An infant with atopic dermatitis and dry skin should be evaluated for CMPA. Many times, the symptoms may be nonspecific warranting milk elimination and diagnostic challenge test desirable.

MAKING A DIAGNOSIS

A detailed history regarding chronological onset of symptoms, introduction of milk and dairy products in infant or maternal diet (in case of breast-fed infant), and cessation of symptoms on milk avoidance warrants thorough investigation to rule out CMPA. Early

Table 2: Symptoms and signs of CMPA in various age groups.

System involved	Infants and toddlers	Older children	Immediate reaction
Gastrointestinal	Dysphagia, regurgitation, colic, abdominal pain, vomiting, anorexia, feed refusal, diarrhea, constipation, failure to thrive, iron-deficiency anemia, occult blood loss	Dysphagia, food impaction, regurgitation, dyspepsia, nausea, vomiting, anorexia, diarrhea, constipation, abdominal pain, iron-deficiency anemia, occult blood loss	Vomiting
Respiratory	Runny nose, wheeze, chronic cough	Runny nose, wheeze, chronic cough	Wheeze, stridor, breathing difficulty
Skin	Urticaria, eczema, swelling of lips or eyelids (angioedema)	Urticaria, eczema, swelling of lips or eyelids	Urticaria, angioedema
General	Anaphylaxis, shock-like symptoms with severe metabolic acidosis, vomiting and diarrhea (FPIES)	Anaphylaxis	Anaphylaxis, FPIES

(CMPA: cow's milk protein allergy; FPIES: food protein-induced enterocolitis syndrome)
Source: Modified from Koletzko S, Niggemann B, Arato A, et al. Diagnostic approach and management of cow's milk protein allergy in infants and children: ESPGHAN GL Committee practical guidelines. J Pediatr Gastroenterol Nutr. 2012;55(2):221-9.

onset symptoms like itching, rashes, cough, respiratory distress, and blood in stools are quiet characteristic of IgE-mediated milk allergy. An atopic march can be characteristically witnessed with more skin manifestations in early infancy followed by respiratory symptoms in younger children.

INVESTIGATIONS

As CMPA could be IgE or non-IgE mediated with a combined reaction in a subset of patients, investigations directing IgE pathway alone may be suboptimal in determining milk allergy. Specific free milk protein IgE may be demonstrated by in vitro measurement of serum-specific IgE, whereas bound IgE may be demonstrated by in vivo skin prick test. Both of these investigations can help in detecting IgE-mediated hypersensitivity with negative results cannot rule out non-IgE mediated CMPA cases. The sensitivity and specificity of specific IgE are 87% and 48%, whereas for skin prick test are 88% and 68%, respectively. Skin prick test can be demonstrated either by using commercial extract or fresh cow's milk. The larger the wheal size (in vivo) or higher the antibody titer (in vitro), the chances of milk protein allergy are higher with longer persistence, hence apart from diagnosis, these tests can also help in prognostication.

Diagnostic Elimination Trial

If suggestive symptoms are present which may or may not be supported by in vitro or in vivo investigations, a diagnostic elimination trial is warranted. A 3–5 days of elimination is sufficient in children with immediate reactions (angioedema, vomiting, eczema exacerbation), whereas up to 2 weeks might be required for patients with delayed reactions (exacerbation of eczema, rectal bleeding). Sometimes prolonged elimination (4 weeks) may be required when chronic diarrhea or faulty growth are suspected manifestations. An improvement in symptoms is suggestive of CMPA and a challenge test followed by reappearance of symptoms will confirm the diagnosis.

Food Challenge Test

If IgE-based investigations are negative and suspicion for CMPA is quite high, a graded oral food challenge (OFC) should be done to prove or disprove milk allergy. OFC is considered gold standard test for diagnosing food allergies. Ideally, a double-blind placebo control food challenge (DBPCFC) test should be performed, but due to practical difficulty in blinding, especially in children, an open-label food challenge is equally informative. In children with delayed reaction, incremental doses of 1, 3, 10, 30 and 100 mL milk may be introduced at 30 minutes interval with close monitoring of vital signs, skin condition, and any gastrointestinal complaints. If severe reactions are expected, then the challenge should begin with extremely small doses like 0.1 and 0.3 mL followed by regular doses. Patients should be observed for a minimum of 2 hours after the maximum dose for any adverse reaction. In case of no reaction, 200 mL/day of milk is advised for next 2 weeks at home with telephonic monitoring for delayed reactions. Milk and dairy products can be freely introduced after 2 weeks, once no immediate or delayed reaction is witnessed. In case of a suspected or proven adverse reaction, the trial should be immediately aborted and the patient should be symptomatically managed with early adrenaline use. A retest may be tried after 6–12 months of elimination period.

Oral food challenge should be performed in hospital settings, preferably with availability of all resuscitation facilities. If there is history of any immediate reaction, possibility of unpredictable reaction (positive specific IgE or skin prick test), and severe atopic eczema (due to difficulty in reaction assessment), it is more important to have all the necessary resuscitation facilities in hand with informed parental consent before proceeding to challenge test. Flowchart 1 suggests a management algorithm of a patient with suspected CMPA.

TREATMENT

Cow's milk protein allergy, once confirmed with various laboratory tests and dietary modifications, should be managed with strict dietary avoidance of milk and dairy products. In case of breast-fed infants, breast milk may be continued while avoiding all milk and milk-containing products from maternal diet. It may take up to 72 hours to clear breast milk antigens ingested by the lactating woman. Mother should be supplemented with calcium supplements (1 g/day) with adequate dietary counseling.

Non-breast-fed babies should be started on extensively hydrolyzed formulas (eHF). eHF are milk formulas where milk protein is present in hydrolyzed oligopeptide (<3,000 Da) form,

Flowchart 1: Algorithm for suspected cow's milk protein allergy.

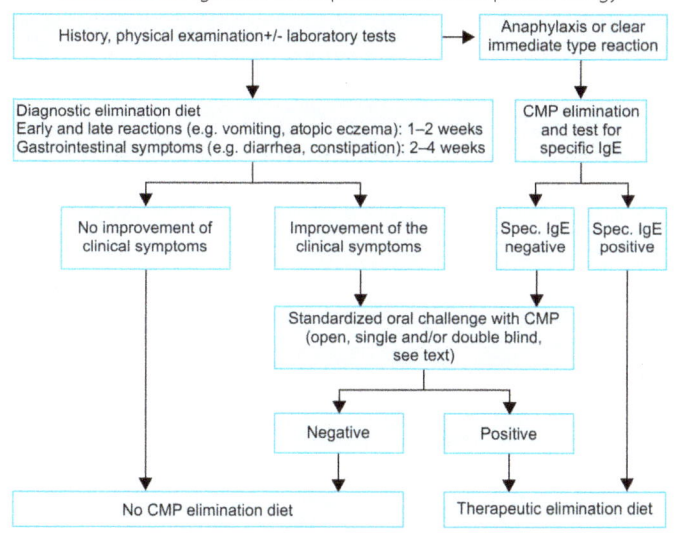

(CMPA: cow's milk protein allergy; IgE: immunoglobulin E)
Source: Koletzko S, Niggemann B, Arato A, et al. Diagnostic approach and management of cow's milk protein allergy in infants and children: ESPGHAN GL Committee practical guidelines. J Pediatr Gastroenterol Nutr. 2012;55(2):221-9.

which is hypoallergenic due to different allergenic protein configuration. Amino acid-based formulas may be required in small percentage of children who might even react to eHF. Prohibiting high cost and bitter taste of hypoallergenic formulas may be the limiting factors in developing countries, where soya-based milk formulas may be a good alternative. About 10–14% of CMPA patients may be sensitive to soya also. Another disadvantage with soya-based formula is high phytate contents which can hamper with absorption of minerals and trace elements. Soya formula is not recommended in infants under 6 months of age.

Hydrolyzed rice formulas may be used in vegan families who are sensitive to both milk and soya protein. There is high degree of cross-reactivity of cow's milk with goat, sheep, buffalo, horse, and camel milk, so these cannot be used. "Milk beverages" derived from almond, coconut, hazelnut, oat, potato, rice or soya are nutritionally inadequate and hence not recommended.

Introduction of extensively heated (baked) CMP-containing products have been tried in the West with mixed results. The tolerance induction using baked milk products and oral immunotherapy are upcoming modalities to combat CMPA, but more robust data is warranted before any recommendation.

RE-EVALUATION

An elimination period can vary from 3 months (negative specific IgE or skin prick test and mild symptoms) to 12 months (high-positive specific IgE or skin prick test and severe symptoms). Approximately, 50% of affected children develop tolerance by the age of 1 year, more than 75% by the age of 3 years, and more than 90%, are tolerant at 6 years of age.

PREVENTION

Maternal intake of cow's milk does not need to be stopped during pregnancy as a precautionary measure to prevent allergy in newborn. Exclusive breastfeeding for at least 4 months and preferably for 6 months is desirable. Exclusive breastfeeding reduces exogenous antigen exposure and provides substances helpful in gastrointestinal mucosa maturation and healthy gut microbiota proliferation. Probiotics and prebiotics may have some role in allergy prevention. CMPA children are at higher risk of developing allergies to other food items, such as egg or peanut. Weaning should be started at 4–6 months of age for future food allergy prevention and a periodic watchful screening is warranted. Delayed weaning beyond 6 months is not recommended.

CONCLUSION

Cow's Milk protein allergy is a common entity with varied presentation. Suspected patients should undergo IgE-based in vitro or in vivo test and OFC under an allergist supervision. More awareness and better diagnostic tools are required for early diagnosis and appropriate management of patients. A controlled therapeutic elimination with adequate dietary supplementation is warranted to prevent malnutrition in the affected individual. Effective tolerance techniques including oral immunotherapy are on the way to strengthen CMPA management.

6.2 FOOD ALLERGY

INTRODUCTION

Food allergy, once thought as a rare clinical entity, is now being considered a serious and often life-threatening health problem. *Food allergy is defined as an adverse health effect arising from a specific immune response that occurs reproducibly on exposure to a given food.* Perceived food allergy is much higher as compared with actual allergy incidence due to attribution of various non-specific symptoms to food items. Perception about food allergy symptoms also varies with cultural and socioeconomic variation, educational status of patient and caregivers and similar complaints in another person in near vicinity.

Food allergy is an immune-mediated process resulting in loss of tolerance to any particular food item. This intolerance could be mediated via IgE and non-IgE-mediated pathways. Some patients may have both pathways occurring simultaneously.

Cow's milk, hen's egg, soy, wheat, peanut, tree nuts, fish and shellfish are the most common food items responsible for 95% of all the food allergies. Every food has its own story, the food allergy symptoms which come early in life go away early, whereas late onset symptoms usually persist for lifelong. In the developed world, allergies to cow's milk and egg are commonly confined to pediatric age group. Characteristically, these allergies are mostly outgrown by late childhood. Similar to developed world, in most of the Asian countries, egg and milk remain the most common food allergens in young children.

EPIDEMIOLOGY

The exact incidence of food allergy is not known, as there exists a large discrepancies between reported and diagnosed allergy cases and self-reported food allergy, leading to over- or underestimation. Estimated prevalence of true food allergy diagnosed by oral food challenge is roughly 3–8% in children and 1–3% in adults in the Western world. The prevalence varies between different geographical locations and has increased in recent years partly due to changing food habits and partly due to better awareness among healthcare practitioners. Substantial data from developing countries is yet to be available.

Most children outgrow their food allergy; the prognosis is generally benign for early onset reactions. A study done in year 1994 reported resolution rates for cow's milk allergy as 45–50% at age 1 year, 60–75% at age 2 years, and 85–90% at age 3 years. However, a similar 2007 study reported non-tolerance to milk protein in 21% of children aged 16 years; these children had persistently elevated cow's milk-specific IgE at all ages. There are more chances of spontaneous resolution of non-IgE-mediated variety, whereas IgE-mediated has potential to last longer probably lifelong. Therefore, prognosis in such cohort of children is usually guarded, and the increased potential for persistence of cow's milk allergy and the effect of specific IgE concentrations or skin prick tests on future outcome may be considered in the counseling of families on expected clinical course. Some children develop tolerance during adolescence.

Likewise, the tolerance to egg allergy has been documented in children with their growth. Rate of resolution of allergy in children were 4% by 4 years of age, 12% by 6 years of age, 37% by 10 years of age, and 68% by 16 years of age. As seen in children with milk allergy, children with elevated levels of egg-specific IgE at all ages, and those with quantitative levels greater than 50 kU/L, were likely to be non-tolerant to egg for their lifetime.

Similar pattern of tolerance is seen in children suffering from wheat allergy. IgE-mediated allergy to wheat showed development of tolerance in 29% by 4 years of age, 56% by 8 years of age, and 65% by 12 years of age. Increased concentrations of wheat IgE or larger wheal size on skin prick test were associated with poor outcomes. True wheat allergy needs to be differentiated with celiac disease as the former is IgE-mediated and later, being gluten intolerance, is IgA mediated.

DIAGNOSIS

Importance of focused history taking, and detailed physical examination cannot be underemphasized. It is rather the most important tool to diagnose food allergy. Carefully taken history should elucidate symptoms, signs, onset and timing, and repeated occurrence of reactions. A symptom diary can help during followup. Usually, general physical examination is unyielding unless done at the time of onset of reaction. But other potential atopic conditions like allergic rhinitis, dermatitis may be picked up, which point towards coexistent food allergy. Food allergy symptoms are not localized to gastrointestinal system alone, a careful search for other system manifestations might provide the vital diagnostic clue.

As mentioned previously, majority of children have IgE-mediated allergy, diagnosis of which is indicated through medical history and physical examination and is confirmed by the presence of allergen-specific IgE (by serum or skin test) and positive food challenge, if necessary. More often than not, detailed history leads to ascertaining of causative food allergen. Moreover, quantity, form of food (whether semi-cooked, raw or cooked), time course of reactions occurring, and other comorbid conditions should be recorded.

Children who develop these clinical symptoms within minutes to 2 hours after ingestion of particular food should be strongly considered harboring food allergy. The symptoms being: Urticaria, angioedema, erythema, pruritus, vomiting, abdominal pain, persistent cough, hoarse voice, wheeze, stridor, respiratory distress, or nasal congestion.

Though less often seen but, if present, cardiovascular symptoms such as hypotension, extreme lethargy, or syncope, also warrant investigation for food allergy, especially if they occur in combination with above mentioned symptoms.

The presence of allergen-specific IgE can be detected by skin prick test or by immunoassay of serum allergen-specific IgE. There are high false-positives with serum-specific IgE tests if total IgE levels are more than 300 kU/L. If results of antigen-specific IgE testing do not correspond with the clinical and food history, a food challenge is indicated.

Food-dependent exercise-induced anaphylaxis requires double hits as "food" and "exercise" in continuation and neither trigger can cause symptoms in isolation.

Skin Prick Testing

It is done by introducing suspected food allergen protein into the superficial layer of skin, and the results are measured within 15–20 minutes by measuring the wheal size. Child should be at least 4–5 days free of anti-histaminics prior to the test. This is a relatively inexpensive test, sensitive but not very specific. Intradermal testing is not advised for testing of food allergy due to increased risk of anaphylaxis. Positive testing alone by skin or blood testing, does not confirm food allergy as neither mode of testing has a high predictive value. A negative test mostly confirms a lack of IgE-mediated hypersensitivity if performed correctly with histamine and normal saline as control tests. Presence of food-specific IgE without a suspicious clinical reaction indicates sensitization but is not always representative of a true allergy. The larger the wheal size, the higher is the chance that the oral food challenge will be positive.

Serum-specific IgE Testing

This test quantifies the amount of free IgE to the allergen-specific protein via an enzymatic assay. It requires blood collection, is independent of effects of anti-histaminics, and is readily available. Analogous to the trends noted with skin prick testing, high food-specific IgE levels have been found to correlate with a likelihood of clinical reaction. Specialists have data at hand with levels that are more than 95% predictive of reaction among children for common allergens such as egg, peanut and milk.

Component-resolved Diagnostics (CRD)

Component resolved diagnostics (CRD) can help in differentiating primary allergen from various cross-reactive allergens. Table 3 shows cross-reactive allergens among pollens and food items. Table 4 highlights various components of food allergens with their risk proportion for causing symptoms.

Table 3: Cross-reactive allergens.

Pollens	Food
Birch	Apple, peach, plum, pear, cherry, apricot, almond, celery, carrot, parsley, caraway, fennel, coriander, soybean, peanut, hazelnut
Ragweed	Cantaloupe, honeydew, watermelon, zucchini, cucumber, banana
Mugwort	Celery, carrot, parsley, caraway, fennel, coriander, mustard, cauliflower, cabbage, broccoli, garlic, onion
Orchard	Cantaloupe, honeydew, watermelon, peanut, potato, tomato
Timothy	Swiss chard, orange

Table 4: High-risk vs low-risk food molecules.

Source	High risk	Low risk
Peanut	Ara h 1, 2, 3, 9	Ara h 8, profilin, CCD
Hazelnut	Cor a 8, 9, 14	Profilin, CCD
Walnut	Jug r 1, 2, 3	Profilin, CCD
Soy	Gly m 5, 6 (4)	Profilin, CCD
Rosaceae fruits	Pru p 3, Mal d 3	Pru p 1, Mal d 1, Profilin, CCD
Wheat	Tri a 14, Tri a 19	Profilin, CCD

(CCD: cross-reactive carbohydrate determinant)

IgG Testing

Food-specific IgG and IgG_4 antibody measurement has no role in diagnosis of food-related allergic disorders. On the contrary, these can be a marker of immune tolerance.

Oral Food Challenge (OFC)

Double-blind placebo control OFC is considered to be the gold standard test for diagnosing food allergies. This test is done either to confirm the diagnosis or to detect tolerance to specific food allergen. In an OFC, the suspected food allergen is delivered to the patient in escalating doses either in an open or blinded fashion. OFC should always be carried out under strict medical supervision, so that any possible adverse reaction can be identified and managed promptly. Double-blind challenge tests are costly and often difficult in practice, and these tests are time and labor intensive too. Single-blind or open food challenges are usually more practical in the clinical setting and can be used to diagnose food allergy with equivocal results. Food challenges have to be done in a facility well equipped with life-saving instruments and a team of qualified personnel. Children with a previous severe food reaction should wait for at least 2 years for re-challenge with same food.

TREATMENT

As of now, no definitive treatment for food allergy exists. Only way to treat is by avoiding suspected allergenic foods and need-based management of symptoms. *Strict avoidance of the causal food/s is the main treatment for food allergy.* Cross-reactive foods need to be identified and avoided. For example, children with an allergy to a particular shellfish (e.g., shrimp, crab, or lobster) should avoid all shellfish, and those with a particular tree nut allergy (e.g., walnut, almond, hazelnut, cashew, pistachio, and Brazil nuts) should avoid all tree nuts unless sensitivity is ruled out by food challenge. Patients allergic to latex should be evaluated for banana, avocado, kiwi, chestnut, potato, green pepper and other fruits and nuts due to risk of cross-reactivity.

At present there are no medications in our armamentarium to prevent IgE-mediated food-induced allergic reactions. For mild non-life-threatening symptoms, antihistaminic agents are used with variable success. But in cases where severe life-threatening reactions (anaphylaxis) occur, adrenaline is the backbone of treatment. Children with a history of severe allergic reactions, can be given epinephrine in response to mild symptoms. Because cases of sudden death have been reported in children who stood up during a severe reaction, children should be nursed in recumbent position and the position be maintained. If symptoms persist or progress, epinephrine dosing can be repeated after 5–15 min. As biphasic reactions are known to occur, children experiencing severe reactions should be transported and managed in hospital facility equipped with emergency care. Box 1 provides indications of using epinephrine in children having food allergy.

Observation is usually recommended for a minimum of 4–6 hours, although children with severe or refractory symptoms might need to be observed for longer period in acute care area or intensive care unit. Systemic corticosteroids are commonly given to prevent biphasic or protracted reactions, but no randomized controlled trials have been done to assess their effectiveness in the management of anaphylaxis.

Box 1: Indications for prescription of self-injectable epinephrine.

- *Absolute indications*
    - Previous cardiovascular or respiratory reaction to a food, insect sting, or latex
    - Previous documented anaphylaxis
    - Exercise-induced anaphylaxis
    - Idiopathic anaphylaxis
    - Food allergy and coexisting persistent asthma
- *Relative indications*
    - Any reaction to small amounts of a suspected food (e.g., airborne food allergen or contact only via skin)
    - History of a previous mild reaction to peanut or a tree nut
    - Distance of home from medical facilities
- *Food allergy reaction in a teenager*

Table 5: Grading of severity of anaphylactic reactions.

Grading	Skin	Gastrointestinal tract	Respiratory	Cardiovascular	Neurological
1. Mild	Itchy eyes or nose, cutaneous pruritus urticaria, flushing	Oral tingling or pruritus abdominal pain, nausea, vomiting	Runny nose, sneezing, throat tightness or tingling, mild wheezing	Tachycardia higher than 15 beats per min	Irritability in young children, reduced activity, increased anxiety
2. Moderate	Diffuse urticaria and angioedema	Severe abdominal pain, repeated vomiting, diarrhea dysphagia	Hoarseness, cough, moderate dyspnea, moderate wheezing	Tachycardia higher than 15 beats per min	Light-headedness, feeling of pending life-threatening event
3. Severe		Profuse diarrhea, loss of bowel control	Severe wheezing, cyanosis or SaO$_2$ <92%, respiratory arrest	Hypotension*, bradycardia, collapse, cardiac arrest	Confusion, loss of consciousness

Severity score is based on the most affected organ system. *Hypotension defined as systolic blood pressure at 1 month to 1 year less than 70 mm Hg, at 1–10 years more than 70 mm Hg plus (age times two) at more than 10 years less than 90 mm Hg. SaO$_2$ = percentage of available hemoglobin that is saturated with oxygen.
Source: Modified from Muraro and colleagues.

Table 5 summarizes classification of severity of anaphylaxis reaction and various systems involved.

RETESTING

As food sensitization can change over the time course, it is prudent to monitor children for tolerance to allergenic food, or development of novel food allergy. It can only be done by repeatedly assessing for development of new symptoms, and to do skin prick test, or serum-specific IgE if required.

The optimum interval for follow-up testing is not known and could depend on the allergenic food. Milk and egg allergies are often outgrown in the first 4–6 years of life, but allergy to peanuts or tree nuts usually persists. For allergy to milk, egg, soy, or wheat, testing every 6–12 months is standard practice in the first 5 years of life. For persistent food allergies beyond 5 years of age, the follow-up testing may be performed every 2–3 years.

PREVENTION

The American Academy of Pediatrics (AAP) published updated recommendations in 2008 reviewing nutritional choices in pregnancy, lactation and in the first year of life which may affect development of atopic disease in infants and children. No definitive conclusions have been found regarding maternal dietary exposures during pregnancy and lactation contributing significantly to the development of food allergy in the infant. Therefore, no adjustments to the maternal diet are recommended at this time. While current evidence does support exclusive breastfeeding in high-risk infants for at least 4–6 months to decrease atopic dermatitis and cow milk allergy in the first two years of life, overall there is little literature supporting the role of breastfeeding in either preventing or delaying the onset of specific food allergies.

Timing of the introduction of complementary or solid foods has also been implicated as a factor in the prevention of food allergy in children. However, there is no evidence to support that delaying introduction beyond 4–6 months of age will affect atopy or development of food allergy. Studies looking at early weaning and the development of food allergy in children have actually found a potential protective effect in early weaning. More recent data also suggest that delaying the introduction of foods considered highly allergenic may, in fact, increase the incidence of allergy to these foods. Complementary feeding should be introduced in infant diet at 4–6 months of age in semi-solid consistency.

Allergies to certain foods (milk, egg, wheat and soy) generally resolve more quickly in childhood than others (peanut, tree nuts, fish and shellfish). Avoid food intake within 2–4 hours of planned exercise for symptom prevention.

EMERGING THERAPEUTICS

In view of possibility of severe fatal reactions secondary to accidental exposure to food allergen and lack of standard treatment guidelines, it has led investigators to find a viable therapeutic option for patients. Therapy can be divided into allergen-specific and allergen-non-specific immunotherapy.

Desensitization is gradual escalation in amount of the allergen needed to induce a reaction whereas tolerance is achieved when reaction does not occur even after taking allergen food as and when required. Tolerance is a long-lasting immunity; while in desensitization, ingestion of allergen must be continued daily else the immunologic changes may be lost. Induction of tolerance would be considered curative for the food allergy.

Allergen-specific therapies include oral immunotherapy (OIT), sublingual immunotherapy (SLIT) and epicutaneous immunotherapy (EPIT). OIT involves introducing the food allergen initially in low oral doses, and typically escalating the dose over a day or two in rapid increment, followed by a slower incremental dose increase over weeks and months.

An alternative form of oral therapy exists for cow milk and egg allergy. Subsets of children who are reactive to unheated or lightly cooked egg and milk have been noted to have tolerance of items containing these allergens that are extensively heated. The food protein is thought to be denatured, with the heat labile protein undergoing a conformational change secondary to the high heat of cooking rendering it to be non-allergenic to some patients. Patients with casein allergy do not tolerate any form of milk as casein is heat stable, whereas allergy to lactalbumin (heat labile protein) creates scope for heated milk in allergic patients.

Similar to OIT, SLIT uses small escalating doses of the food allergen; however, doses are given under the tongue via an extract vehicle. Studies have shown SLIT thus far to be quite safe yet concerns for its efficacy exist as SLIT is unable to achieve the high doses that appear to be necessary in OIT to induce desensitization.

For any type of immunotherapy against food allergens, the consensus is yet to be achieved and no immune tolerance technique is currently recommended.

CONCLUSION

Food allergy is still an important health concern as there are no specific guidelines for diagnosis and management and the prevalence is rising steadily. It is prudent for clinicians to have a high index of suspicion, and to establish proper diagnosis with the currently available diagnostic tests. Avoidance of the offending allergen and prompt treatment of acute reactions are the current mainstays of food allergy management.

SUGGESTED READING

1. Baker MG, Sampson HA. Phenotypes and endotypes of food allergy: A path to better understanding the pathogenesis and prognosis of food allergy. Ann Allergy Asthma Immunol. 2018;120(3):245-53.
2. Boyce JA, Assa'ad A, Burks AW, et al. Guidelines for the diagnosis and management of food allergy in the United States: report of the NIAID-sponsored expert panel. J Allergy Clin Immunol. 2010;126:S1-58.
3. Burks AW, Jones SM, Wood RA, et al. Oral immunotherapy for treatment of egg allergy in children. N Engl J Med. 2012;367:233-43.
4. Caffarelli C, Baldi F, Bendandi B, et al. EWGPAG. Cow's milk protein allergy in children: a practical guide. Ital J Pediatr. 2010;36:5.
5. Calvani M, Miceli Sopo S, Giorgio V. Oral immunotherapy in food allergy: how difficult to weigh its risks and benefits? J Allergy Clin Immunol. 2011;128:250-251. [online] Available from https://www.jacionline.org/article/S0091-6749(11)00567-7/abstract [Accessed December 2018].
6. Comberiati P, Cipriani F, Schwarz A, et al. Diagnosis and treatment of pediatric food allergy: an update. Ital J Pediatr. 2015;41:13. [online] Available from https://ijponline.biomedcentral.com/articles/10.1186/s13052-014-0108-0 [Accessed December 2018].
7. Gupta R, Sheikh A, Strachan DP, et al. Time trends in allergic disorders in the UK. Thorax. 2007;62:91-7.

8. Koletzko S, Niggemann B, Arato A, et al. Diagnostic approach and management of cow's Milk protein allergy in infants and children: ESPGHAN GL Committee practical guidelines. J Pediatr Gastroenterol Nutr. 2012;55(2):221-9.
9. Lifschitz C, Szajewska H. Cow's milk allergy: evidence-based diagnosis and management for the practitioner. Eur J Pediatr. 2015;174:141-50.
10. Longo G, Berti I, Burks AW, et al. IgE-mediated food allergy in children. Lancet. 2013;382:1656-64.
11. Motala C, Hawarden D. Diagnostic testing in allergy. SAMJ. 2005;95(7):531-4. [online] Available from http://www.samj.org.za/index.php/samj/article/download/3584/2428 [Accessed December 2018].
12. Perry TT, Matsui EC, Kay Conover-Walker M, et al. The relationship of allergen-specific IgE levels and oral food challenge outcome. J Allergy Clin Immunol. 2004;114:144-9.
13. Prescott S, Allen KJ. Food allergy: riding the second wave of the allergy epidemic. Pediatr Allergy Immunol. 2011;22:155-60.
14. Robinson R, Kumar R. The effect of prenatal and postnatal dietary exposures on childhood development of atopic disease. Curr Opin Allergy Clin Immunol. 2010;10(2):139-44.
15. Robison RG, Food allergy: Diagnosis, management & emerging therapies: Indian J Med Res. 2014;139:805-13.
16. Rona RJ, Keil T, Summers C, et al. The prevalence of food allergy: a meta-analysis. J Allergy Clin Immunol. 2007;120:638-46.
17. Sampson HA, Aceves S, Bock SA, et al. Food allergy: a practice parameter update-2014. J Allergy Clin Immunol. 2014;134(5):1016-25.
18. Sicherer SH, Sampson HA. Food allergy. J Allergy Clin Immunol. 2010;125 (suppl 2):116-25.
19. Vandenplas Y. Prevention and management of cow's milk allergy in non-exclusively breastfed infants. Nutrients. 2017;9(7):731.

Skin Allergies

CHAPTER 7

7.1 URTICARIA

INTRODUCTION

Itchy skin lesions are common presenting complaints in a busy pediatric practice. Almost 25% of population have at least one episode of urticaria in their lifetime. These are often symptomatically managed with "over-the-counter" antihistaminic medications. Mostly, symptoms are short lasting without any significant recurrence but sometimes these persists for longer duration and have a huge clinical and financial burden on patient and care-givers. Both prolonged symptoms and desired medications have significant negative impact on quality of life. There is an immediate need for rationale management approach of this common condition.

PATHOPHYSIOLOGY

Urticaria is recognized by appearance of itchy wheals on the superficial skin which is sudden in onset. It may be associated with angioedema. The salient features of typical lesions are:
- Wheal and flare: Swelling of variable size and shape with surrounding erythema (more visible in fair skinned individuals)
- Pruritus: Itch is the characteristic finding, sometimes it may be so intense giving burning sensation
- Transient nature: Rashes are short lasting and usually disappear in 1–24 hours.

Mast cells are principal mediator of inflammatory reaction. Vasodilation and plasma leakage happen due to histamine, various leukotrienes, and prostaglandins release.

ACUTE URTICARIA

If the urticarial rashes resolve within 6 weeks of onset, they are labeled as acute. These are mostly viral triggered itchy rashes which require symptomatic management in form of antihistaminics. Other potential causes are certain medications, foods, stress, parasitic infections, insect venom, and contact allergens like latex. Half of the patients have unknown etiology and one-third of acute urticaria patients ultimately develop chronic urticaria. Often, rashes resolve within a week time but sometimes there are periods of waxing and waning up till 6 weeks.

CHRONIC URTICARIA

Rashes are persistent or recurrent (for >6 weeks) with varied etiologies. 0.5–5% of patients are suffering from chronic urticaria. Adult females are most commonly affected. Apart from physical and spontaneous reasons, others like infections (4%), food (4%), additives (2.65%), aeroallergens (2.2%), and drugs (1.6%) could be potential triggers.

Classification

As per the recent European Academy of Allergy and Clinical Immunology (EAACI) guidelines, urticarial rashes may be classified as:
- Spontaneous: The rashes may resolve soon or may be long lasting
- Inducible: This includes cold or heat contact, delayed pressure, solar, dermographic, and vibratory types
- Others: These could be aquagenic, cholinergic, contact and exercise induced.

DIFFERENTIALS OF URTICARIA
- Vasculitis—painful lesions lasting more than 48 hours, discoloration left after healing

- Systemic mastocytosis—multisystem involvement (liver, spleen, lymph nodes, and bone marrow)
- Atopic dermatitis—highly pruritic with dry skin and lichenification in chronic cases
- Bullous pemphigoid—skin blisters, autoimmune
- Erythema multiforme—type IV hypersensitivity to certain infections and medicines, usually self-limiting
- Familial cold autoinflammatory syndrome—recurrent signs of systemic inflammation (fever, rash, joint pain), triggered by cold, starts in early infancy, and last life long
- Fixed drug eruptions—blisters with residual pigmentation during healing, usually occur after medication
- Subacute cutaneous lupus erythematosus—nonscarring photosensitive skin condition
- Pruritic urticarial papules and plaques of pregnancy—in third trimester of first pregnancy
- Muckle-Wells syndrome—recurrent hives with hearing loss, amyloidosis may develop
- Schnitzler's syndrome with monoclonal immunoglobulin G kappa gammopathy—chronic nonpruritic hives, periodic fever, bone and joint pain, swollen lymph glands, hepatosplenomegaly.

DIAGNOSTIC EVALUATION

- History: Focused clinical details can give an important clue for targeted laboratory investigations and management plan. The following points should be enquired:
  - Time of onset of disease
  - Frequency and duration of wheals
  - Diurnal variation
  - Shape, size, and distribution of wheals
  - Associated angioedema
  - Associated subjective symptoms
  - Family and personal history regarding urticaria, food or respiratory allergy

- Previous or current allergies, infections, systemic diseases
    - Psychosomatic and psychiatric illnesses
    - Surgical implantations and events during surgery
    - Gastric and intestinal complaints
    - Symptoms exacerbation by physical agents or exercise
    - Use of drugs—nonsteroidal anti-inflammatory drugs, injections, immunizations, hormones, laxatives, suppositories, ear- and eye drops, and alternative system medicines (Homeopathy, Ayurveda, Unani)
    - Observed correlation with food
    - Cyclical exacerbation or resolution with menstrual cycle
    - Smoking exposure (passive or active)
    - Type of work (occupational exposure)
    - Hobbies
    - Stress
    - Occurrence in relation to weekends, holidays, and foreign travel
    - Impact on quality of life
    - Previous therapy and response to therapy.
- Relevant physical examination
- Investigations:
    - Baseline—complete blood count, liver function test, kidney function test, C-reactive protein, erythrocyte sedimentation rate (ESR), urine routine and microscopy
    - Specific—as per the history and physical examination:
        - Vasculitis—immunoglobulin levels, antinuclear antibody, immune complex, and skin lesion biopsy
        - Infections—serologic studies for hepatitis C virus (HCV), HBV, HAV, Epstein-Barr virus (EBV), *Mycoplasma Pneumoniae*; relevant cultures, fecal antigen for *Helicobacter Pylori* or urea breath test
        - Allergic—IgE (total or specific), skin tests, eosinophil count, challenge, elimination test, and tryptase levels
        - Hereditary angioedema—C3, C4, C1 esterase inhibitor, genetic analysis (mutations in C1-inhibitor gene—*Serping 1* gene on chromosome 11)

- Physical—methacholine test, running test, ice cube test, ultraviolet and visible light exposure, dermatographism, pressure test, and warm water immersion test
- Autoimmune chronic urticaria—autologous serum skin test (ASST) and basophil histamine release test (BHRT)
- Others—free T_3, free T_4, thyroid-stimulating hormone (TSH), thyroid autoantibodies, and celiac screening.

MANAGEMENT

Treatment of urticaria is usually symptomatic with antihistaminic drugs. Acute urticaria is short lasting and usually resolves with in 1 week of onset, however, chronic urticaria is difficult to manage. Following steps are suggested for management in case of urticaria:

- Level I:
    - Elimination of possible eliciting factors
    - Nonsedating second generation H_1 antihistaminics (nsAH)
    - If symptoms persist even after 2 weeks—go to level II.
- Level II:
    - Up dosing of nsAH (× up to 4 times)
    - Add another second generation H1 antihistamine
    - Add H_2 antagonist
    - If symptoms persist after another 4 weeks of therapy—go to level III.
- Level III:
    - Add leukotriene antagonist or change to another nsAH
    - Add first generation antihistaminic at bed time
    - If symptoms still persist after another 1–4 weeks—go to level IV.
- Level IV:
    - Immunomodulators (like Cyclosporine), $H_1 + H_2$ blocker, anti-IgE antibody
    - Thyroxine supplements—if hypothyroid or antithyroid antibody positive

- Vitamin D
- Plasmapheresis
- Autologous whole blood injection—in adults with refractory chronic urticaria.

*During exacerbations, systemic steroids may be added for 3-7 days at all levels.

*Referrals—Dermatologist, Allergist, and Immunologist.

7.2 ANGIOEDEMA

INTRODUCTION

Angioedema was initially described in 1586 and thereafter many terminologies like giant urticaria, Quincke's edema, and angioneurotic edema have been given to describe this. Isolated angioedema is fairly uncommon in pediatric population, many a times it is associated with urticaria. 40% of children with urticaria are affected with associated angioedema at some times of their life span, while standalone angioedema affects only 6.65% of all urticarial patients.

PATHOPHYSIOLOGY

Acute attacks of angioedema occur from increased permeability of tissue capillaries in skin and mucosa followed by plasma leak and edema formation. Any body part may be involved like limbs, face, throat, trunk, bowel, and genitals. The characteristic features are:
- Rapid onset, appreciable swelling of lower dermis and subcutaneous tissue
- Minimal to no itch, sometimes pain may be there
- Mucosa frequently affected
- Slowly resolves over 72 hours.

All attacks involving upper part of the body (above shoulders) must be considered serious as they may involve larynx and thus potentially life-threatening. The chemical mediators involved could be either histamine or bradykinin.

Histaminergic angioedema may be dictated by an immunoglobulin E- (IgE) or non IgE-mediated pathway. A thorough diagnostic work-up yields allergic etiology in few patients only. The attacks are associated with itching and usually respond to antihistaminics and steroids.

Bradykinin-mediated reactions are due to either enhanced production or reduced degradation and thus activation of endothelial cells leading to tissue edema formation. Several mechanisms like complement, coagulation, and contact pathways may be responsible for this derangement. Response to antihistaminic is questionable.

CLASSIFICATION

As per the etiology, angioedema may be classified as:
- Mast cell mediated
- Hereditary angioedema type 1 (HAE-1), HAE-2, HAE with normal C_1 inhibitor (HAE-nC_1-INH)
- Acquired (C_1-INH deficiency from a secondary cause)
- Angiotensin-converting enzyme (ACE) inhibitor induced
- Idiopathic.

Mast Cell Mediated

Mast cell mediators (histamine, heparin, leukotriene C_4, and prostaglandin D_2) are mainly responsible for increase in vascular permeability. It is usually associated with pruritus. It could be IgE-mediated (food, drugs, stinging insect, latex and contact to vegetables and saliva), direct mast cell-mediator release (opiates, muscle relaxants, and radiocontrast agents), and perturbations in arachidonic acid metabolism within mast cells (aspirin and other nonsteroidal anti-inflammatory drugs).

Hereditary Angioedema

It is an autosomal dominant condition with C_1 inhibitor deficiency, either absolute (due to reduced production) or relative (due to lack of function), which results in vascular leakage. Type I is most common (85%) with low C_1-INH levels and function whereas rest cases are attributed to low function alone (type II). In HAE-nC_1-INH, there is gain of function mutation in factor XII and thus increased production of kinin. HAE is more common in adolescent females with a positive family history in 75% of patients. Rest may be affected due to de novo mutation of *C_1-INH* gene.

Acquired Angioedema

These are much less common and found in older age group (fourth decade of life). Most cases are associated with B cell lymphoproliferative disorders [acquired angioedema (AAE) type I] where as some have autoantibody against C_1-INH (AAE type II). As bradykinin plays major role in AAE, antihistaminics and steroids have limited role in management.

ACE Inhibitor-induced Angioedema

About 0.1–6% of patients, who are using ACE inhibitors for any medical indications, suffer from angioedema within first week of starting therapy. Sometimes, it may occur after months to years of drug intake. It is more common in females, smokers, and African-American population. It is predominantly bradykinin mediated.

DIAGNOSIS

Common clinical symptoms are non-itchy swelling of skin and submucosa involving face, extremities, abdomen, laryngeal edema, and asphyxiation. Lesions above shoulders have higher risk of laryngeal involvement and are potential life-threatening. Almost half of the patients with HAE have experienced at least 1 laryngeal episode in their lifetime. Patients with HAE may also have spasmodic abdominal pain, gastrointestinal upset, and intestinal obstruction.

Patients with associated urticaria should be investigated as per the recommendations for urticaria diagnosis. Isolated angioedema patients should undergo special investigations prior to starting treatment:

Table 1: Comparison of HAE and AAE.

	Family history	Complement levels/laboratory findings		
		C_4	C_1-INH antigen	C_1-INH function
HAE-1	Yes	↓	↓	↓
HAE-2		↓	Normal or ↑	↓
HAE-nC1-INH	Yes	Normal	Normal	Normal
AAE	No	↓	Normal or ↓	↓

(AAE: acquired angioedema; HAE: hereditary angioedema; nC_1-INH: normal C_1 inhibitor)
Source: Kanani A, Betschel SD, Warrington R. Urticaria and angioedema. Allergy Asthma Clin Immunol. 2018;14:115-27.

- C_4 (natural substrate for C_1) level
- C_1q level
- C_1-INH antigen
- Function of C_1-INH.

Table 1 depicts comparison of HAE and AAE. Patients with AAE should be worked up for B-cell lymphoproliferative disorders.

MANAGEMENT

- Acute attacks:
    - C_1-INH replacement therapy—dose as 20 units/kg rapid intravenous push
    - Icatibant: It is a bradykinin receptor blocker. The recommended dose is 30 mg subcutaneously
    - Ecallantide: It is an inhibitor of plasma kallikrein (enzyme responsible for bradykinin release).
- Short-term prophylaxis—should be used during anticipated trigger exposure for example physical trauma, examination time, stressful life events, medical or dental procedure.
    - C_1-INH replacement: It may be given within 24 hours of an anticipated procedure. The dose will be 1,000 units for an adult

- Attenuated androgens: Danazol (2.5–10 mg/kg/day) should be started 5 days prior to anticipated procedure and to be continued till 3 days after the trigger.
- Long-term prophylaxis—should be used in patients who have predisposing factors like two or more attacks per month, recurrent laryngeal attacks, or who are less responsive to treatment during acute attacks.
    - C1-INH replacement—1,000 units every 3–4 days
    - Attenuated androgens: They increase C_4 and C_1-INH levels. Adverse effects like virilization serum transaminases abnormalities, menstrual irregularities, excessive hair growth, decreased libido, weight gain, vasomotor symptoms, lipid abnormalities, and depression should be monitored.

Flowchart 1 suggests management algorithm for angioedema.

7.3 ATOPIC DERMATITIS

INTRODUCTION

It is a chronic skin ailment with periodically recurring inflammation. Disrupted epithelial barrier associated with dysregulated immune functions predisposes atopic dermatitis (AD) in susceptible individuals. The characteristic features are dry, scaly skin lesions with constant itch occurring mostly in early childhood. *Staphylococcus aureus* is a common colonizer. Its prevalence is around 10–20% of all the children, in United States. People living in urban states are more commonly affected than rural area. AD has significant effect on sleep, quality of life, school performance, self-esteem of children, and family dysfunction. Available medications like antihistaminics alone are insufficient for appropriate management, creating a need for other effective techniques.

PATHOPHYSIOLOGY

Atopic dermatitis is a multifactorial disease with genetic, environmental, and immunologic factors as predominant

Skin Allergies 189

Flowchart 1: Management algorithm for angioedema.

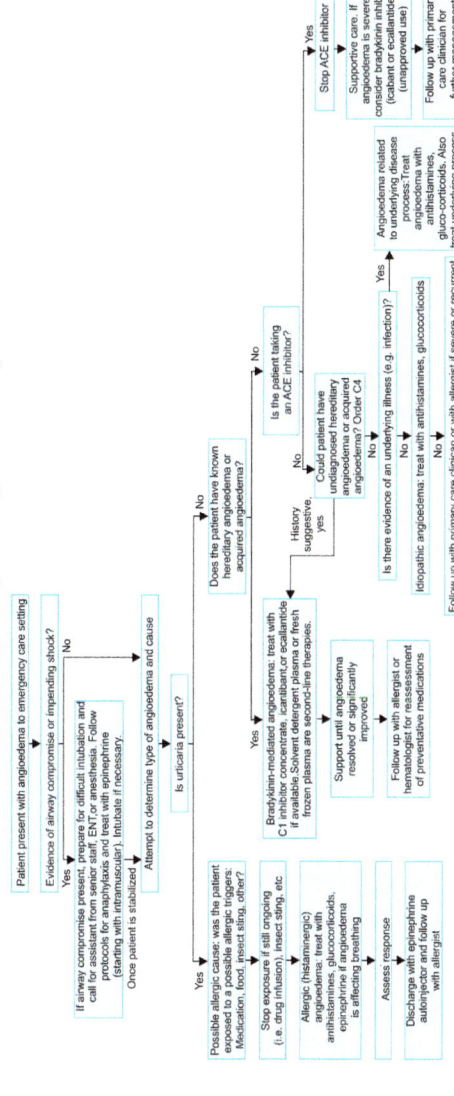

(ACE: angiotensin-converting enzyme)

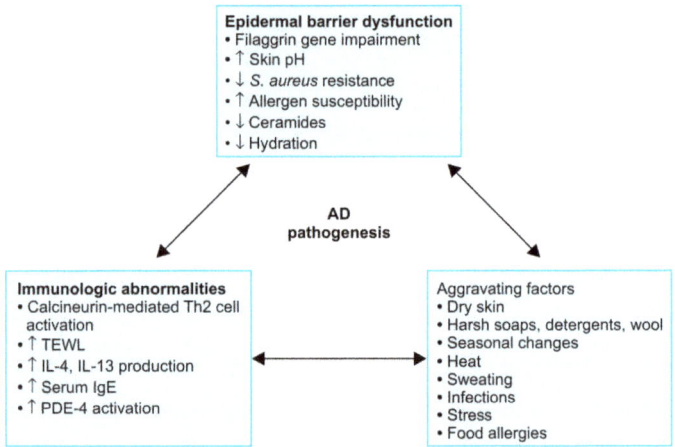

Fig. 1: Pathophysiology of AD.
(AD: atopic dermatitis; IgE: immunoglobulin E; IL: interleukin; PDE-4: phosphodiesterase 4; TEWL: transepidermal water loss; Th2: T helper type 2)
Source: Sayaseng KY, Vernon P. Pathophysiology and management of mild to moderate pediatric atopic dermatitis. J Pediatr Health Care. 2018;32:S2-S12.

contributors (Fig. 1). Family history of atopy, early onset (within infancy), and filaggrin (*FLG*) gene mutation are predictors of severe disease. Air pollutants, ozone levels in living area, and ultraviolet (UV) radiation exposure have strong positive relationship with development of AD. Serum immunoglobulin E (IgE) levels are commonly raised.

Skin barrier disruption is the key element in pathophysiology of AD. Several genetic diseases contribute to skin barrier dysfunction. Loss-of-function mutations of *FLG* gene causes disturbed keratinization and loss of natural moisturizing factor, thus leads to atopic triad viz AD, allergic rhinitis and asthma. Interleukin (IL-4) and IL-13 are mostly responsible for inflammation and pruritus in AD. Intense pruritus leads to further epithelial disruption due to scratching, which promotes progression of the disease. Transepidermal water loss and barrier dysfunction enhances disease activity and food/environmental allergen sensitization by increased penetration.

Skin excoriation due to severe itching leads to superinfections, the most common culprit being *S. aureus*.

DIAGNOSIS

Detailed history is the most important guide in suspecting a diagnosis of AD. Personal or family history of atopy along with repeated episodes of itchy skin lesions and dryness of skin is highly suggestive of the disease. In acute conditions, the skin is erythematous, scaly, and excoriated, whereas lichenification and loss of pigmentation occurs in chronic phase. Papules and spongiotic vesicles are hallmark of severity of condition.

Location of skin involvement varies with different age groups. Face, upper and lower limbs, and trunk are commonly affected in infancy, antecubital and popliteal areas with wrists and ankles are involved in toddlers (1-3 years of age), whereas, extensor aspects of limbs are more commonly involved in older children and adolescents.

Common trigger factors could be certain foods (milk and egg) or aeroallergens (house dust mite and cockroaches). A careful history and other associated system involvement like rhinitis and asthma might help in delineating the particular cause.

Several diagnostic criteria have been described in the literature, among which, "Hanifin and Rajka" criteria are most commonly used.

"Hanifin and Rajka" Diagnostic Criteria for Atopic Dermatitis

- Major features:
    - Pruritus
    - Characteristic morphology and distribution
    - Facial and extensor involvement in infants and children; flexural involvement with lichenification in adults

- Chronic or relapsing course
- Personal or family history of atopy, including asthma, allergic rhinitis, and AD.
- Minor features:
  - Early age of onset
  - Xerosis
  - Palmar hyperlinearity, ichthyosis, and keratosis pilaris
  - Immediate skin test reactivity and elevated serum IgE
  - Cutaneous infection, including *S. aureus* and herpes simplex virus
  - Nipple eczema
  - Cheilitis
  - Pityriasis alba
  - White dermatographism and delayed blanching
  - Perifollicular accentuation
  - Anterior subcapsular cataracts
  - Itch when sweating
  - Nonspecific hand or foot dermatitis
  - Recurrent conjunctivitis
  - Dennie-Morgan folds
  - Keratoconus
  - Facial erythema or pallor.

DIFFERENTIAL DIAGNOSIS

- Contact dermatitis
- Seborrheic dermatitis
- Drug reactions
- Infantile psoriasis
- Scabies
- Nutritional deficiencies—zinc/biotin
- Acrodermatitis enteropathica
- Netherton syndrome
- Ichthyosis vulgaris
- Peeling skin disorder

- Severe dermatitis, multiple allergies, and metabolic wasting syndrome
- Primary immunodeficiency diseases and Omenn syndrome
- Lymphocytic-variant hypereosinophilic syndrome (HES)
- Cutaneous T-cell lymphoma.

TREATMENT OF ACUTE FLARES

Topical corticosteroids and immunomodulators (calcineurin inhibitors and PD-4 inhibitors) reduce skin inflammation. Skin condition and delivery of medication can affect absorption and efficacy of drugs used. Humid conditions, occlusive dressings, and breached epidermis increase the absorption of percutaneously applied medications. Molecules with molecular weight of less than or equal to 500 Da can penetrate normal or abnormal skin barriers. Other properties of medication dispensing vehicle and their efficacy are elaborated in Table 2. Figure 2 demonstrates the

Table 2: Vehicles in topical medications.

Potency	Vehicle	Consistency/appearance	Composition	Recommended application sites
Maximum	Ointments	Translucent, greasy	Oil base	All, except intertriginous areas
	Creams	Smooth, silky	Oil and water mixture	All
	Lotions and solutions	Thin, watery, clear	Water and alcohol base	Scalp, hairy areas
	Gels	Jelly-like	Glycol and water mixture	Scalp, hairy areas
	Aerosols	Spray	Medication suspended in a base, pressurized	Scalp, moist lesions
Minimum	Foams	Frothy	High water content	Scalp, hairy areas

Source: Modified from Sayaseng KY, Vernon P. Pathophysiology and management of mild to moderate pediatric atopic dermatitis. J Pediatr Health Care. 2018;32:S2-S12.

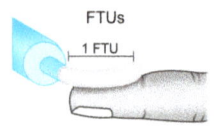
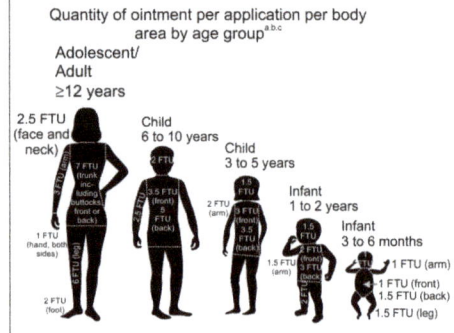

FTU = amount of ointment expressed from a tube with a 5 mm diameter nozzle measured from the distal skin crease to the tip of the palmar surface of an adult's index finger (~0.5 g)

1 FTU = adequate amount of ointment for "thin and even" application to an area of skin equal ~2 adult hands* (fingers together)

Moisturizer[c]	Basic management			
Infant child	100 g/week			
	150–200 g/week			
Adolescent/adult	500 g/week			
Ointment	Acute Treatment 2-times daily	Maintenance treatment		
		1–2 times weekly	2–3 times weekly	1–2 times daily
Infant	60–100 g/week	10 g/month	15 g/month	75 g/month
Child	125–250 g/week	20 g/month	30 g/month	150 g/month
Adolescent/adult	260–300 g/week	40–60 g/month	60–90 g/month	300–450 g/month
Cream[b]	Acute treatment 2-times daily	Maintenance Treatment		
		1–2 times weekly	2–3 times weekly	1–2 times daily
Infant	60–110 g/week	15 g/month	20 g/month	100 g/month
Child	140–275 g/week	25 g/month	35 g/month	175 g/month
Adolescent/adult	290–330 g/week	45–70 g/month	70–100 g/month	350–500 g/month

Fig. 2: Topical application amounts.
(FTUs: fingertip units)
[a]Measurements are relative to adult hand/finger size.
[b]Creams used should be 10% more than ointments.
[c]Moisturizer may be required in increased amount.
*Monthly estimates for two to three times per week application.

Source: Eichenfield LF, Boguniewicz M, Simpson EL, et al. Translating Atopic Dermatitis Management Guidelines into practice for Primary care Providers. Pediatrics. 2015;136: 554-65.

amount to be applied at the affected area. One fingertip unit (FTU) is the quantity of ointment expressed from a dispensing tube with 5 mm diameter nozzle measured from distal skin crease to the tip of the palmar surface of an adult's index finger. This quantitates to approximately 0.5 g and sufficient for thin and even application to 2 adult hands (with fingers).

- *Topical corticosteroids*:
  - Molecular weight of 200 Da helps in easy subcutaneous penetration
  - Twice daily application for 2 weeks on the affected areas usually suffice
  - Categorized in seven categories with group I being the most potent (Table 3)

Table 3: Topical steroid potency chart.

Class of potency	Drugs
I (Super potent)	• Clobetasol propionate (0.05%) cream, ointment • Betamethasone dipropionate (0.05%) ointment • Halobetasol propionate (0.05%) ointment
II (Potent)	• Betamethasone dipropionate (0.05%) lotion • Mometasone furoate (0.1) ointment • Desoximetasone (0.25%) cream, ointment
III (Upper mid-strength)	• Fluticasone propionate (0.05%) ointment • Betamethasone valerate (0.1%) cream
IV (Mid-strength)	• Mometasone furoate (0.1%) cream • Triamcinolone (0.1%) ointment
V (Lower mid-strength)	• Fluticasone propionate (0.05%) cream • Desonide (0.05%) lotion
VI (Mild)	• Aclometasonedipropionate (0.05%) cream, ointment • Desonide (0.05%) gel • Clobetasone butyrate (0.05%) cream • Fluocinolone acetonide (0.025%) ointment, shampoo
VII (Least potent)	• Hydrocortisone acetate (0.5%, 1%, and 2.5%) lotion, ointment

Source: Modified from Sayaseng KY, Vernon P. Pathophysiology and management of mild to moderate pediatric atopic dermatitis. J Pediatr Health Care. 2018;32:S2-S12.

- Monitor for local adverse effects—striae, telangiectasia, generalized hypertrichosis, skin atrophy, increased risk of cataract, and glaucoma (if applied in periorbital areas)
- Systemic steroids—not recommended.
- *Topical calcineurin inhibitors*:
  - As the molecular weight is near 800 Da, these agents do not cross the dermis
  - Improve skin clearance and reduces itch by suppressing calcineurin-mediated activation of T helper type 2 (Th2) cells
  - Available as tacrolimus 0.03% concentration ointment for children 2–15 years of age and 0.1% for older patients
  - Can be used on whole body including face and intertriginous areas
  - No risk of skin atrophy
  - No evidence for theoretical risk of lymphoma
  - Transient burning may be experienced by some patients, at the site of application, which settles in few days.
- *Phosphodiesterase 4 (PDE-4) inhibitors*:
  - PDE-4 inhibitors (crisborole) has been approved by Food and Drug Administration (FDA) for mild-to-moderate AD in children more than 2 years
  - Suppresses proinflammatory cytokines Th1 and Th2
  - Inhibits tumor necrosis factor-alpha.
- *Biologics*:
  - Soluble receptors, monoclonal antibodies and cytokines [recombinant interferon, antitumor necrosis factor (TNF)] and inhibitors of IgE/IL-5 pathway—lack sufficient evidence
- *Immunosuppressant*:
  - Cyclosporin A—recommended for severe refractory AD
  - Azathioprine and methotrexate—optimal dose and duration unclear.
- *Antimicrobials*:
  - Oral antibiotics may be suggested for secondary bacterial infections

- Intranasal mupirocin may be advised along with bleach bath.
- *Antihistamines*:
  - Diphenhydramine, hydroxyzine, and cyproheptadine—may be helpful to relieve itching
  - Fexofenadine, cetirizine and loratadine—helpful in comorbid allergies.
- *Probiotics*:
  - Blocks Th2-mediated immune responses, thus reduces allergic hypersensitivity.
- *Phototherapy*:
  - May be used as second-line in refractory cases
  - Narrow-band UVB—indicated in children more than 6 years of age.
- *Allergen immunotherapy*:
  - Indicated in sensitization to house dust mites
  - Favorable safety profile.

SKIN CARE

- *Moisturizing agents*:
  - Unscented moisturizers at least twice daily
  - Take caution with natural oils (e.g. coconut oil), which may act as sensitizer in some individuals.
- *Bathing practices*:
  - Neck folds, axillae, and diaper areas should be cleaned daily
  - Avoid hot water and prolonged bathing
  - Promote lukewarm water for 15 minutes of bath.
- *Dilute bleach baths*:
  - Sodium hypochlorite in bath reduces skin *S. aureus* concentration
  - One-eighth to one-fourth cup of concentrated bleach should be mixed in full bathtub (40 gallons water) (1 gallon = 3.785 liters)
  - Soak for 5–10 minutes only followed by rinsing with fresh lukewarm water.

- *After flare maintenance therapy*:
  - Apply topical corticosteroids or calcineurin inhibitors one to two times per week as preventive measure in case of frequent relapses.
- *Patient/caregiver education*:
  - Avoid triggers—excessive bathing, no moisturizers, less humid environment, emotional stress, xerosis, hyperthermia, scents, solvents, and detergents
  - Apply topical medications (occlusive ointments) first, immediately after bath, followed by moisturizers
  - Wet wrap therapy—two-to-three times a week; uncontrolled wet wrap therapy may result in skin maceration, folliculitis, and enhanced absorption of corticosteroids and thus its local side effects.

NONPHARMACOLOGICAL MEASURES

- *Role of foods*:
  - Therapeutic or diagnostic elimination diets may be recommended in case of proven or suspected food allergy.
- *Role of environmental triggers*:
  - Avoidance measures for mechanical and chemical irritants—wool, irritant soaps, toiletries containing alcohol or perfumes
  - Antidust mite measures—specialized protective coatings, vacuum cleaning, dehumidifiers, and sun exposure of infested curtains/pillow covers/bed sheets
- *Textiles*:
  - Avoid irritating fabric.
- *Balneotherapy*:
  - Immersion of body or parts in bathtubs or pools of mineral water
  - May be adjuvant in long-term management of AD
  - *Other beneficial factors*: Relaxing spa environment, warm climate, increased sun exposure, and therapeutic education program.

Skin Allergies

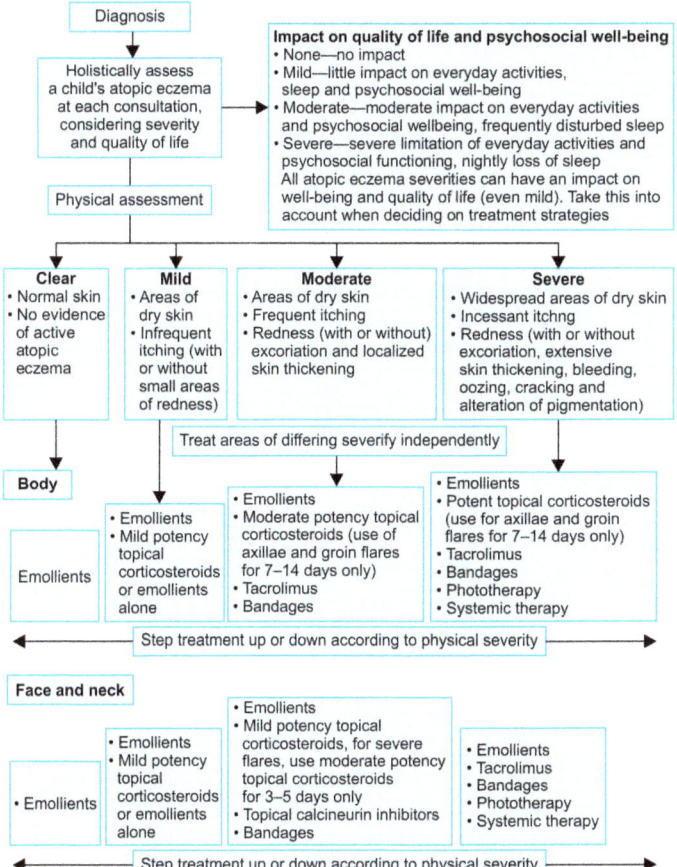

Flowchart 2: Approach to a child with atopic dermatitis.

*Flowchart 2 depicts an approach to a child with atopic dermatitis.

WHEN TO REFER TO A SPECIALIST?

- Refractory AD despite conventional treatment
- Involvement of face or skin folds

- Associated comorbidities—attention deficit hyperactivity disorder, autism, anxiety, and depression
- Effect on quality of life—chronic itching and sleep disturbances.

SUMMARY

Atopic dermatitis is a complex disease with epithelial disintegrity in genetically predisposed individuals. Significant itchy skin lesions are the characteristic features. Allergen identification and its avoidance measures play important role along with appropriate skin care and topical medicines. Early suspicion and timely referral to a specialist is warranted in refractory cases.

7.4 CONTACT DERMATITIS

INTRODUCTION

As per the recent estimate, dermatitis prevalence has been reported about 20% in western world. This includes both atopic and contact dermatitis (CD). CD alone contributes to 4–7% of all patients visiting for dermatological problems. Hand dermatitis, the most common reason to seek to a physician/allergist/dermatologist, accounts for approximately 2% cases at any given time and 20% lifetime risk in any individual. Occupational skin diseases (OSDs) ranks second after musculoskeletal problems as per UK EPIDERM (experience of dermatologists) surveillance data with dermatitis being the most prominent among all, contributing to 79% of all OSD.

Substances like nickel (14.5%), fragrance (3.7%), cobalt (2.2%), hydroxyisohexyl cyclohexene carboxaldehyde (1.4%), and paraphenylenediamine (PPD) (1%) are common causes for CD in Europe. Figures from India are sparse due to under recognition and under reporting of this emerging entity.

DEFINITION

Contact dermatitis is a type of skin inflammation, which is characterized by erythema and vesiculation in acute phase and dryness, lichenification, and fissuring in the chronic phase.

TYPES

- *Subjective irritancy*: Characterized by idiosyncratic stinging reaction, commonly involving face, with no visible changes over skin. Common cosmetic and sunscreen constituents may be responsible for subjective irritancy.
- *Acute irritant CD*: Mild to marked irritation after single large or frequent brief exposures to strong irritants or caustic agents.
- *Chronic (cumulative) irritant CD*: It happens after repetitive exposure of less potent irritants, which could be either "wet" like detergents, organic solvents, soaps, weak acids, and alkalis or "dry" like low-humidity air, heat, powders, paper, cardboard, and dust.
- *Allergic CD*: Some allergens produce allergic skin reaction, in previously sensitized individuals, by type IV (delayed type) hypersensitivity immune mechanism.
- *Phototoxic, photoallergic, and photoaggravated CD*: Certain allergens, after application, when exposed to ultraviolet (UV) rays produces allergic manifestations on skin. These allergens or UV rays are unable to produce symptoms, when exposed in isolation.
- *Systemic CD*: It happens after systemic administration of a chemical, to which an individual is already exposed. Drug hypersensitivities are common example.
- *Protein CD*: It occurs after long-term handling of proteinaceous substances like foods and animal danders. It is usually mediated by early (type I) hypersensitivity with positive skin prick test.

PATHOPHYSIOLOGY

- *Irritant CD*: Almost 80% of all CD reactions are due to irritant nature of causative agents. It directly causes epidermal damage and dermal inflammation leading to a variety of symptoms ranging from simple dryness (xerosis) to caustic lesions (burns). Severity and extent of lesions will directly depend upon chemical nature and concentration of product, frequency

- *Allergic CD*: Allergenic substances (usually nonproteinaceous) called as haptens, bind to tissue proteins to form complete allergen or complete antigen and then processed by dendritic cells (DCs) followed by migration to regional lymph nodes. DCs present allergens to CD8+ and CD4+ T cells, which have effector and regulatory functions, respectively. B-cells are instructed to produce immunoglobulin M (IgM) antibodies. Specific T cells reach to skin by blood circulation leading to completion of sensitization process. During subsequent exposure to similar antigenic substance, released IgM (from B-cells) and activated T cells binds to allergen-protein complex and leads to complement activation with release of various inflammatory and chemotactic factors viz interferons-γ (IFN-γ), interleukin 2 (IL-2), and IL-17. These cytokines destroy keratinocytes and stimulates new cell recruitment in the skin, in turn causing eczematous lesions. Three elements are key factors for any allergic CD; haptens, antigen presenting DC, and hapten specific T cells. Figure 3 summarizes all the events during allergic CD. Table 4 differentiates salient characteristics between irritant and allergic CD.

Skin irritation and skin damage is the initial step in both irritant and allergic CD. If the process limits itself to superficial damage and dealt by innate immunity only, it restricts itself to irritant variety, whereas if it triggers adaptive immunity leading to sensitization, in predisposed individuals, and produces delayed hypersensitivity manifestations, it causes allergic CD. In acute conditions, it is characterized by erythema and vesiculation whereas dryness, lichenification, and fissuring of skin predominates in chronic phase of the disease.

Irritant CD involves innate (nonspecific) immunity, whereas adaptive or acquired (specific) immunity have major contribution in allergic CD (Table 5).

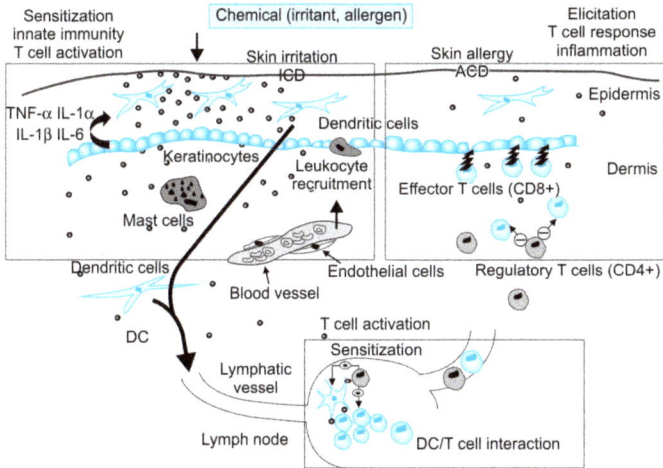

Fig. 3: Pathophysiology of allergic contact dermatitis.
(DC: dendritic cell; IL: interleukin; TNF-α: tumor necrosis factor- α)
Source: Nosbaum A, Vocanson M, Rozieres A, et al. Allergic and irritant contact dermatitis. Eur J dermatol. 2009;19(4):1-8.

Table 4: Allergic versus irritant contact dermatitis (CD).

Characteristics	Allergic CD	Irritant CD
Skin lesions	Anywhere over body surface	Limited to contact site
Predominant symptoms	Itching	Burning
Surface appearance	Vesicles and bullae	Dry and fissured skin
Epidemiology	Affects some subjects out of all who handle the product	Affects majority of subjects handling the product
Histology	Spongiosis and exocytosis	Epidermal necrosis
Patch test	Positive (eczematous reaction)	Negative
Skin immunology	Presence of activated T cells	No activated T cells
Blood immunology	Presence of specific T cells	No specific T cells

Table 5: Innate and adaptive immunity.

Innate immunity	Adaptive immunity
Present in multicellular organism	Present in vertebrates
Immediate response (3–12 hours)	Delayed response (3–5 days)
Constitutive effector functions (inflammation and phagocytosis)	Inducible effector functions (proliferation, activation, maturation, and differentiation)
Granulocytes, natural killer cells, monocytes, macrophages, and dendritic cells	T and B lymphocytes
Receptors are (pattern recognition receptors) (PRR)—hundreds of specific receptors bind to conserved molecular structures shared by large groups of pathogens	Receptors are B-cell receptor (BCR) and T-cell receptor (TCR) for antigen—immediate repertoire (10^{14}–10^{18} TCR), produced by somatic recombination
No memory, no affinity maturation	Memory and affinity maturation present
Recognition of danger signals	Recognition of "non-self" antigens versus "self" antigens (positive and negative clonal selection)

MAKING A DIAGNOSIS

As allergen avoidance is the only definite treatment available for CD, every possible effort should be made for its identification. Detailed history is the initial prerequisite before proceeding towards any diagnostic testing or suggesting specific avoidance measure. Some of the salient points to be covered in the history are:

- History of atopic dermatitis in infancy or early childhood
- Personal history of asthma or nasal symptoms
- Family history of atopy
- Site of onset of initial symptoms and mode of progression—allergic CD symptoms appear 1–4 days after contact with the causative allergen
- Any history of local application—cosmetics, personal-care products, medication, clothing, bandages, gloves, goggles, etc.
- History of relevant wash products and shampoos
- Relationship to activity—hairdressing, holiday, home improvement, painting, decorating, recreation or sport
- Severity of symptoms at work and home
- Relationship with environmental change or sunlight exposure

- Frequency of hand washing should be asked in hand dermatitis
- Temporal association of exposure to suspected allergen and onset of symptoms
- History of itching suggests allergic CD.

DIAGNOSTIC TESTS

After a detailed history and relevant physical examination, diagnosis of CD needs to be confirmed by certain laboratory parameters. Allergen specific T cells may be detected in patient's blood with ELISPOT assay (enzyme-linked immunospot), though the sensitivity and specificity are quite low. Patch testing (an in vivo technique) is considered as gold standard for diagnosing allergic CD with sensitivity and specificity in between 70% and 80%.

Patch Testing

- *Principle*:
    - Patch test is an in vivo reproduction of type IV or delayed hypersensitivity reaction in an already sensitized person.
- *Indications*:
    - Chronic or persistent dermatitis
    - Uncontrolled or partially controlled dermatitis despite medications.
- *Prerequisites*:
    - Patient/caregiver counseling regarding the expected reactions of the test like a positive patch test might flare up underlying dermatitis/eczema or may cause temporary pigmentation
    - Careful avoidance of UV ray's exposure for 6 weeks, systemic immunosuppressants for 3 months, and biological agents for 6 months before attempting patch test.
- *Dermatologist/allergist should be aware about limitations of patch testing*:
    - False-positive—due to high concentration of test allergens/irritants, pressure reaction of filling chambers, and testing at the time of active dermatitis

- False-negative—due to inadequate allergen concentration, inability of the vehicle to release sufficient quantity of allergen, prior UV light exposure, daily intake of prednisolone more than or equal to 10 mg in adults, other immunosuppressants and insufficient occlusion or contact time.
- *Procedure*:
  - Specific allergens are applied on the skin in a standardized concentration in an appropriate vehicle and under occlusion. This test is usually carried out on the back or sometimes on the outer aspect of upper arms of patient.
  - Many preprepared patches like "thin-layer rapid-use epicutaneous (TRUE)" and "Epiquick" tests are available with Finn chambers preloaded with standard allergens in predetermined concentration. Table 6 depicts allergen panel included in commercially available "TRUE" test.

Table 6: TRUE test allergen panel.

Panel 1.1	Panel 2.1	Panel 3.1
Nickel sulfate	p-tert-butylphenol formaldehyde resin	Diazolidinyl urea
Wool alcohols	Epoxy resin	Imidazolidinyl urea
Neomycin	Carba mix	Budesonide (Rhinocort)
Potassium dichromate	Black rubber mix	Tixocortol-21-pivalate
Caine mix	Methylchloroisothiazolinone/methylisothiazolinone	Quinolone mix
Fragrance mix	Quaternium-15	
Colophony	Mercaptobenzothiazole	
Paraben mix	p-Phenylenediamine	
Negative control	Formaldehyde	
Balsam of Peru	Mercapto mix	
Ethylenediamine dihydrochloride	Thimerosal	
Cobalt dichloride	Thiuram mix	

(TRUE: thin-layer rapid-use epicutaneous)

Table 7: Allergens associated with early and late reactions.

Reactions	Allergens
Early (at 48 hours)	Balsam of Peru resin (*Myroxylon pereirae*), benzoyl peroxide, carba mix, cinnamic alcohol, cocamidopropyl betaine, fragrance mix, imidazolidinyl urea, thiuram mix, and wool alcohol
Maximum on day 5, resolved by day 7	Fragrance mix, methyldibromo glutaronitrile phenoxyethanol, octyl gallate, balsam of Peru, benzalkonium chloride, benzoic acid, and disperse blue
Late (days 6–7)	Dyes (paraphenylenediamine), medications (neomycin, caine mix, and topical steroids), metals (nickel sulfate, gold sodium thiosulfate, palladium chloride, potassium dichromate, and cobalt chloride), preservatives and glues (dodecyl gallate, p-tert-butylphenol formaldehyde resin, methylchloroisothiazolinone, epoxy resin, ethylenediamine dihydrochloride, mercapto mix, and thimerosal)

- Patches may be customized as per the requirement of allergens, to be tested, but the concentrations may vary, creating high possibility of false-positive or false-negative reactions.
- Reactions are read at least 20 minutes after patch removal.
- Test readings should be taken at day 2, day 4, and day 7 completion after application of patch. Allergens associated with early and late reactions are enumerated in Table 7.
- *Reading and interpretation*:
  - Always correlate patch test results with clinical symptomatology.
  - International Contact Dermatitis Research Group has issued recommendations for scoring the patch test reactions (Table 8).
- *Photopatch testing*:
  - After a routine patch testing (in duplicate at two sites simultaneously), one side is irradiated with ultraviolet A (UVA) (with 5 J/cm^2) and readings are compared 48 hours later.

Table 8: Patch test reaction scoring.

Symbol	Morphology	Interpretation
-	No reaction	Negative
?	Erythema only and no infiltration	Doubtful reaction
+	Erythema, infiltration, and possibly discrete papules	Weak-positive reaction
++	Erythema, infiltration, papules, and vesicles	Strong-positive reaction
+++	Erythema, infiltration, and confluent vesicles	Extreme-positive reaction
ir	Different types of reactions (soap effects, vesicles, blister, and necrosis)	Irritant reaction
nt		Not tested

- *Open-patch testing*:
  - It is commonly used where skin manifestations are not clearly demarcated to one type of hypersensitivity. Contact urticaria, protein CD, and other potential irritants or sensitizers are assessed. It is usually performed on forearm, upper outer arm or scapular areas. Application site is regularly assessed for the initial 30-60 minutes (for immediate hypersensitivity) and at 3-4 days post-application (for delayed hypersensitivity). Tested irritant may be reapplied periodically to check for combination effect.

COMMON CAUSES

- *Metals*:
  - Nickel—most common cause as commonly found in jewellery
  - Chromate—common occupational contact allergen, found in cement and affect construction workers. Other potential sources could be leather, bleaching agents, paints and printing solutions
  - Cobalt.

- *Cosmetics and skin care products*:
    - Perfumes are the most common culprits
    - Nail polish, nail polish remover, and other nail care products
    - Preservatives, active or category-specific ingredients, excipients, emulsifiers, and sunscreens.
- *Clothes and shoes*:
    - Lesions are commonly located in axilla due to allergen release from the textiles after coming in contact with sweat and friction
    - Chrome, adhesives (paratertiary butylphenol formaldehyde resin) and resin in leather articles.
- *Drugs*:
    - Local antibiotics, antiseptics, and anesthetics
    - Due to topical drug, by the vehicle or by a preservative.
- *Plants*:
    - Family Liliaceae, Alstroemeriaceae, and Compositae
    - Urushiol is the most common cause of allergic CD, which is present in poison ivy and poison oak. Among exposed persons, 70% become sensitized.
- *Natural rubber latex (NRL)*:
    - May cause type I hypersensitivity, irritant or allergic CD
    - For type I hypersensitivity, skin prick test may be useful
    - For irritant or allergic CD, use test or patch test may be done. Use test involves application of a glove that has been soaked for 20 minutes in water or saline and monitoring for reactions to happen.

MANAGEMENT

- *Avoidance*:
    - Culprit allergens and irritants needs to be avoided as much as possible
    - Personal protective equipment (gloves, masks, goggles, and cap) help in limiting occupational exposure

- Rubber or polyvinyl chloride household gloves, with an inner cotton liner may be useful. A glove may be protective for limited time only
- Occupation change as last resort.
- *Protection*:
  - Using gloves in hand dermatitis—rubber or polyvinylchloride gloves with cotton lining are recommended for general household work
  - Barrier creams—efficacy less certain
  - pH optimization—healthy skin has an acidic pH between 4.6 and 5.6. Alkaline pH caused by repeated exposure of soap, bleach, solvents, and tap water disrupts the epidermal barrier and predisposes toward irritant CD. Either hyperacidification or hydrophobic skin-protectant products could be potentially helpful in preventing from alkaline shift.
- *Substitution*:
  - Replace soaps and detergents with emollients
  - Using thiuram-free gloves, isothiazolinone-free creams/cleansers in allergic patients.
- *Treatment*:
  - First line—topical steroids and topical tacrolimus; systemic steroids may be required for a short-term in widespread systemic distribution
  - Second line—phototherapy and systemic immunomodulators like methotrexate and mycophenolate mofetil
  - Third line—psoralen plus UVA, cyclosporine and alitretinoin in chronic hand dermatitis, and azathioprine in chronic actinic dermatitis
  - Supportive—cool compresses, calamine lotion, colloidal oatmeal bath, antihistaminics, antibiotics, and moisturizers.
- Hyposensitization—oral hyposensitization to urushiol and nickel has been tried in research projects.
- Immunomodulators—macrolactams have been tried in certain centers in CD.

- *Education*:
  - Regular education programs, both for healthcare providers and patients, should be planned.

PREVENTION

- Avoid scratching the eczematous area
- Avoid all triggering agents
- Wash skin immediately with soap and water if exposed to a triggering substance
- Use sunscreen [without para-aminobenzoic acid (PABA)]
- Wear gloves, long sleeves, pants, and boots while working outdoors
- Use fragrance-free products
- Cover nickel containing objects with clear nail polish
- Use barrier cream to block certain allergens like poison ivy.

PROGNOSIS

- 25% of all occupational CD completely heal over 10-year period after adequate avoidance and treatment measures
- 50% patients have partial response and remaining 25% do not respond
- Long-term prognosis for occupational CD is poor
- Poor prognosis depends upon severity and extent of dermatitis at presentation
- Dermatological allergies are quite common. An algorithmic approch, appropriate diagnosis and targeted management is the key to success.

SUGGESTED READING

1. Cicardi M, Aberer W, Banerji A, et al. Classification, diagnosis, and approach to treatment for angioedema: consensus report from the Hereditary Angioedema International Working Group. Allergy. 2014;69(5):602-16.
2. Eberting CL, Blickenstaff N, Goldenberg A. Pathophysiologic treatment approach to irritant contact dermatitis. Curr Treat Options Allergy. 2014;1:317-28.

3. Eichenfield LF, Boguniewicz M, Simpson EL, et al. Translating atopic dermatitis management guidelines into practice for primary care providers. Pediatrics. 2015;136(3):554-65.
4. Ferrante G, Scavone V, Muscia MC, et al. The care pathway for children with urticaria, angioedema, mastocytosis. World Allergy Organ J. 2015;8(1):5.
5. Fonacier L, Bernstein DI, Pacheco K, et al. Contact dermatitis: A practice parameter—update 2015. J Allergy Clin Immunol Pract. 2015;3:S1-39.
6. Galli E, Neri I, Ricci G, et al. consensus conference on clinical management of pediatric atopic dermatitis. Ital J Pediatr. 2016;42:26.
7. Johnston GA, Exton LS, Mohd Mustapa MF, et al. British Association of Dermatologists' guidelines for the management of contact dermatitis 2017. Brit J Dermatol. 2017;176:317-29.
8. Kanani A, Betschel SD, Warrington R. Urticaria and angioedema. Allergy Asthma Clin Immunol. 2018;14:59.
9. Lyons JJ, Milner JD, Stone KD. Atopic dermatitis in children: clinical features, pathophysiology and treatment. Immunol Allergy Clin North Am. 2015;35(1):161-83.
10. Machado Martins LE, dos Reis VM. Immunopathology of allergic contact dermatitis. An Bras Dermatol. 2011;86(3):419-33.
11. Nosbaum A, Vocanson M, Rozieres A, et al. Allergic and irritant contact dermatitis. Eur J Dermatol. 2009;19(4):1-8.
12. Saint-Mezard P, Rosieres A, Krasteva M, et al. Allergic contact dermatitis. Eur J Dermatol. 2004;14:284-95.
13. Sánchez-Borges M, Asero R, Ansotegui IJ, et al. Diagnosis and treatment of urticaria and angioedema: a worldwide perspective. World Allergy Organ J. 2012;5(11):125-47.
14. Sayaseng KY, Vernon P. Pathophysiology and management of mild to moderate pediatric atopic dermatitis. J Pediatr Health Care. 2018;32(2):S2-12.
15. Silverberg NB. A practical overview of pediatric atopic dermatitis, part 1: epidemiology and pathogenesis. Cutis. 2016;97(4):267-71.

Other Allyergies

8.1 ALLERGIC CONJUNCTIVITIS

INTRODUCTION

Allergic diseases of eye are very common and the incidence has dramatically increased over the past few decades both in developed and developing countries. Many factors, such as changing genetics, rising air pollution, intrusion of pets in homes, and early childhood exposure to various allergens are the key contributors to rising eye allergies.

Allergic conjunctivitis could be seasonal, perennial, vernal and atopic keratoconjunctivitis. Giant papillary conjunctivitis (GPC), a non-allergic form is also commonly found, and is due to minor trauma through contact lenses and ocular prosthesis.

TYPES OF ALLERGIC CONJUNCTIVITIS

Seasonal and Perennial Allergic Conjunctivitis

- These are most common presentations for allergic conjunctivitis, especially in children, affecting 15–20% of the population at least once in their lifetime. Targeted allergens can be demonstrated mostly of the time in these clinical varieties. These are mediated by IgE-based mechanism (Type 1 hypersensitivity) within 20–30 minutes of allergen exposure. There is increased concentration of histamine, tryptase, prostaglandins, and leukotrienes in tears of affected individuals which is due to mast cell activation.
- Seasonal symptoms are caused by airborne pollens and mostly occur in the spring and summer time with high pollen concentration in the environment. Characteristic features of both seasonal and perennial variety are itching, redness, and conjunctival swelling (Fig. 1).

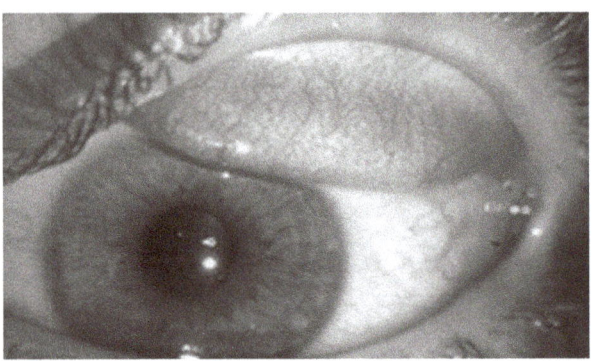

Fig. 1: Conjunctival swelling and chemosis in seasonal allergic conjunctivitis
(For color version, see Plate 18).
Source: Rosa ML, Lionetti E, Reibaldi M, et al. Allergic conjunctivitis: a comprehensive review of the literature. Ital J Pediatr. 2013;39:18.

Vernal Keratoconjunctivitis

- This type of conjunctival inflammation is more common in warm weather seasons. It is characterized by chronic allergic inflammation of the ocular surface with overexpression of mast cells, eosinophils, neutrophils, Th2-dervied cytokines, chemokines, adhesion molecules, growth factors, fibroblasts, and lymphocytes. The typical symptoms could be itching, photophobia, redness, swelling, and eye discharge. The characteristic sign is "cobblestone-like" swellings (Fig. 2) on upper tarsal conjunctiva. Trantas dots (Fig. 3) represent clumps of necrotic eosinophils, neutrophils, and epithelial cells and these dots appear during active stage of the disease.

Atopic Keratoconjunctivitis

- It is considered as eye counterpart of atopic dermatitis and leads to chronic inflammation of the eye surface and eyelid. Eyelid skin is usually chemotic with a sandpaper-like texture (Fig. 4). Conjunctival scarring with Trantas dots may be present. Patients may develop cataract in this variety of conjunctivitis.

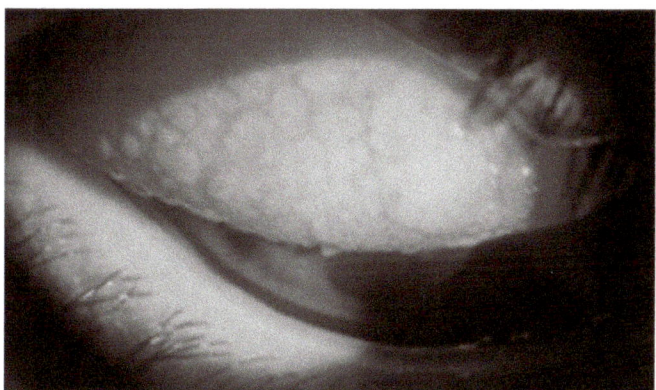

Fig. 2: Cobblestone-like appearance in vernal conjunctivitis *(For color version, see Plate 18).*

Source: Rosa ML, Lionetti E, Reibaldi M, et al. Allergic conjunctivitis: a comprehensive review of the literature. Ital J Pediatr. 2013;39:18.

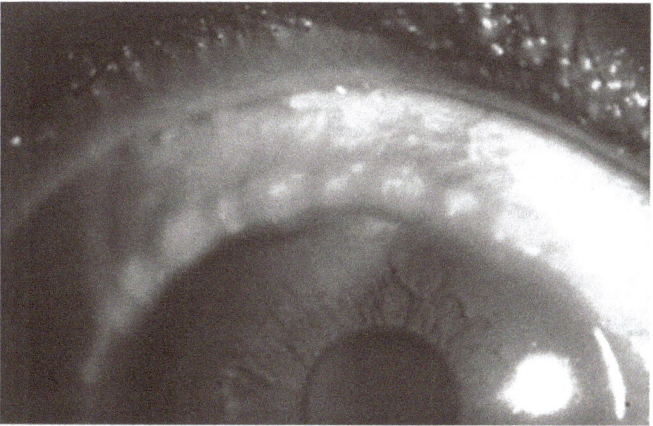

Fig. 3: Horner-Trantas dots *(For color version, see Plate 18).*

Source: Sanchez MC, Parra BF, Matheu V, et al. Allergic conjunctivitis. J Investig Allergol Clin Immunol. 2011;2:1-19.

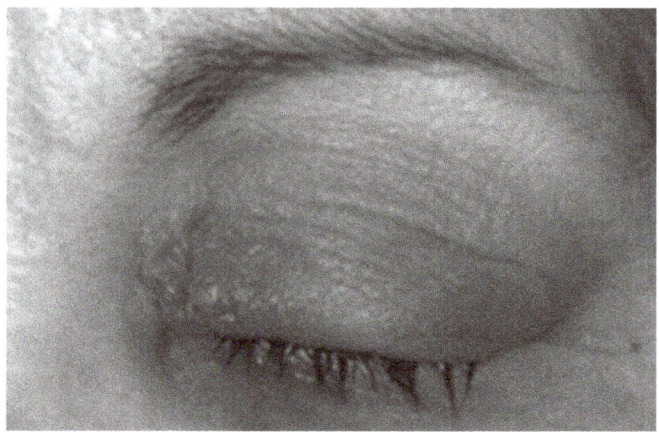

Fig. 4: Sandpaper-like texture of eyelid skin *(For color version, see Plate 18).*
Source: Rosa ML, Lionetti E, Reibaldi M, et al. Allergic conjunctivitis: a comprehensive review of the literature. Ital J Pediatr. 2013;39:18.

Contact Allergy

- It is a delayed type (type 4) hypersensitivity response through interaction of antigens with release of cytokines. These are usually incomplete which combine with skin proteins to make them complete allergens, e.g. poison ivy, poison oak, neomycin, nickel, latex, atropine and its derivatives. As it is delayed reaction, symptoms might peak by 2–5 days after the exposure.

DIAGNOSIS OF ALLERGIC CONJUNCTIVITIS

History and clinical examination are most important in making the diagnosis. Allergen identification may be helped by skin or serum-specific IgE testing. Conjunctival challenge test is rarely required to confirm the diagnosis. Differentials of ocular allergy are compared in Table 1.

Table 1: Differential diagnosis of ocular allergy.

	Seasonal allergic conjunctivitis	Perennial allergic conjunctivitis	Vernal keratoconjunctivitis	Atopic keratoconjunctivitis	Giant papillary conjunctivitis
Personal/family history of atopy	Common	Common	Possible	Constant	Possible
Age	Children/Adults	Children/Adults	Children	Adults	Adolescents/Adults
Gender	M = F	M = F	M > F	M > F	M = F
Seasonal	Spring	Perennial	Perennial/Summer	Perennial	Spring
Corneal involvement	No	No	Yes	Yes	No
Vision involvement	Minimal	Minimal	Mild	Severe	Minimal
Papillary hypertrophy	No	No	7–8 mm Limbus affected	<1 mm	>1 mm
Periocular skin involvement	Edema	Edema	Edema	Dermatitis	Edema
Exposure to topical drugs	No	No	No	No	No
Contact lens wearer	No	No	No	No	Yes
Serum IgE	Elevated	Elevated	Variable	Greatly elevated	Variable
Eosinophils in swab	Frequent	Very frequent	Characteristic	Characteristic	Not frequent
Goblet cells	Increased	Increased	Increased	Decreased	Variable
Skin tests	Positive	Positive	Nonspecific	Positive	Variable
Other atopic diseases	Rhinitis, asthma	Rhinitis, asthma	Variable	Dermatitis, asthma, rhinitis	Variable
Response to anti-allergic drugs	Good	Good	Low	Low	Variable
Response to topical steroids	Constant	Constant	Constant	Constant	Constant

TREATMENT

- Allergen avoidance—remains mainstay of the preventive steps.
- Cold compresses.
- Artificial tear drops or gel—act as barrier to inflamed conjunctiva.
- Antiallergics:
  - H_1 topical anti-histamines like levocabastine hydrochloride—require 6 hourly dosing and may cause local irritant effect.
  - Decongestants combined with H_1 anti-histaminies—help by local vasoconstriction and reducing inflammation; side effects are burning or eye stinging, rebound hyperemia or conjunctivitis medicamentosa.
  - Mast cell stabilizers—these can be used for prophylactic purpose.
  - Multi-model antiallergic agents—these exert multiple pharmacological actions like histamine receptor antagonism, mast cell stabilization, and suppression of eosinophil activation. Commonly available agents are olopatadine, ketotifen, azelastine, epinastine, and bepotastine.
  - Non-steroidal anti-inflammatory drug (NSAIDs)—these help in reduction of hyperemia and pruritus and have an adjunctive role.
  - Corticosteroids—most potent agents in patients with severe allergy as these exert immunosuppressive and antiproliferative effects. The notable adverse effects are delayed wound healing, secondary infection, elevated intraocular pressure, and formation of cataract.
- Allergen-specific immunotherapy—targeted immunotherapy is quite effective.

8.2 LATEX ALLERGY

INTRODUCTION

Natural rubber latex (NRL) is obtained from the sap of *Hevea brasiliensis* tree. After harvesting NRL, it undergoes various manufacturing processes (e.g. heat vulcanization and cross-linking with polyisoprene) to form either latex products or dry natural rubber. Latex products, those made by dipping method like gloves, condoms, balloons, and catheters are highly allergenic as sulfur heat vulcanization process is relatively short and performed at lower temperature, which is not enough to reduce latex allergenicity. Products made from crepe rubber (like shoe soles) are unlikely to cause allergic reaction. Protein content of dry natural rubber is low minimizing the allergic property; simultaneously additives like thiurams, carbamates, and mercaptobenzothiazole are responsible for contact dermatitis.

TYPES OF LATEX ALLERGY

Three types of clinical reactions can occur related to latex:
1. *IgE-mediated allergic reaction (Type I hypersensitivity)*: This is true latex allergy caused by NRL protein exposure in sensitive subjects. Exposure through skin, mucosal surface or inhalation could be among the possible routes. Symptoms can develop within 30 minutes to 2 hours of exposure. There could be generalized hives, angioedema, rhinitis, conjunctivitis, asthma or fatal anaphylaxis. The allergenic proteins in latex may be leached on the cornstarch powder in gloves, spread of which is responsible for respiratory exposure to patients and workers in the surrounding area.
2. *Contact dermatitis (Type IV hypersensitivity)*: It is usually due to multiple chemicals used during latex processing like thiuram, carbamate, and mercaptobenzothiazole. Clinical symptoms are usually localized to contact area mostly hands or feet. Symptoms usually take 24–48 hours to develop after contact. Erythematous rash, papules, vesicles, and oozing are characteristic features. Life-threatening manifestations are rare.
3. *Irritant dermatitis*: Nonimmune-mediated localized itch is the pathognomonic feature. It is usually caused by frequent skin washing, sweating and or irritation from powder lubricants during persistent contact.

TYPES OF LATEX ALLERGENS

Thirteen different types of allergens are known. The important allergens are characterized as:
- *Hev b 1* and *3*: Main allergen in spina bifida
- *Hev b 5* and *6*: Main allergen in healthcare workers
- *Hev b 2, 4, 7* and *13*: Secondary but relevant allergen in healthcare workers
- *Hev b 6.02* and *7*: Verified cross-reactivity with fruits
- *Hev b 8, 11* and *12*: Pan-allergens with unknown cross-reactivity with fruits.

WHO ARE AT RISK OF DEVELOPING LATEX ALLERGY?

- Healthcare workers including dental practice staff
- Carers such as residential care home staff
- Cleaners and housekeepers
- Hairdressers
- Caterers who wear gloves at work
- Motor mechanics
- People working in the electrical industry
- Balloon entertainers
- Patients who had a number of operations, e.g. spina bifida
- People with certain food allergies like banana, avocado, tomato, potato, kiwi, and chestnut.

PREVALENCE OF LATEX ALLERGY AMONG VARIOUS RISK GROUPS

- Patients with spina bifida: 20–70%
- Healthcare professionals: 10–15%
- Other professionals exposed to latex: 10–12%
- Individuals with history of atopy and latex exposure: 36%
- General population with history of atopy: 8–17%
- General population without history of atopy: 1–6%.

CLINICAL MANIFESTATIONS

- *Contact urticaria*: The most common manifestation after latex protein exposure is recurrent acute attacks of chronic eczema. Xeroderma could be nonspecific irritant symptom. NRL is most common cause of contact urticaria.
- *Angioedema*.
- *Allergic rhinitis and asthma*: These occur via exposure of NRL through inhalational route and commonly found in those individuals who are frequently exposed to latex environment like healthcare professionals. Latex contributes to 2.5–10% of all the cases of occupational asthma.
- *Systemic reactions*: Latex is second most common cause of intraoperative anaphylaxis after muscle relaxants. 27% of anaphylactic reactions following anesthesia in children are attributed to latex with higher incidence in younger age group. Latex reaction occurs during the maintenance phase of anesthesia, while muscle relaxants and opiates cause problems during induction phase, in sensitized individual. Latex proteins can also be transferred through food handling with gloved hands in the industry.
- *Latex-fruit syndrome*: The reaction is due to cross-reactivity between latex proteins and certain foods. About 50% of NRL allergic subjects demonstrate cross-reactivity to one or more fruits, whereas 10% of fruit allergic individuals may cross-react to NRL. Table 2 enumerates various food items with different levels of cross-reactivity.

Table 2: Degree of association of fruits with latex allergy.

Degree of Association	Fruits or food items with cross-reactivity to latex allergen
High	Banana, Avocado, Chestnut, Kiwi
Moderate	Apple, Carrot, Celery, Papaya, Potato, Tomato, Melons
Low or undetermined	Pear, Peach, Plum, Cherry, Pineapple, Strawberry, Fig, Grape, Apricot, Passion fruit, Nectarine, Mango, Rye, Wheat, Hazelnut, Walnut, Soybean, Peanut, Buckwheat, Dill, Oregano, Sage, Sweet pepper, Cayenne pepper, Shellfish, Sunflower seed, Citrus fruits, Coconut, Chick pea, Lychee, Zucchini, Persimmon

DIAGNOSIS OF LATEX ALLERGY

A good history focusing on presence of other allergies, atopy, previous operations, medical procedures, belonging to high-risk group, latex product exposure, and reactions to certain fruits (kiwi, chestnut, avocado and banana) should be enquired. Clinical findings may be supplemented by in vitro (specific IgE) or in vivo (skin prick or patch test). Flowchart 1 demonstrates the working algorithm for latex allergy management.

- Skin tests:
    - Prick tests: These have sensitivity of 93% and specificity of 100% for type 1 latex hypersensitivity.

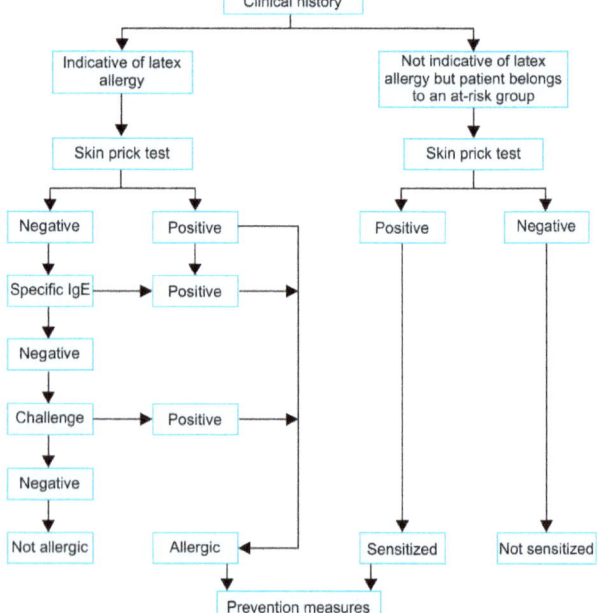

Flowchart 1: Diagnostic algorithm for latex allergy.

Source: Cabanes N, Igea JM, de la Hoz B. Latex allergy: position paper. J Investig Allergol Clin Immunol. 2012;22(5):313-30.

- Patch tests: These are useful for detecting type 4 hypersensitivity reactions to latex additives like mercaptobenzothiazole, N-1-paraphenylenediamine, and mixture of substances (carba mix, para-phenylenediamine mix, and thiuram mix).
- Serum-specific IgE: The sensitivity and specificity vary between 97–100% and 33–83%, respectively.
- Flow cytometry: Though with a sensitivity of 93% and specificity of 91.7%, this technique is not used widely, due to higher cost.
- Challenge test: These are indicated in situations where clinical history is non-coherent with laboratory tests.
- Rubbing test: Diagnostic yield is very low due to high rate of false positivity and non-standardized allergen extract.
- Glove use test: Appearance of erythema, pruritus, and blisters or respiratory symptoms are considered as positive test result:
  - Step 1: Place the fingertip of glove over the dampened finger for 15 minutes to 2 hours. Proceed to step 2 if test results are negative.
  - Step 2: Complete powdered glove is put on one hand with a vinyl or nitrile glove on other hand as control.
  - Limitations: Difficulty in blinding favors the false-positive results. False-negative results may be documented in patients who have avoided latex for a long time.
- Specific bronchial challenge test: Aqueous latex extract (with a nebulizer or in a chamber with aerosolized glove extract) or dust aerosol generated by shaking gloves may be used for challenge tests. These tests have limited practical value.

Diagnosis of Food Allergies Associated with Latex Allergies

Prick-prick test (skin prick test using the fresh fruits) with relevant fruits in patients with latex allergy have 80% sensitivity. Flowchart 2 simplifies the diagnostic algorithm.

Flowchart 2: Diagnosis and treatment of latex-fruit allergy syndrome.

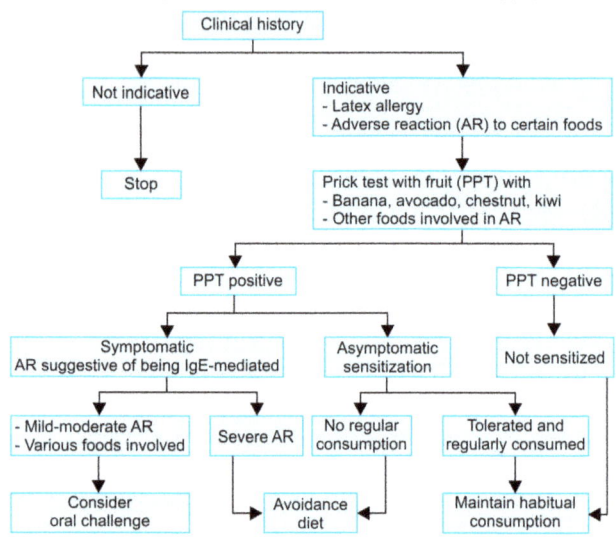

(PPT: prick-prick test with fresh fruit)

Source: Cabanes N, Igea JM, de la Hoz B. Latex allergy: position paper. J Investig Allergol Clin Immunol. 2012;22(5):313-30.

TREATMENT

- Symptomatic treatment.
- Specific immunotherapy: As per the available limited literature, with parenteral and sublingual route, immunotherapy is not widely recommended for latex allergy.
- Patient education:
  – Avoid latex-containing products
  – Using alternative products like gloves though alternative material might jeopardize user safety. Table 3 enumerates many characteristics of different types of available gloves
  – Wear a medical identification bracelet: This might be helpful in emergency cases for making aware the rescuer about your allergic status

Table 3: Characteristics of different varieties of gloves.

	Latex	Nitrile	Neoprene	Vinyl
Resistance	5	5	5	1
Biological protection	5	5	5	2
Chemical protection	4	5	5	1
Elasticity	5	3	4	1
Comfort	5	2	4	3
Sensitivity	5	2	4	3
Price	3	2	1	5

5—maximum score (in price, the cheapest); 1—minimum score (in price, the most expensive)

Source: Cabanes N, Igea JM, de la Hoz B. Latex allergy: position paper. J Investig Allergol Clin Immunol. 2012;22(5):313-30.

- Avoid high-risk fruits (*see* Table 2)
- Avoid food which is prepared or served by food handlers wearing latex gloves
- Avoid occupations like nursing, dentistry, surgeon, hairdressing or food preparation.

- Prevention:
  - Labeling: Correct labeling of all latex products is warranted
  - Primary prevention:
    - Preventive steps should be taken in children with high risk, e.g. spina bifida
    - Correct and rational use of latex gloves is recommended in healthcare settings and dentist's offices
    - Use of unpowered gloves and those with low protein content need to be promoted.
  - Secondary prevention:
    - In sensitized and allergic individuals—avoidance is the most appropriate step
    - Use latex-free gloves like nitrile gloves

- Avoid items with latex:
  - Everyday items: Erasers, rubber bands, rubber balloons, condoms, contraceptive cap, hot water bottles, latex pillows, baby teats/dummies, stress balls, washing-up gloves, carpets, adhesives including hair glue, underwear elastic, sports equipment (basketballs, hand grips and gym mats), swimming cap and goggles, calculator, and remote control buttons.
  - Medical equipment: Examination and surgical gloves, oral and nasal airways, endotracheal tubes, intravenous tubing, surgical masks, rubber aprons, injection ports, wound drains catheters, bungs and needle sheaths on medicines, dental dams, anesthesia masks, syringes, blood pressure cuffs, stethoscopes, tourniquets, electrode pads, surgical masks, and consumer items.
- Preparation of surgical theater and preoperative period:
  - Procedure or surgery should be scheduled first thing in the morning when the latex allergen in the air is minimum.
  - Remove all products containing latex from the operating room, a day before surgery.
  - Cleaning staff should not wear latex gloves.
  - The surfaces should be cleaned again on the day of surgery to remove any suspended allergen.
  - The mattress should be protected with double bed sheet.
  - Cover all monitoring devices, cables/tubes (oximeter, blood pressure, electrocardiogram) to avoid direct contact with the skin.
  - Products sterilized in ethylene oxide must be rinsed before use. Residual ethylene oxide may cause allergic reaction in a latex-sensitive patient.

Box 1: Contents of cart in operating room with latex-free supplies.

- Latex-free procedure and surgical gloves
- Bandages and dressings
- Glass syringes
- Ampoules
- Disposable pressure cuff
- Stethoscope
- Oxygen mask and nebulizer with gender tape for adjustment
- Ventilation system
- Neoprene bags
- Plastic masks
- Ambu bag
- Endotracheal tube of polyvinyl chloride (PVC) without sleeve
- Bracelets for patient identification
- Poster to identify the operating room
- Epinephrine injection kit

Source: Vargas A, Foncea C, Astorga P. Latex allergy: overview and recomendations for the perioperative management of high-risk patients. J Head Neck Spine Surg. 2017;1(1):555552.

- A cart with latex-free supplies (Box 1) should be available inside the operating room.
- Operating room should be equipped to handle any anaphylactic reaction.
- Arm should be covered with cotton mesh before applying blood pressure cuff or stethoscope.
- Elastic cap and gender boot should be worn by the patient.
- Intraoperative preparation:
  - Surgical and nursing team should wear latex-free gloves.
  - Minimize the traffic inside operating room.
  - Latex-free or glass syringes should be used.
  - Medications should be preferred in glass ampoules. If glass ampoules are not available, remove the rubber stoppers rather than piercing them before medicine preparation.
  - Medications should be prepared immediately prior to their administration.

- Postoperative period:
  - Room and medication preparation should be same as that of intraoperative period.

UNRESOLVED ISSUES

- Deeper understanding of latex allergy progression in general population needs to be explored.
- Varied response to different latex proteins needs to be interpreted.
- Clinical efficacy of preventive steps needs to be determined.
- Role of genetic polymorphisms associated with latex allergy should be evaluated.
- Whether latex eradication leads to allergy cure in an individual needs to be answered.
- Role of specific immunotherapy needs to be investigated in the latex allergy.

8.3 ADVERSE DRUG REACTIONS

INTRODUCTION

Any noxious, unintended, undesired, and abnormal effect after ingestion/application/administration of a particular drug is labeled as adverse drug reaction (ADR). ADRs can happen at therapeutic or preventive doses. As per the recent estimates, 15.1% of the patients sustained ADRs during their hospitalization and 6.7% of patients experienced serious reactions.

TYPES OF ADVERSE DRUG REACTIONS

- *Type A*: Predictable reactions occurring in most normal patients, given sufficient dose and duration of therapy (Table 4). These are quite common and are related to the known pharmacologic actions of the drug (e.g. side effects, overdose, and drug interactions). These reactions account for 75–80% of all ADRs.

Table 4: Type A drug reactions.

Drug reaction	Examples
Overdose	• Hepatic failure (Acetaminophen) • Metabolic acidosis (Aspirin)
Side effects	• Nausea, headache (Methylxanthines) • Oral thrush or vaginal candidiasis (Glucocorticoids) • Nephrotoxicity (Aminoglycosides)
Secondary or indirect effects	• Diarrhea due to alteration in gastrointestinal bacteria after antibiotics • Phototoxicity (Doxycycline or Thiazide diuretics)
Drug interactions	• Macrolide antibiotics increasing theophylline, digoxin, or statin blood levels

Table 5: Type B drug reactions.

Drug reactions	Examples
Intolerance*	• Tinnitus after Aspirin intake
Idiosyncrasy**	• In G6PD deficiency: Antioxidant drugs (e.g. Dapsone, Chloroquine) cause hemolytic anemia • In TMPT deficiency: Toxicity during azathioprine therapy • Pseudoallergic reaction—with NSAIDs
Immunologic drug reactions*** (Drug Allergy)	• Anaphylaxis: β-lactam antibiotics • Photo-allergy: Quinidine • Immune-mediated thrombocytopenia: Heparin • Serum sickness: Antivenom preparation • Vasculitis: Phenytoin • Stevens-Johnsons syndrome: Trimethoprim-sulfamethoxazole • Drug-induced hypersensitivity syndrome: Allopurinol in HLA-B58:01 individuals

(G6PD: glucose-6-phosphate dehydrogenase; NSAIDs: nonsteroidal anti-inflammatory drugs; TPMT: thiopurine methyltransferase)
*Side effects at subtherapeutic doses.
**Drug effect not attributable to known pharmacologic properties of drug and not immune-mediated, usually caused by abnormalities of metabolism, excretion or bioavailability.
***Including various IgE and non-IgE mediated immunologic phenomenon (Table 6).

- *Type B*: Drug hypersensitivity reactions restricted to a small subset of the general population (Table 5), accounting to 20–25% of the patients with ADRs. The reactions are rare, unpredictable,

Table 6: Immunologic drug reactions.

Type of immunologic drug reaction	Incidence	Signs and symptoms	Timing	Common culprit drugs	Diagnostic testing available?
IgE, mast cell and basophil mediated Type I Gell and Coomb	Common	Urticaria, angioedema, bronchospasm, laryngeal edema, nausea, vomiting, hypotension, shock	Immediate—seconds to two hours after last dose. Faster and more severe upon re-exposure	β-lactam antibiotics (penicillins and cephalosporins), muscle relaxants, foreign proteins (e.g. rituximab), platinum-based chemotherapy (e.g. cisplatin)	Immediate—serum tryptase levels. Later—skin prick test and intradermal testing
Antibody-mediated (IgG and IgM) cell destruction Type II Gell and Coombs	Uncommon	Hemolytic anemia, thrombocytopenia, neutropenia or agranulocytosis	Delayed—days to weeks after beginning therapy, faster upon re-exposure	β-lactam antibiotics, NSAIDs, quinidine, methyldopa, ticlopidine	Direct Coombs, tests for antiplatelet antibodies, tests for antineutrophil antibodies
Immune complex-mediated tissue damage Type III Gell and Coombs	Uncommon	Serum sickness, serum sickness-like reactions, vasculitis, drug fever, acute glomerulonephritis	Delayed—weeks to months after beginning therapy. Faster on re-exposure	β-lactam antibiotics, sulfonamide antibiotics, sirolimus/ tacrolimus	No direct test available. Patterns of clinical or laboratory findings and biopsy may be helpful
T-cell mediated Type IV Gell and Coombs	Common	Prominent skin findings ± other organ involvement – Exanthematous eruption, DRESS/DiHS, AGEP	Delayed at least 24–48 hours or even weeks after beginning therapy	β-lactam antibiotics, sulfonamide antibiotics and sulfasalazine, minocycline, phenytoin, carbamazepine, lamotrigine, allopurinol, nevirapine	Variable. In-vitro lymphocyte activation test for DRESS syndrome
Unclassified		Drug-induced lupus, Fixed drug eruption			Patch testing may be useful

(AGEP: acute generalized exanthematous pustulosis; DRESS/DiHS: drug rash with eosinophilia and systemic symptoms/drug-induced hypersensitivity syndrome; IgE: immunoglobulin E; IgG: immunoglobulin G; IgM: immunoglobulin M; NSAIDs: nonsteroidal anti-inflammatory drugs)

Table 7: Pseudoallergic drug reactions.

Drug	Clinical reaction	Presumed mechanism
Aspirin and other nonsteroidal anti-inflammatory drugs	Exacerbations of rhinitis, asthma (in patients with Aspirin-exacerbated respiratory disease), urticaria, angioedema	Inhibited prostaglandin production and enhanced leukotriene production
Opiates	Pruritus, urticaria	Direct stimulation of mast cells and/or basophils causing release of mediators
Vancomycin	Flushing during infusion	Direct stimulation of mast cells and/or basophils causing release of mediators
Radiocontrast media	Anaphylaxis, shock	Unknown mechanism
Ciprofloxacin	Urticaria	Direct stimulation of mast cells and/or basophils causing release of mediators
Local anesthetics	Syncope	Vasovagal reflex
Protamine	Hypotension, pulmonary hypertension	Unknown mechanism
Choline	Pruritus, urticaria	Unknown mechanism
Isoniazid	Hepatitis	Unknown mechanism

dose independent, unrelated to pharmacologic actions, and occur only in susceptible individuals.
- *Pseudoallergic (anaphylactoid) reactions*: These are due to direct release of mediators from mast cells and basophils (Table 7).

RISK FACTORS FOR ALLERGIC REACTIONS TO DRUG/S
- Age—more in young and middle-aged adults
- Gender—females are more predisposed
- Genetic polymorphisms in human leukocyte antigen (HLA)
- Viral infections—human immunodeficiency virus (HIV), herpes virus, and Epstein-Barr virus (EBV) increase the risk of drug reactions by certain immunologic mechanisms

- Drug-related factors—pharmacodynamics and pharmacokinetics of a drug affect host predisposition for drug allergies:
  - Topical, intramuscular, and intravenous routes have high risk than oral route
  - Prolonged high doses or frequent doses are riskier than large single dose
  - High molecular weight compounds and hapten-forming drugs are more immunogenic.

SIGNS AND SYMPTOMS OF IMMEDIATE ALLERGIES TO DRUGS

- Skin—warmth, flushing, itching, urticaria, and angioedema
- Eyes, ears, nose—eye or nose itching, tearing, conjunctival injection and/or edema, periorbital edema, rhinorrhea, nasal congestion, and sneezing
- Mouth—itching or tingling of lips, tongue or oral mucosa, metallic taste, angioedema of lips, and tongue or uvula
- Throat—itching, sense of constriction or swelling in throat, change in voice quality, hoarseness, difficulty swallowing, drooling, and stridor
- Lungs—shortness of breath, chest tightness, repetitive cough, wheezing, and drop in oxygen saturation or cyanosis
- Cardiovascular—light headedness, faintness, dizziness, tachycardia, syncope, palpitation, tunnel vision, hypotension, and cardiac arrest
- Gastrointestinal—nausea, vomiting, abdominal pain, and diarrhea
- Gynecologic—vaginal itching, uterine cramps, and bleeding
- Neurologic—anxiety, sense of impending doom, altered mental status, and seizures.

DIFFERENTIAL DIAGNOSIS OF DRUG ALLERGY

- IgE-mediated drug allergy—urticaria, angioedema, anaphylaxis, and bronchospasm:
  - Carcinoid syndrome

- Insect bites/stings
- Mastocytosis
- Asthma
- Food allergy
- Scombroid fish poisoning
- Latex allergy
- Infections (EBV, hepatitis A, B, C, and gastrointestinal parasites).
- Non-IgE-mediated reactions—exanthema, drug rash with eosinophilia and systemic signs (DRESS), Stevens-Johnson syndrome (SJS), and toxic epidermal necrolysis (TEN):
  - Acute graft-versus-host disease
  - Kawasaki disease
  - Still's disease
  - Psoriasis
  - Insect bites/stings
  - Viral infection
  - Streptococcal infection.

APPROACH TO A PATIENT WITH SUSPECTED DRUG ALLERGY

- *History*:
  - Is the presentation consistent with drug hypersensitivity?
  - Are the signs and symptoms suggestive of an immunologic response (i.e. drug allergy)?
  - Is the drug to which the patient was recently exposed known to cause such symptoms, or does it usually cause pseudo-allergic reactions, e.g. NSAIDs?
  - What were the symptoms and signs?
  - How severe is the reaction and what organ systems are involved?
  - How long ago did the reaction took place?
  - Did the patient require medical treatment or hospitalization because of the reaction?
  - Why was the medication taken?

- The dose and route of medication taken.
- Had the patient taken the medication on a previous occasion?
- Was the patient taking other concurrent medications when the reaction occurred?
- Were any of these newly started?
- The timing of onset of the reaction (from initiation of the drug).
- Any treatment given and response to that treatment (including duration of reaction).
- Has the patient received that medication or a related medication again since the reaction? If so, were there recurrent symptoms?
- Any prior or subsequent history of exposure to other agents in that class, and presence or absence of any associated reactions.

- *Testing for immediate reactions*:
  - Markers of anaphylaxis: Serum tryptase levels should be collected between 15 minutes and 3 hours after symptom onset. Sample should be transported to the laboratory in a frozen state.
  - Skin testing for drug-specific IgE: This is done to evaluate type I allergic reactions. The suspected medication should not cause direct mast cell degranulation (opioids, quinolones, and vancomycin). Commonly tested drugs are β-lactam antibiotics, neuromuscular blockers, radio-contrast dyes, local anesthetics, thiobarbiturates, and monoclonal antibodies.
  - The negative predictive value of skin test with penicillin is very high (if tested for both major and minor antigens).
  - For rest of the antibiotics, negative result does not exclude allergy, as patient may be allergic to drug metabolite or metabolite/protein complexes.
  - In vitro tests: No proven role.

- *Testing for delayed reactions*:
    - Patch testing—may be useful in patients with maculopapular exanthem, acute generalized exanthematous pustulosis, DRESS, and flexural exanthema.
    - Intradermal testing with delayed readout—slightly more sensitive than patch testing. It should only be done if a commercially available injectable form of the drug is available.
    - In vitro testing: Lymphocyte transformation/activation tests and drug-induced cytotoxicity assays. These are still considered as research tools.
- *Graded challenge (Drug provocation test)*:
    - Appropriate for a patient who is *unlikely to be allergic* to a particular drug. These can be used to exclude the drug allergy with a very high negative predictive value.

MANAGEMENT

- *General measures*:
    - All suspected drugs must be stopped with immediate effect.
    - Anaphylactic reactions should be anticipated, diagnosed, and appropriately managed.
    - Patients should be taught regarding anaphylaxis recognition and self-administration of epinephrine.
- *Individual preventive measures*:
    - A list of drugs, to be avoided and to be given as an alternate, should be provided to the individuals.
    - Slow injection and pretreatment with glucocorticosteroids and H_1-antihistamines should be given as premedication for non-allergic reactions, whereas these might not be beneficial to prevent IgE-mediated drug allergy.
- *Drug desensitization*:
    - Classical desensitization is most successful for type I (IgE-mediated) hypersensitivity though variable success to several other types of immunologic and non-immunologic drug reactions has been witnessed.

- It should be considered when the offending drug is essential and when no suitable alternative is available, like:
    - Sulfonamides in HIV-infected patients
    - Quinolone in cystic fibrosis patients
    - Allergy to anti-tuberculosis drugs in tuberculosis
    - Allergy to tetanus vaccine
    - Hemochromatosis with allergy to deferoxamine
    - Aspirin and NSAID hypersensitivity in patients with cardiac, rheumatic disease or selected cohort of asthma.

ASPIRIN-EXACERBATED RESPIRATORY DISEASE

Diagnosis

- *Samter's triad*: Asthma, chronic rhinosinusitis with nasal polyposis.
- Acute exacerbation after ingestion of NSAID typically begins 30 minutes to 3 hours after ingestion. It could be dose related with severe symptoms after large dose ingestion. Urticaria and/or angioedema occur in 15% of Aspirin-exacerbated respiratory disease (AERD) patients.

Management

- Medications: Leukotriene-modifying agents (Montelukast, zafirlukast, zileuton)
- Surgery: Polypectomy
- Aspirin desensitization.

Aspirin Desensitization

Mechanism of action:
- Reduces the expression of leukotrienes.

Indications:
- Nasal polyposis that worsen or recur after surgery despite optimal medical management.
- Other conditions requiring daily use of NSAIDs.

Procedure:
- If sinus surgery/polypectomy is required, schedule desensitization 2–4 weeks after surgery.
- Obtain informed consent, baseline vital signs, and spirometry.
- Pre-medication: Montelukast in the morning on the day of planned desensitization—it reduces lower respiratory tract symptoms.
- Vital signs, FEV_1 (or peak flow), and clinical assessment prior to each dose and with symptoms.
- Treatment of reactions—antihistamines, salbutamol, and epinephrine (as and when required).
- Lower respiratory tract reaction—15% decrease in the FEV_1 from baseline FEV_1.
- After successful desensitization, start daily aspirin 650 mg twice daily.
- Subsequent desensitization is performed if Aspirin is missed for more than 48 hours (Table 8).
- Most patients take 2 days. One may adjust the dose and/or extend the dosing interval based on patient history and assessment.
- If reaction occurs, observe the patient for minimum 3 hours.
- When stabilized, repeat provoking dose; escalate if tolerated (Provoking dose is usually 81 mg).

Table 8: Suggested desensitization protocol.

Time	Aspirin dose
0 hours	20.25 mg
2 hours	40.5 mg
4 hours	81 mg
6 hours	162 mg
8 hours	325 mg

TAKE-HOME MESSAGES

- Drug allergy involves various immunologic mechanisms and can have varied symptomatology.
- Diagnosis depends on detailed history, skin testing, and graded challenges.
- Skin is the most frequently affected organ; however, multi-organ dysfunction may occur.
- Drug avoidance is the definite treatment.
- Drug tolerance/desensitization procedures may be considered if a particular drug cannot be avoided.

8.4 INSECT VENOM ALLERGY

INTRODUCTION

Stinging insects are an important yet under-recognized cause of hypersensitivity in humans. About 5–7.5% of the population is affected at least once in their lifetime with some form of systemic reaction due to insect sting. The incidence is much higher in beekeepers, up till 32%. The risk of anaphylaxis is higher in subsequent exposures with previous history of insect venom anaphylaxis. Fatal anaphylaxis due to insect venom accounts for 0.03–0.48 per million inhabitants per year and 20% of all anaphylaxis. The anaphylaxis risk is lower in children.

CLASSIFICATION OF STINGING INSECTS

Three families of Hymenoptera order of insects are mainly responsible for venom hypersensitivity (Flowchart 3):
1. Formicidae: Fire ants
2. Vespidae: Yellow jackets, hornets, and paper wasps
3. Apoidea: Honey bees and bumblebees.

IDENTIFICATION OF INSECTS

Most of the time, patients are unable to provide clues regarding the type of stinging insect, thus demanding the need for knowing demographic and individual insect characteristic (Fig. 5 and Table 9).

Flowchart 3: Taxonomic tree of stinging insects.

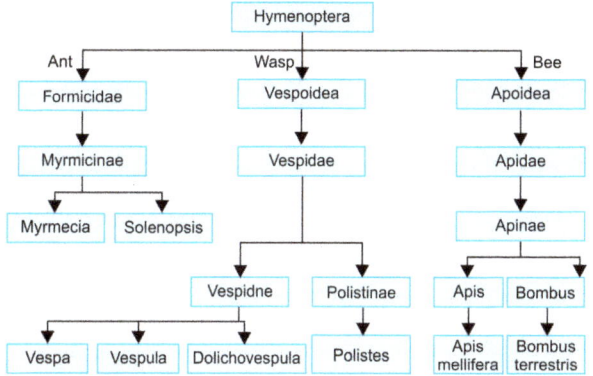

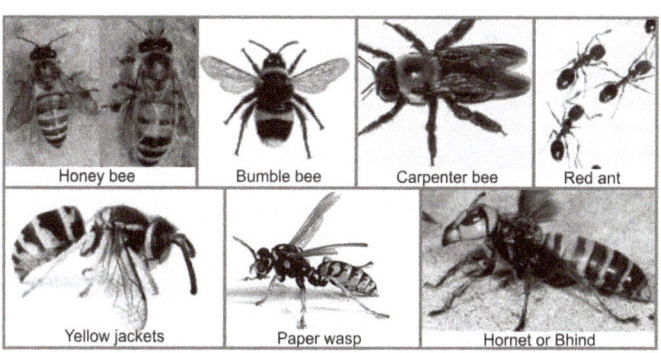

Fig. 5: Images of culprit insects *(For color version, see Plate 19).*
Source: Ludman SW, Boyle RJ Stinging insect allergy: current perspectives on venom immunotherapy. J Asthma Allergy. 2015;8:75-86.

RISK FACTORS FOR SEVERE REACTIONS

- Male sex
- Old age
- Raised baseline tryptase levels

Table 9: Habits and habitat of insects.

Common name	Typical number of adults in a nest	Solitary, but many can occur in the same area	Will sting in defense of the nest	Will not sting unless handled or pinched	Nest	Principal food
Honey bee	Thousands		✓		Wax coombs in hollow trees, building voids, or manmade hives	Pollen and honey made from nectar
Bumble bee	Dozens		✓		Wax pots in the ground or other cavities	Pollen and honey made from nectar
Carpenter bee	One	✓		✓	Tunnels in wood trim, fences and decks	Pollen and nectar
Yellow jackets	Hundreds to thousands		✓		Paper combs hidden by envelope and attached to vegetation or buildings	Insects, nectar, and ripe fruit
Paper wasps	Dozens		✓		A single, exposed paper comb with cells open at the bottom	Insects (often caterpillars), nectar
Hornet	Hundreds		✓		Brittle, brown combs, with or without envelop, in hollow trees or building voids	Insects (often bees and yellow jackets), ripe fruit, sap

- Patient on angiotensin-converting enzyme (ACE) inhibitors or beta blockers
- Physical exercise around sting time
- Eosinophilia
- Nonsteroidal anti-inflammatory drug ingestion.

APPROACH TO A PATIENT WITH INSECT HYPERSENSITIVITY

Flowchart 4 depicts a working algorithm for patients with insect hypersensitivity.

- *Box 1*: Specific detailed history and physical examination:
  - Small or large local reaction, systemic reaction, and anaphylaxis
  - Try to identify the responsible insect:
    - Patient's activity at the time of sting
    - Location of the person at the time of sting
    - Visual identification of the insect
    - Presence of a stinger (honey bees) or sterile pustule (imported fire ant sting).
- *Box 2*: Was there an anaphylaxis reaction?
  - Small local reaction—redness, swelling, itching, and pain
  - Large local reaction:
    - Increase in size for 24–48 hours
    - Swelling of more than 10 cm in diameter contiguous to the site of the sting
    - 3–10 days to resolve.
  - Systemic reaction or anaphylaxis.
- *Box 3, 3A, and 3B*: Was there a dermal reaction (cutaneous systemic or large local)?
  - Local pain and swelling—cold compresses, oral antihistamines, and analgesics.
  - Large local reactions—as above plus oral steroids, antibiotics if evidence of infection.
  - Special circumstances—relative risk of anaphylaxis, anticipated effect in quality of life.

Flowchart 4: Approach to a patient with insect hypersensitivity.

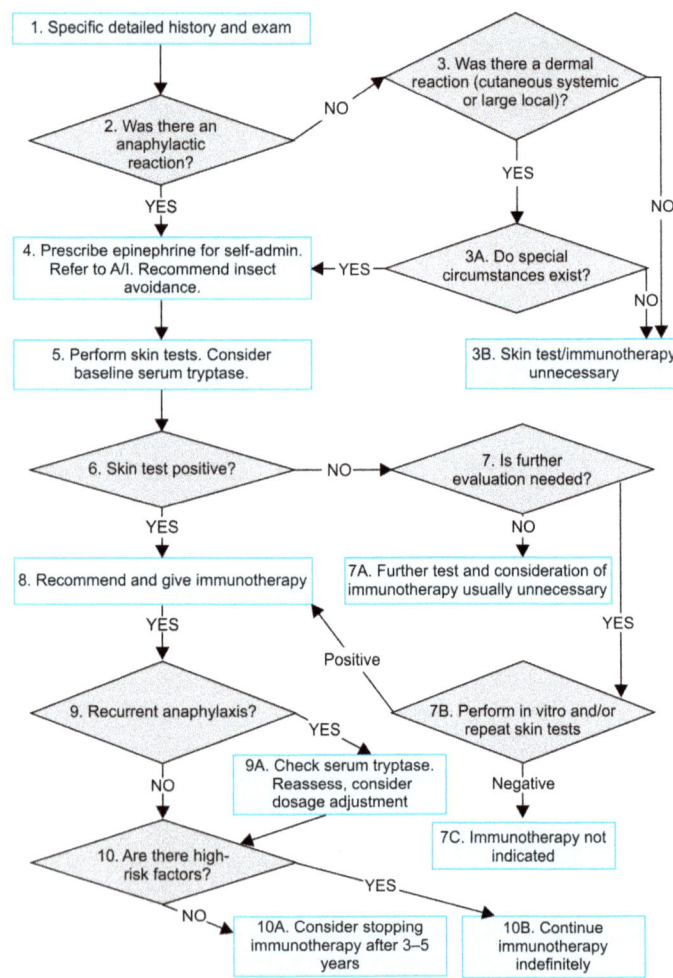

Source: BK Golden D, Demain J, Freeman T, et al. Stinging insect hypersensitivity. A practice parameter update 2016. Ann allergy asthma immunol. 2017;118:28-54.

- *Box 4*: Prescribe epinephrine for self-administration/refer to an allergist-immunologist/recommend insect avoidance:
  - Proper instruction about administration and use should be given.
  - Carry a medical identification—bracelet or necklace.
  - Measures for avoiding insect stings (Table 10).
- *Box 5*: Perform skin or in vitro testing and consider measuring basal serum tryptase:
  - Detection of all potentially relevant sensitivities requires testing with all the commercially available bee and vespid venoms and might include fire ant extracts when patient has exposure to fire ant stings.
  - Specific IgE sensitivity for insect venom is lower than skin prick testing.
  - Basal serum tryptase should be done in all patients who are candidates for venom immunotherapy (VIT)—an abnormal result is associated with severe anaphylaxis to

Table 10: Measures to avoid insect stings.

Effective measures	Ineffective measures
Avoid preparing, grilling, or eating outdoors	Avoiding fragrances
Avoid flowering plants	Avoiding brightly colored or floral clothing
Avoid drinking from straws, open cans or bottles outdoors	Using insect repellents
Remove fallen fruit or per feces	Running, flailing the arms
Cover trash cans	
Watch for nests in bushes or in the ground when mowing	
Avoid going outdoors barefoot	
When gardening, wear long sleeves, long pants and gloves. Tuck shirt into pants and pants into socks to prevent tick bites	

Source: BK Golden D, Demain J, Freeman T, et al. Stinging insect hypersensitivity. A practice parameter update 2016. Ann Allergy Asthma Immunol. 2017;118:28-54.

Table 11: Cross-reactivity of different insects for venom hypersensitivity testing.

	Honeybee	Yellow jacket (YJ)	Hornet	Wasp	Imported fire ant (IFA)
Honey bee	++++	+	+/-	-	-
YJ	+	++++	+++	++	+/-
Hornet	+/-	+++	++++	++	+/-
Wasp	-	++	++	++++	+/-
IFA	-	+/-	+/-	+/-	++++

Source: BK Golden D, Demain J, Freeman T, et al. Stinging insect hypersensitivity. A practice parameter update 2016. Ann Allergy Asthma Immunol. 2017;118:28-54.

stings, increased risk of systemic reactions during VIT, and greater risk of sting anaphylaxis after stopping VIT.

- *Box 6*: Positive skin or in vitro test response?
  - There is no absolute correlation between the skin reactivity or the level of venom-specific IgE and the severity of the reaction to a sting.
  - In vitro cross-reactivity of Hymenoptera venoms (Table 11).
- *Box 7, 7A, 7B, and 7C*: Is further evaluation needed?
  - Skin testing is most reliable and preferred diagnostic method.
  - If skin test negative, other tests may be warranted—serum-specific IgE, repeat skin tests, and basal serum tryptase levels.
- *Box 8*: Recommend and give VIT
  - Venom extracted from venom sacs is used commonly for VIT against wasps, hornets, jumper ants, and honey bees. Whole-body extract is used for VIT against fire ants.
  - Venom immunotherapy reduces the risk of systemic reactions in stinging insect-sensitive patients with an efficacy of up to 98%.
  - Goal of VIT is primarily to prevent life-threatening reactions.
  - Venom immunotherapy has also shown promising results in reduction of large local reactions.

- Venom immunotherapy injections are administered weekly, beginning with 0.1-1 µg and increasing to 100 µg of each venom (1 mL of venom extract—100 µg, 1 mL of mixed vespid venom—300 µg).
- The interval between maintenance dose injections—4 weekly during 1st year followed by 6-8 weekly.
- Contraindications of VIT are:
  - Malignancy
  - Severe asthma
  - Immunological conditions
  - Chronic heart and lung disease
  - Severe hypertension
  - Patient on β-blockers, tricyclic antidepressants, monoamine oxidase inhibitors, and ACE inhibitors
  - Pregnancy.
- *Box 9*: Recurrent anaphylaxis:
  - If anaphylaxis reoccurs due to same insect, for which the patient is on VIT, increase the injection dose to 200 µg.
  - If different or unknown insect—further testing warranted.
  - Measure basal serum tryptase levels as failure of VIT may be due to underlying mast cell disorders (Box 9A).
- *Box 10, 10A, and 10B*: Are there high-risk factors? Consider stopping VIT after 3-5 years:
  - Ideally, VIT should be continued indefinitely especially in high-risk patients.
  - Venom immunotherapy may be stopped after 3-5 years, a decrease in serum venom sIgE to insignificant levels or conversion to a negative skin test result.
  - Risk factors for relapse are:
    - Very severe reaction to previous stings
    - Elevated basal tryptase level
    - Systemic reaction during VIT
    - Less than 5 years of VIT
    - Honey bee anaphylaxis
    - Frequent exposure.

LONG-TERM MANAGEMENT FOLLOWING A SYSTEMIC VENOM ALLERGIC REACTION

High-risk activities should be reduced or supervised. Patients should be prescribed and demonstrated adrenaline auto-injectors use. Methods for sting removal should be taught and availability of anti-histamines, bronchodilators, and corticosteroids should be ensured.

UNANSWERED AREAS AND SCOPE FOR FUTURE RESEARCH

- Efficacy of sublingual immunotherapy
- Optimal duration of venom immunotherapy for prolonged treatment effect
- The role of sting challenge before or after immunotherapy and effect on quality of life
- Impact of venom immunotherapy in children and adolescents on quality of life
- Development of improved diagnostics for venom allergy.

SUGGESTED READING

1. Anaphylaxis Campaign. (2016). Latex Allergy Factsheet. [online]. Available from https://www.anaphylaxis.org.uk/wp-content/uploads/2016/08/Latex-2016-version-8-with-final-amendment-AS-comms-approval.pdf [Accessed December 2018].
2. Berger WE, Granet DB, Kabat AG. Diagnosis and management of allergic conjunctivitis in pediatric patients. Allergy Asthma Proc. 2017;38(1):16-27.
3. Bielory L, Meltzer EO, Nichols KK, et al. An algorithm for the management of allergic conjunctivitis. Allergy Asthma Proc. 2013;34:408-20.
4. BK Golden D, Demain J, Freeman T, et al. Stinging insect hypersensitivity. A practice parameter update 2016. Ann Allergy Asthma Immunol. 2017;118:28-54.
5. Cabanes N, Igea JM, de la Hoz B. Latex allergy: position paper. J Invetig Allergol Clin Immunol. 2012;22(5):313-30.
6. Demoly P, Adkinson NF, Castells M, et al. International Consensus (ICON) on Drug Allergy. Allergy. 2013.

7. Khan DA, Solensky R. Drug Allergy. J Allergy Clin Immunol. 2010;125: S126-37.
8. Ludman SW, Boyle RJ. Stinging insect allergy: current perspectives on venom immunotherapy. J Asthma and Allergy. 2015;8:75-86.
9. Rosa ML, Lionetti E, Reibaldi M, et al. Allergic conjunctivitis: a comprehensive review of the literature. Ital J Pediatr. 2013;39:18.
10. Sanchez MC, Parra BF, Matheu V, et al. Allergic conjunctivitis. J Investig Allergol Clin Immunol. 2011;2:1-19.
11. Solensky R. Drug Allergy: An updated practice parameter. Annals of Allergy, Asthma & Immunology. 2010;273:e1-78.
12. Vargas A, Foncea C, Astorga P. Latex allergy: Overview and recommendations for the perioperative management of high-risk patients. J Head Neck Spine Surg. 2017;1(1):1-6.
13. Warrington R, Silviu-Dan F. Drug allergy. Allergy Asthma Clin Immunol. 2011;7:S10.

Approach to an Allergic Patient

INTRODUCTION

The diagnosis of allergic disorders begins with a thorough clinical history and physical examination. A suggested history provides the clue for the possibility of allergy and responsible allergens, which directs for either in vivo skin testing or in vitro serological assays and/or provocation challenge tests as confirmatory measures for the detection of immunoglobulin E (IgE)-mediated reactions. Clinical history is the most important pointer and the derived information may be supplemented with the available allergy tests. Once the medical, family, and environmental histories identify a temporal association between allergic symptoms and allergen exposures, allergic disease may be suspected. Firm diagnosis requires confirmation by selected tests that are performed to verify the patient's production of specific IgE antibody.

MEDICAL HISTORY

The approach is similar to the standard medical history and should follow the local sequence of presenting complaints, history of presenting complaint, past medical history, drug history, social history, family history, and review of systems.

The hallmark symptoms of IgE-mediated reaction/s include sneezing, pruritis, urticaria, angioedema, bronchospasm, hypotension, tachycardia and rarely full-blown anaphylaxis. Some patients may experience nonspecific symptoms, such as nausea, vomiting, gastrointestinal disturbance and headache. Rarely myocardial infarction and seizure may occur in conjunction with anaphylaxis as a consequence of severe anaphylaxis. The severity of systemic reactions may be graded according to the

Table 1: Classification of the severity of immunoglobulin E-mediated allergic reaction (Mueller 1990).

Mueller grading	Clinical features
Grade I	Generalized urticaria, itching, malaise, anxiety
Grade II	Any of the above plus two or more of the following: angioedema, chest constriction, nausea, vomiting, diarrhea, abdominal pain, and dizziness
Grade III	Any of the above plus two or more of the following: dyspnea, wheezing, stridor, dysarthria, hoarseness, weakness, confusion, and feeling of impending disaster
Grade IV	Any of the above plus two or more of the following: fall in blood pressure, collapse, loss of consciousness, incontinence, and cyanosis

Source: Mueller UR. Clinical presentation and pathogenesis. In: Mueller UR, editor. Insect sting allergy. Stuggart: Gustav Fischer; 1990, p. 33-65.

Mueller classification (Table 1). IgE-mediated reactions are caused by mast cell degranulation and occur soon after (maximum up to 2 hours) allergen exposure. On the other hand, non-IgE-mediated reactions are usually delayed and seldom lead to anaphylaxis.

- *Urticaria*: It is well-demarcated, raised, and erythematous rash with a pale center and is often associated with intense itching. It may occur with or without angioedema. It may also be seen in a number of nonallergic disorders. According to the European Association of Allergology and Clinical Immunology (EAACI), urticaria can be categorized into acute (<6 weeks) or chronic (>6 weeks). Cholinergic urticaria, which is a type of physical urticaria, mainly occurs in the armpits, groins, and lower limbs. Eczematous and maculopapular rashes are often T-cell mediated and a photosensitive rash is suggestive of lupus and drug reaction, which should not be confused with urticaria.
- *Angioedema*: It is characterized by deep tissue swelling affecting the mucocutaneous junction. It is acute and nonpersistent but once established, angioedema may take up to several days to resolve. Facial and lip swellings, though vivid, do not have any life-threatening consequences whereas oropharyngeal swelling could compromise the airway and warrant the use of adrenaline.

Trigger of Symptoms

Establishing a link between a potential trigger and the patient's reactions is an essential part in the allergy history. One should try to identify whether the culprit allergen could consistently reproduce the symptoms within a similar time frame. The lack of symptoms and temporal consistency could steer away from an allergy diagnosis.

Importance of Cofactors

Although the mechanism is not clear, it is well known that cofactors like nonsteroidal anti-inflammatory drugs (NSAIDs), exercise, alcohol, stress, and menstruation can potentially trigger or exacerbate symptoms of allergy. Patients with salicylate intolerance may develop upper respiratory symptoms and/or bronchospasm (asthma, salicylate intolerance, and nasal polyps—Samter's triad) in response to NSAID/s and aspirin. Exercise-induced allergy or food-dependent exercise-induced anaphylaxis should be considered when patient's symptoms are clearly associated with the presence of cofactors. The connection between symptoms and physical factors such as pressure, change in temperature, solar exposure, and even contact with water are well-described in specific disorders such as symptomatic dermatographism, cholinergic urticaria, cold urticaria, solar urticaria, and aquagenic urticaria, respectively.

Disease Progression and Severity

Progression may be suggested by change in frequency, duration or severity of symptoms, or a need for increased medication requirement for symptom control, or a delay in response to the same medications as compared with previous episodes.

Past Medical History

Atopic diseases such as eczema, asthma, and rhinitis often occur in clusters within affected families with variable penetrance suggesting a genetic predisposition to these conditions. Moreover, the "allergic march" hypothesis proposed a link between the development of eczema to allergic rhinitis to asthma. It is important to establish the duration of allergy symptoms to guide the decision on implementing secondary prevention of asthma; such as immunotherapy for allergic rhinitis as literature provides some evidence of early immunological intervention for the prevention of asthma.

Treatment or Drug History

Angiotensin-converting enzyme inhibitors (ACEIs) are well recognized causes of spontaneous angioedema by promoting the accumulation of bradykinin. Its effect may last up to 6–8 weeks following the withdrawal of treatment. NSAIDs may cause intolerance and lower the threshold of other allergic reactions. The use of beta blocker may induce refractory anaphylaxis. Use of steroids (short or long term, topical or systemic), antihistaminics, and tricyclic antidepressants should be taken into account before considering for in vivo skin prick test. Therefore, it is important to take in-depth medication history for better management of allergic disorders.

Social and Occupational History

Details of an individual's housing or indoor environment may be helpful in diagnosing perennial allergic rhinitis. Damp humid environment fosters the growth of mold and house dust mite. Information regarding pets and hobbies would be useful. Smoking history (active or passive, indoor or outdoor) is important in the evaluation of rhinitis and asthma.

Family History

In addition to atopic diseases, hereditary angioedema and periodic fever syndromes are genetic disorders that follow Mendelian inheritance. A family (pedigree) tree marking the atopic individuals would be useful in establishing the diagnosis in index case and simultaneously for the identification of other allergic patients in the family.

Table 2: Differential diagnosis based on various allergic symptoms.

Predominant feature	Differential diagnoses
Urticaria	• Type I hypersensitivity • Idiopathic • Physical (aquagenic, cold, solar, cholinergic, exercise induced) • Urticarial vasculitis • Periodic fever syndrome
Urticaria and angioedema	• Type I hypersensitivity • Chronic idiopathic
Angioedema	• Type I hypersensitivity • Oral allergy syndrome (type I hypersensitivity) • Angiotensin-converting enzyme inhibitor induced • Idiopathic • Hereditary • Acquired
Rhinitis	• Seasonal allergic rhinitis (type I hypersensitivity) • Perennial allergic rhinitis (type I hypersensitivity) • Nonallergic (chronic rhinosinusitis) • Nasal polyps
Asthma	• Allergic asthma to common aeroallergens (type I hypersensitivity) • Nonallergic • Occupational (type I hypersensitivity) • Aspirin/nonsteroidal anti-inflammatory drug hypersensitivity • Sulfite hypersensitivity
Anaphylaxis	• Type I hypersensitivity—foods, drugs, insect sting, etc. • Drug induced • Exercise induced • Food-dependent exercise-induced (type I hypersensitivity) • Idiopathic
Other rashes	• Delayed hypersensitivity • Stevens-Johnson syndrome • Toxic epidermal necrolysis • Drug reaction with eosinophilia and systemic symptoms (DRESS)
Others	• Eosinophilic gastrointestinal or respiratory diseases

Based on various symptoms, there could be many differentials of allergic disorders (Table 2), which should be kept in mind.

PHYSICAL EXAMINATION

If the patient is asymptomatic, the physical examination may reveal no or minimal findings, yet the medical history can be compatible with allergy. Examination will need to be tailored to the patients complaint, as well as their age and other factors. Examination begins with vital signs, anthropometric measures (weight, height, body mass index) followed by system-specific screening. Table 3 enumerates common salient findings as per different systems in patients with allergic disorders.

Characteristic Signs of Allergic Disorders

- *Allergic shiners*: Dark circles under the eyes; this is due to increased blood flow near the sinuses.

Table 3: Findings on physical examination in an allergic person.

Body system	Salient findings
Eyes	Excessive lacrimation, erythema of the bulbar conjunctiva, cobblestoning of the tarsal conjunctiva, and dermatitis of the eyelids
Nose	Transverse crease, turbinate edema and pallor or bluish discoloration, discharge, polyps, nasal septal deviation or perforation
Sinuses	Tenderness, purulent drainage from sinus ostia
Oropharynx	Mouth breathing, dental malocclusion or overbite or postnasal drip, cobblestoning of the oropharyngeal wall, halitosis, and hypertrophied tonsils or adenoids
Ears	Tympanic membrane dullness, redness, retraction, and perforation or lack of mobility
Neck	Neck vein distension, adenopathy or tenderness
Chest	Deformity, altered percussion, egophony, audible wheezing, abnormal sounds on auscultation, and chest wall tenderness
Heart	Gallops, rubs or murmurs
Abdomen	Tenderness, distension or mass
Extremities	Tenderness, erythema, and signs of a connective tissue disorder
Neurologic	Weakness, impaired cognition or thought process including difficulty in recall or understanding their disease
Skin	Rashes, dermatographism, and infection

- *Dennie-Morgan lines*: Extra skin fold or line under the lower eyelids. These lines are named after the name of the doctor, who first noticed the relationship between this extra fold of skin and an allergic tendency.
- *Allergic salute*: Children hand seems to be scratching the nose constantly giving an expression of saluting. This is due to continuous nasal pruritus.

WHO NEEDS TO BE TESTED?

- Patients with recurrent or persistent symptoms
- Patient with moderate to severe symptoms
- Patients in which controllers and preventers need to be continued or escalated.

SUGGESTED READING

1. Allergic Rhinitis and Its Impact on Asthma guidelines.
2. Bischoff SC. Food allergy and eosinophilic gastroenteritis and colitis. Curr Opin Allergy Clin Immunol. 2010;10(3):238-45.
3. GINA guidelines on asthma and beyond.
4. Zuberbier T, Bindslev-Jensen C, Canonica W, et al. EAACI/GA2LEN/EDF guideline: definition, classification and diagnosis of urticaria. Allergy. 2006;61:316-20.

Allergy Testing: Allergen Identification

CHAPTER 10

INTRODUCTION

Different modalities of allergy testing are available now-a-days. Any single technique is not complete in itself. It has its own benefits and limitations. We need to understand the basics of allergic reaction and identification techniques of various tests. This will help in customizing appropriate test to individual patient.

BASIS OF ALLERGY TESTING

There are two sequential steps in allergic reactions: sensitization and re-exposure (Fig. 1).

Sensitization

In genetically predisposed individuals, T-cells are activated via first time exposure of antigen (allergen) through antigen presenting

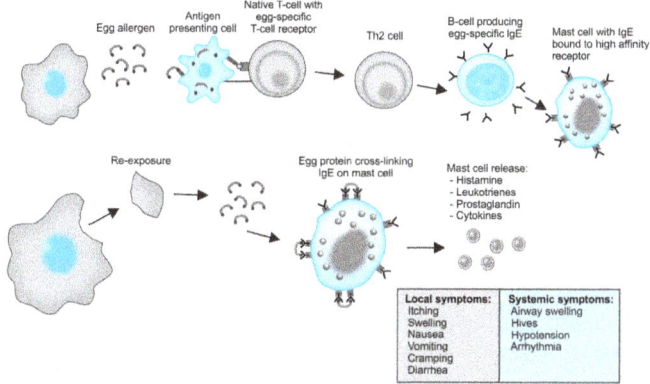

Fig. 1: Sensitization and re-exposure reactions to egg allergen.

cell (APC). The differentiated T-cells are responsible for class switching of the B-cell through various interleukins like IL-4 and IL-13. This process lead to IgE production (type I hypersensitivity) and release in circulation. Circulating free IgE get attached to the high affinity FcεRI receptor on the surface of mast cells and basophils. The process, where the specific IgE are bound to the mast cells, is labeled as sensitization.

Re-exposure

Whenever a second exposure to the offending allergen happens, the allergen binds to specific IgE on the mast cells to activate it. The mast cell activation causes massive release of histamine and other preformed allergy mediators. These cytokines are responsible for clinical symptoms, which could vary from asymptomatic to severe anaphylactic reaction.

The detection of released IgE or mast cell mediators forms the basis of allergy testing.

DIAGNOSIS OF TYPE I HYPERSENSITIVITY

Allergic disorders are suspected on the basis of nature of chief complaints, detailed relevant history, knowledge about environmental exposure and a minor contribution from physical examination (Chapter 9). A suggested history provides the clue for the possible allergens, which directs for either in vivo testing [skin prick test (SPT), intradermal test, challenge and provocation tests] or in vitro (total and specific IgE estimation) assays for the detection of IgE mediated hypersensitivity reactions. There are other surrogate markers of the allergic reactions, which might help in diagnostic evaluation in certain circumstances.

LABORATORY TESTS

Any laboratory test should be carefully selected based on its relevance (after taking detailed history and focused physical examination) and operational issues (cost, risk of anaphylaxis, time required) in management (allergen avoidance and immunotherapy) of any given patient. Laboratory diagnosis revolves around detection of IgE (free or bound) and the released cytokines (histamine and others). Laboratory tests focusing on functional (e.g. spirometry, peak expiratory flow rate, flexible rhinolaryngoscopy) and structural (e.g. radiographs) aspects can aid in better management of a patient in that particular episode but have limited role in disease remission or prevention. The tests which can make an impact on disease modification (either by allergen avoidance or immunotherapy) will be discussed here.

In Vitro Test

Total IgE

Ishizakas and Hornbrook detected IgE molecule for the first time in 1966. This can specifically recognize allergens that are typically proteins, e.g. the dust mite Der P1, cat Fel d1 or components from grass, weed, tree pollens and certain foods. These proteins are responsible for immediate (type I hypersensitivity) reactions. Reexposure of culprit allergen causes release of various mediators like histamine, leukotriene, and certain cytokines which are responsible for clinical manifestations in individual organs like respiratory system(asthma, sinusitis, otitis media), eye (conjunctivitis), skin (dermatitis) and gastrointestinal system (food allergies).

Total IgE levels are neither sensitive nor specific for the diagnosis of allergy. Patients with parasitic infestations, immunodeficiencies (e.g. AIDS, hyper IgE syndromes, etc.), Epstein-Barr virus (EBV) infection, rheumatological conditions (rheumatoid arthritis) and history of smoking may have raised IgE levels, on the contrary a normal IgE level does not rule out allergic disorders.

The only role of total IgE, from allergy perspective, is in cases where humanized monoclonal anti-IgE (omalizumab) is planned for treatment of atopic condition. If the level is in between 30 and 700 kIU/L then the total IgE level can be used to calculate the dose or assess the efficacy of omalizumab. Patients with conditions like refractory allergic bronchopulmonary aspergillosis and chronic urticaria, require anti-IgE therapy. In general, total IgE has very limited role in either diagnosing or ruling out an allergic disorder.

Specific IgE

Allergen specific IgE (sIgE) obviates the false-positive total IgE in disorders other than allergies. Is it based on the radioallergosorbent test (RAST), a technique of solid phase assay which consists of incubating a patient's serum with a preactivated allergen, conjugated to a cellulose paper disk. sIgE, if present in the serum, will bind to the respective allergens on the paper disk while rest of the antibodies are washed away. Bound IgE is then detected by the addition of a radiolabeled (I^{125}) antihuman IgE directed toward the Fc receptor. The amount of bound radiolabeled antihuman IgE is measured in a gamma counter in quantitative manner. Over past 50 years, radiolabeled techniques have been changed to enzyme conjugated antihuman IgE antibody methods.

Allergen specific IgE is a good tool when compared to total IgE for detection of individuals with type I hypersensitivity. However because of the nonstandard commercial allergen extract compositions, the interassay variation between manufacturers can be significant. Thus the results from one assay cannot be compared to the results from another analytical system, highlighting importance of monitoring with same laboratory in follow-up. Another major drawback in sIgE estimation includes the potential for false-positives with high total IgE levels, likely caused by non-specific binding to test allergen as per concentration gradient of free IgE molecules. All these techniques detect the free sIgE levels only and not the bound IgE thus sIgE may not accurately reflect the biological and clinical relevance of the IgE associated with mast cells and basophils.

Component Resolved Diagnostics

Crude allergen extracts, containing many allergenic and less/nonallergenic components, were used conventionally for sIgE estimation. Some of these components are structurally homologous with other environmental allergens. For example, individuals who are positive for sIgE to birch pollen may also show elevated IgE to peanut and hazelnut. Using crude allergens to detect sIgE, therefore, has the potential to yield falsely elevated sIgE to one of the allergen when individual was actually allergic to other allergen and test became positive due to cross reactivity of similar antigens in between two different allergens. To combat this problem, recombinant allergens as well as individual allergenic proteins for a given allergen have been manufactured, which can be used in component resolved diagnostic (CRD) tests to more accurately diagnose allergy. For instance, Ara h1, 2, 3 and 9 are allergenic proteins of peanut with high risk to allergy whereas Ara h8 has very low risk. Peanut, hazelnut, walnut, soya, wheat and rosacea fruits, all share profilin and cross reactive carbohydrate determinant (CCD) as common protein allergens, but these are having very low risk for clinically significant allergies. The high risk component allergenic proteins for peanut are (Ara h 1, 2, 3, 9), hazelnut (Cor a8, 9, 14), walnut (Jug r1, 2 , 3), soya (Gly m5, 6), wheat (Tri a14, 19) and rosacea fruits (Pru p3, Mal d3), respectively.

In Vivo Test

Skin test

Allergy skin testing (AST) is an established diagnostic procedure which has been in vogue for more than one and a half century, first elaborated by Charles Harrison Blackley in 1860s in his research activities on "hay fever". It detects the presence of bound IgE attached to mast cells and basophils. It acts like a second exposure to the offending allergen (in minute quantities under controlled conditions) to the sensitized person, thus releasing histamine and other cytokines responsible for immediate wheal and flare. In other words, skin test is a mini-allergen test and it reproduces the actual reaction in the patient. Skin test is considered as "gold standard" for diagnosis of IgE-mediated allergic disorders. Table 1 highlights the major differences between skin test (in vivo) and serum IgE (in vitro) tests.

Table 1: Head-to-head comparison between serum specific IgE and allergy skin test (AST).

sIgE test	Skin test
Points favoring sIgE	
Widely available	Requires an allergist or an experienced person
Little cooperation required	Patient cooperation warranted
No risk of any reaction to patient	Slight risk of systemic reaction present
Can be done if patient on any drugs (antihistaminics, steroids, etc.)	Patient should be off antihistaminics and antidepressants.
Can be done soon after anaphylaxis or in acute exacerbation	Requires a time gap after anaphylaxis or acute exacerbation
Can be done with any skin condition	Area of normal skin is required
Laboratory standardization required	No standardization at present
Points favoring skin test	
Minor pain during venesection	Minor discomfort, painless, bloodless
Results takes at least 48 hours	Result available in 20 minutes
Not directly meaningful to patient, not adding any value to allergen avoidance measures	Results are visible and compelling to patients; may have value in ensuring compliance with allergen avoidance and immunotherapy
Detect free IgE only, so detects hypersensitivity	Based on bound IgE and released cytokines, detects clinically relevant hypersensitivity (allergy)
Reasonably good sensitivity	Better sensitivity for clinically important allergies
Many food allergens, drugs and rare pollens are not available for testing	Can extemporaneously prepare allergens and do prick-prick testing
Chances of false-positive with high total IgE levels	No interference from high total IgE
Costly assay	Cost effective

The basic purpose of AST is to introduce minimal amount of the antigen into the most superficial skin layer (epidermis) through stratum corneum. There are two types of AST: epicutaneous and intradermal, the difference between the two has been shown in Table 2.

Table 2: Epicutaneous vs intradermal skin tests.

Parameter	Epicutaneous AST	Intradermal AST
Safety	Very safe	Some risk
Technique	Simple	Complicated
Reliable	More	Less
False-positives	Less	More
Clinical correlation	High	Low
Number of ST/sitting possible	Many	Few
Patient comfort	Good	Less
Painful to patient	Minimal to no pain	Painful
Reproducibility	Poor	Good
Sensitivity	Good	Very high

Epicutaneous AST or commonly called as *skin prick test* is widely used for allergen identification with good clinical correlation.

Technique of epicutaneous allergy skin testing: Forearm and upper back are the most commonly used sites for SPT. A small drop of antigen (allergen) is placed on the skin and a sharp instrument is passed through the drop, penetrating the skin at approximately 45°. The device is then lifted quickly, creating a minute break in the epidermis. Approximately 0.3 µL of fluid is introduced into the skin at a depth of 1 mm just beneath the stratum corneum (in the epidermis only). In this area, only superficial touch receptors are present while blood vessels and pain receptors are lying deep in the dermis, thus this test is pain and blood free if done properly. We have renamed this test as *skin-touch test (STT)* based on true nature of the test and non scary name for pediatric patients. After allergen deposition, it diffuses down in to dermis where it gets attached to IgE bound on mast cells releasing histamine and other cytokines which are responsible for wheal and flare type of reaction.

Prick-prick test: If the commercial extract of a suspected allergen is not available, than the crude extract can be pricked prior to skin prick to test for that allergen. As AST is epicutaneous, there is no risk of infections by this method.

Number of skin prick test needs to be performed: The number of test allergen varies with individual patient, availability of standard allergen extracts and healthy test area. It should be based on patient's age, history, location, exposure to allergens, genetic tendency and socioeconomic factors. "Less is more" should be the rule. Skin testing for only a few major and clinically relevant allergens is usually sufficient.

Who should be tested?

A person with history of occasional symptoms will not be a good candidate for AST as allergen avoidance or immunotherapy is not warranted in person with infrequent symptoms. Patients with moderate-to-severe symptoms and/or persistent symptoms should be tested for allergen identification. Repeated uncontrolled symptoms requiring frequent reliever medications would be another cohort of patients who need to be evaluated.

Selection of antigens for allergy skin testing: There is no general rule regarding selection of the allergens for AST. The knowledge about local flora is important in the selection of inhalant allergens. Mostly the selection of antigens is guided by patient's history, demographic factors and occupational exposure. Inhalants, ingestant (foods) and injectable (venoms) are the important groups of allergens. Inhalants could be indoor (house dust, house dust mites, cockroaches, pets and fungal spores) or outdoor (tree, grass and weed pollens and fungal spores).

Prick devices: Various types of prick devices can be used (Figs. 2 and 3). Single tip devices have better control but have to be used many times. Flexibility is limited with multi-test devices with an advantage of testing several allergens simultaneously.

Interpretation of skin-prick test or skin-touch test: Limited number of allergens are tested on patient's forearm or back with positive (histamine) and negative (normal saline) controls. Negative control is considered as acceptable, if wheal through saline prick is between 0–3 mm in diameter; more than that suggests dermatographism (baseline reactivity of the skin) demanding invalidity of the test.

Allergy Testing: Allergen Identification

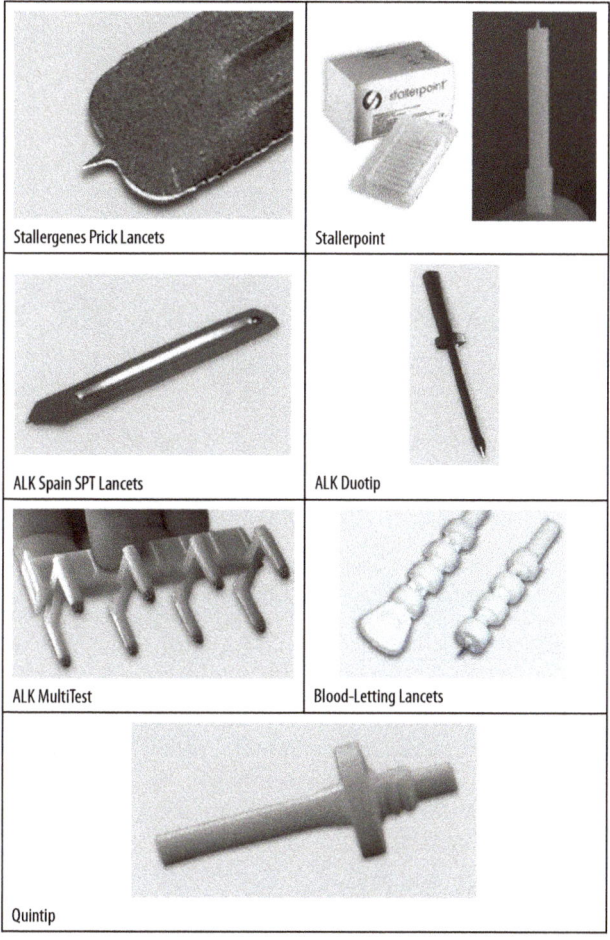

Fig 2: Lancet to be used for allergy skin testing (AST)
(For color version, see Plate 19).

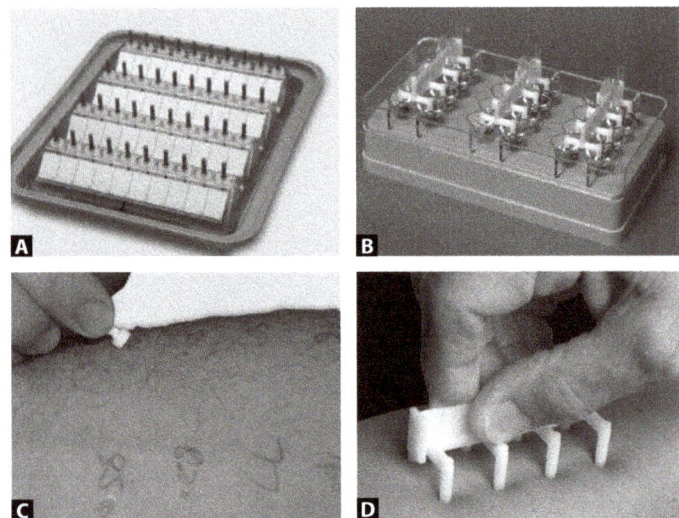

Figs. 3A to D: Lancets and multi-test devices for allergy skin testing (AST): (A) Duotips in tray containing extracts, waiting for use; (B) Multi-test devices in tray containing extracts, waiting for use; (C) Drops applied to skin being pricked with a blood lancet (prick and lift technique); (D) Multi-test device applied to skin *(For color version, see Plate 20).*

Positive control with histamine has to be equal to or more than 3 mm than the negative saline control for validity of the test. Any reaction equal to or more than 3 mm of negative control (saline) is considered positive AST. Figures 4A to E show SPT (STT) at an allergy clinic in North India.

Factors influencing allergy skin testing:
- *Medications*: Following medications should be stopped prior to AST to prevent false-negative test:
  - Antihistaminics (H_1 blockers)—48 hours
  - Astemizole—60 days
  - Ketotifen—5 days
  - Tricyclic antidepressants—2 weeks

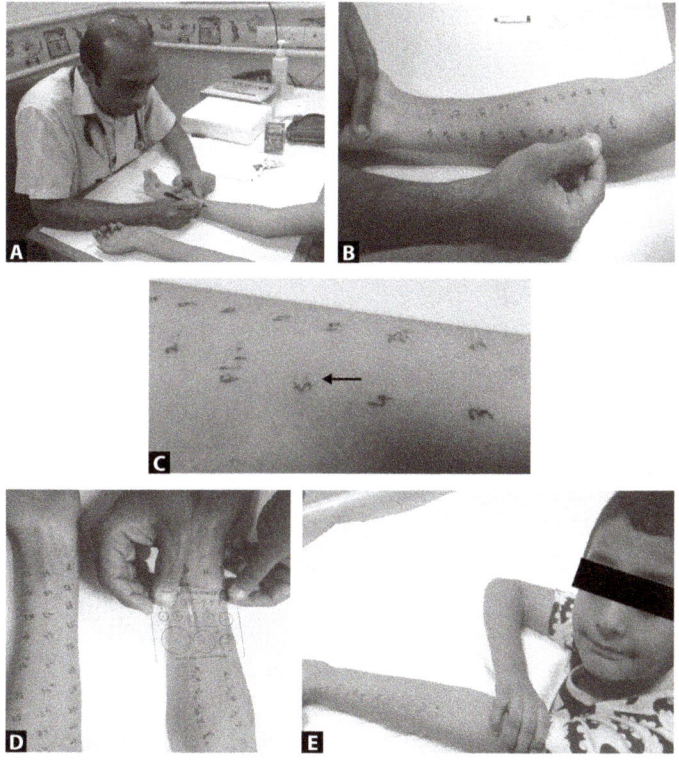

Figs. 4A to E: Skin prick test or skin-touch test (STT) at an allergy clinic. (A) Marking on forearm for allergen identification; (B) STT with lancet; (C) Wheal and flare reaction (marked by arrow); (D) Measurement of allergic reaction and (E) Child after STT (a blood less pain less procedure) *(For color version, see Plate 20).*

- Short-term steroids—no effects
- Long-term steroids—2 weeks
- Long-term topical steroids—2–3 weeks.
- *Age*: There is no lower age limit for AST, though it is preferable beyond 4 months of age. The skin reactivity generally declines with age, especially after 65 years.

- *Area of the body*: The mid and upper back are more reactive (33%) than the lower back for wheal and flare reaction after the SPT. The back as a whole is more reactive (53%) than the forearm. There should be at least a gap of 5 cm away from the wrist and 3 cm away from antecubital fossa, on the forearm, for better skin reactivity.
- *Distance between two pricks*: The recommended gap between two contiguous test sites should be a minimum distance of 2 cm. This gap is advised to minimize the chances of merging of two nearby wheals in case of strong reactions and thus reducing false-positives and false-negatives.

Correlation of allergy skin testing: Researchers comparing sIgE with AST have found 80% correlation for inhalant allergens whereas this is much lesser for food allergens. Size of wheal and chances of allergic asthma have shown a positive correlation. The decline in AST reactivity has been demonstrated after 3 years of allergen immunotherapy.

Patch Test

During the atopic patch test (APT), intact protein allergens are applied epicutaneously followed by evaluation of the induced eczematous skin lesions during a periodic assessment over next 7 days. The APT is based on type IV hypersensitivity reaction. Benefits of APT over AST are that: it can be tested at a younger age, low risk of anaphylaxis and better specificity. APT can detect cellular component of hypersensitivity which is a major limitation for AST. Lower sensitivity than AST, more time consuming and limited number of antigen detection at one time are some of the disadvantages of APT. It is recommended for adverse reactions to metals, cosmetics, etc.

Provocation Test

A small quantity of a suspected allergen is introduced, through natural route, to the patient under strict monitoring. Such types of challenges are useful when history is inconclusive, and none of the in vitro or in vivo tests are supporting the diagnosis. These tests should be done in allergist office with the availability of all the resuscitation facilities. Allergens are administered in gradually increasing doses to monitor for any untoward effect. Observation should be done for sufficient time period.

Food Challenge

Food challenges are considered to be the "gold standard" tests for detecting adverse reactions to food items. Immune mechanisms, including IgE and non-IgE mediated, are best detected by challenge tests. Oral food challenges may be open, single-blind or double-blind placebo controlled. In double blind placebo controlled food challenge (DBPCFC) tests, the test food item is masked with another food item (called as "vehicle" food) and then administered in gradually escalated doses. The active food and an equivalent amount of placebo are given in random order and both tests are performed in a controlled manner. DBPCFC though an ideal and recommended test, but not feasible in most of the circumstances due to difficulty in blinding of all the qualities of a test food item viz. color, odor, taste, consistency, temperature, etc. A single-blind challenge, in which patient or attendant is unaware but physician knows about the contents of test material, is sufficient as a screening tool for reactivity, especially in children. An open feeding trial, to rule out rare false-negative challenges, may be considered if the result of the blinded challenge is inconsistent with the clinical history. Significant reduction of sIgE during follow-up of a food allergic patient, may signal the appropriate time for performing diagnostic food challenge.

Elimination diet: A trial elimination for at least 6–12 weeks of the suspected food(s) should be tried prior to food challenge. It may be of three forms:
1. Elimination of one or several suspected foods.
2. Elimination of all but a defined group of allowed foods.
3. An elemental diet consisting of hydrolyzed formula or amino acid-based formulas in infants. The symptoms should resolve

once culprit food is eliminated from the diet and they should reappear once the particular food is reintroduced. These elimination diets alone are seldom diagnostic of food allergies.

Nasal Provocation Test

It is an extremely helpful method, though not standardized and less practiced, when there is any discordance between medical history and the result of AST and/or serological tests. Test allergen extract is applied over anterior part of the inferior turbinate, with consequent allergic reaction development. Technique standardization, allergen type, dose of allergen and form of allergen administration (drops, nebulized form) are among the several difficulties during this test. It should be performed after a pharmacological washout period (H_1 antihistaminics, benzodiazepines, corticosteroids and mast cell stabilizers). Aqueous solution or lyophilized powder should be administered unilaterally, in varying concentration. Dose response should be evaluated and compared to pretest saline challenge to rule out the possibility of possible irritant effect.

Bronchial Challenge Test

This test is also called as methacholine or histamine challenge test, done for asthma diagnosis. Both drugs provoke bronchoconstriction, which can be quantified by spirometry. Histamine causes nasal and bronchial mucus secretion and bronchoconstriction via H_1 receptor, whereas methacholine acts on M_3 receptors. This test is routinely not recommended and is absolutely contraindicated in patients with severe airway obstruction. Aortic aneurysm is relative contraindication due to risk of rupture by hypertension during spirometry.

Alternative Techniques

There are certain other upcoming methods with questionable utility.

Cytotoxic Food Testing (Bryan's Test)

The fundamental principle behind this test is that in vitro mixing of patient's blood (leukocytes) with an antigen, to which that person is allergic, results in injury to cells. Patient's blood drops are added to a dried food extract solution on a microscope slide. Slide is examined timely for "cytotoxic effects", which can be documented as disintegration of cells. The test has not got utility due to lack of correlation with clinical allergy.

Provocation Neutralization

During provocation procedure, the patient is asked to report any symptom that develops after various concentrations of suspected allergens are administered under the tongue or injected into the skin. Several concentrations (in dilutions) are given until a dose is found that "neutralizes" the self-reported symptoms. The neutralizing dose, given periodically, helps in immune tolerance generation. This test is not recommended, nowaday, due to lot of subjective and objective variations.

Kinesiology

George J Goodheart, in 1964, initiated a pseudoscientific system of muscle-testing and therapy, known as applied kinesiology. Its basic notion is that every organ dysfunction is accompanied by a specific muscle weakness, which enables diseases to be diagnosed through muscle-testing procedures.

Iridology

It is a noninvasive study of the iris through the analysis of their color, texture and structure. It can provide valuable information about the body's constitutional strengths and weaknesses, levels of inflammation, toxemia and the efficiency of eliminative systems and organs.

Electrodermal/Vega Testing

It is a bioenergetic regulatory technique, originated from acupuncture and homeopathy. Ill health begins on an informational/energetic level and, therefore, symptoms of an imbalance of energy can and do occur long before any evident pathological morphology. The vega technique measures this bioenergetic phenomenon by recording the change in skin conductivity after application of a small voltage.

Pulse Test

Arthur F Coca, in 1956, demonstrated significant increase in pulse rate in patients after ingesting particular food item, to which they were suspected to be allergic. This was probably due to stress response for the particular food allergen. This method cannot differentiate between food allergy and sensitivity.

Reflexology

A specialized massage technique is used for presumed healing, concentrating on reflex areas in feet, which reflect particular organs of the body. It is a relaxing method of stimulating the body's self-healing properties.

Hair Analysis

Hair can be analyzed in two ways. First of all, the hair is tested for toxic levels of heavy metals, such as lead, mercury, cadmium, selenium, chromium, manganese and magnesium. These heavy metals have no scientific value on allergic diseases. Another hair test is called "dowsing", in which a dowser swings a pendulum over the hair and an allergy is diagnosed if an altered swing is noted.

IgG Enzyme-linked Immunosorbent Assay-based Test

This test measures IgG and IgG4 antibodies to various foods which should not be confused with IgE based RAST and Immuno-CAP. IgG antibody development is a normal response to food, we eat, which indicate exposure but not sensitization. This test is not useful for allergy detection rather high IgG levels could be protective.

CONCLUSION

Diagnosis of allergy is mostly dependent on detailed focused history with a small contribution from physical examination. Pharmaceutical industries are flooded with lot of allergy tests, we need to be vigilant in choosing the appropriate one for individual patient. While choosing the allergen panel, exposure history and local environment of the patient should be kept in mind. "Less is more" should be the dictum, regarding number of allergens to be tested.

SUGGESTED READING

1. ASCIA (2016). Skin Prick Testing for the diagnosis of allergic disease: A manual for practitioners. [online] Available from https://www.allergy.org.au/images/stories/pospapers/ASCIA_SPT_Manual_March_2016.pdf [Accessed December 2018].
2. Blaiss MS. Approach to the allergic patient. In: Liberman P, Anderson J, editors. Allergic Diseases Diagnosis and Treatment. Totowa, NJ: Humana Press, Inc.; 1997. pp. 15-26.
3. Dreborg S. Diagnosis of food allergy: tests in vivo and in vitro. Pediatr Allergy Immunol. 2001:12:24-30
4. Gosepath, J.; Amedee, RG. & Mann, WJ. (2005). Nasal provocation testing as an international standard for evaluation of allergic and non-allergic rhinitis. Laryngoscope, Vol.115, No.3, (March 2005), pp. 512-6, ISSN 0023-852X
5. Hamilton RG. Laboratory Diagnosis of Human Allergic Disease. In: Leung DYM, Sampson H, Geha R, Szeflar (Eds). Pediatric Allergy: Principles and Practice, 2nd edition. Amsterdam: Elsevier BV; 2016. pp. 240-9.
6. Knight, Vijaya, Ronald Harbeck. In vitro Laboratory Tests for the Diagnosis of Allergy. In: Vedanthan PK, Nelson HS, Agashe SN, Katial R (Eds). Textbook of Allergy for the Clinician. Florida: CRC Press; 2014. pp. 47-52.
7. Oppenheimer J, Nelson HS. Skin testing: a survey of allergists. Ann Allergy Asthma Immunol. 2006;96:19-23.
8. Portnoy J. Diagnostic testing for allergies. Ann Allergy Asthma Immunol. 2006;96:3-4.
9. Portnoy J. What do allergy skin tests really mean? Ann Allergy Asthma Immunol. 2002;89:335-6.
10. Roberts G, Lack G. Diagnosing peanut allergy with skin prick and specific IgE testing. J Allergy Clin Immunol 2005;115:1291-6.
11. Tripathi A, Booth BH. Diagnosis of immediate hypersensitivity. In: Grammer LC, Greenberger PA (Eds). Patterson's Allergic Diseases, 6th edition. Philadelphia, PA: Lippincott Williams & Wilkins; 2002. pp. 145-57.
12. Vedanthan PK. Allergy Skin Testing. Textbook of Allergy for the Clinician, Florida: CRC Press;2014. pp. 36-46.

CHAPTER 11
Allergy Testing: Supportive Investigations

INTRODUCTION

Allergy testing and allergen identification needs to be supported by structural and functional assessment of the involved system. This helps in stage characterization, optimizing treatment and monitoring the disease progression. Allergic airway diseases (rhinitis and asthma) needs to be classified in different stages as per the Allergic Rhinitis and its Impact on Asthma (ARIA) and Global Initiative for Asthma (GINA) guidelines respectively. There are various modalities available for the same.

STRUCTURAL ASSESSMENT

Nasal Endoscopy

It can be a useful adjunct for visualization of nasal cavity and upper airways in an allergic patient. Table 1 enumerates various findings at different locations.

Indications for nasal endoscopy are:
- Nasal obstruction (particularly unilateral)
- Unexplained headache
- Facial pain
- Epistaxis
- Persistent rhinorrhea
- Sinusitis
- Earache, recurrent or chronic otitis media
- Regional adenopathy
- Reassessment of postsurgical patient
- Chronic cough
- Atypical asthma

Table 1: Findings of upper airways.

Region	Findings
Mucosa	• Mucus (clear or purulent), color (affected by vascular changes), inflammation, cobble-stoning, mucosal atrophy
Nasal cavity • Turbinate • Septum • Polyps • Paranasal sinuses	 • Bony or mucosal hypertrophy, compression effect from septal deviation, surgical resection, clefting (horizontal and sagittal), polypoidal extension, degeneration, Concha bullosa • Deviation, dislocation, perforation, spurs, maxillary ridge • Arising from paranasal sinuses, turbinate degeneration, mucocele • Direct inspection
Nasopharynx and Oropharynx • Choana • Torus, eustachian tube orifice • Adenoids • Pharyngeal wall • Malignancies	 • Atresia or stenosis • Cystic degeneration, edematous obstruction, postsurgical scarring • Adenoiditis, Rathke's pouch cyst hypertrophy, anterior herniation through choana • Osteophytes, carotid aneurysm, constrictor muscle spasm • Carcinomas originating in Rosenmuller's fossa
Oropharynx, Hypopharynx, Larynx • Posterior tongue • Lingual tonsils • Epiglottis • Glottis • Arytenoids • Vocal cords	 • Cystic circumvallate papillae, mucocele • Hypertrophy • Edema, positional deformity • Erythema, edema, laryngocele • Contact ulcers, edema • Contact ulcers, webs, paralysis, nodules, polyps, vocal cord abduction syndrome

- Dysphagia
- Hoarseness.

Bronchoscopy

Bronchoscopy has no direct role in allergy or asthma diagnosis, but it is sometimes useful in structural assessment of lower airways taking bronchoalveolar lavage and ruling out other differentials

in a child with recurrent respiratory symptoms. It might help in following conditions:
- Structural assessment of lower airway for any extrinsic or intrinsic compression or mucosal inflammation
- Foreign body aspiration
- Airway malacias or stenosis
- Bronchoalveolar lavage for infectious etiology
- To rule out other asthma mimickers.

FUNCTIONAL ASSESSMENT

Spirometry

It measures the volume of breath inhaled or exhaled and the time required to perform the maneuver. Flowchart 1 demonstrates the steps of spirometry interpretation. Figures 1A and B depict graphical representation of obstructive and restrictive lung functions.

Impulse Oscillometry

Principle
- Computer-driven loudspeaker output to apply bursts of square wave oscillometry pressures of multiple frequencies to patient's airway and analyzing pressure-flow relationship using spectral analysis.
- These sound waves travel over the normal tidal breaths of patients making it convenient to be used in small noncooperative children, during sleep or ventilation or when conventional spirometry method is unable to explain the clinical symptoms of patient.
- Mathematical analyses of impedance (Zrs) is done, which consists of resistance (Rrs) and reactance (Xrs) at individual frequency.

Parameters to Measure
- Impedance (Zrs): Depends on Rrs and Xrs
- Resistance (Rrs): Depends on pressure and flow received at transducer

Flowchart 1: Systematic interpretation of spirometry.

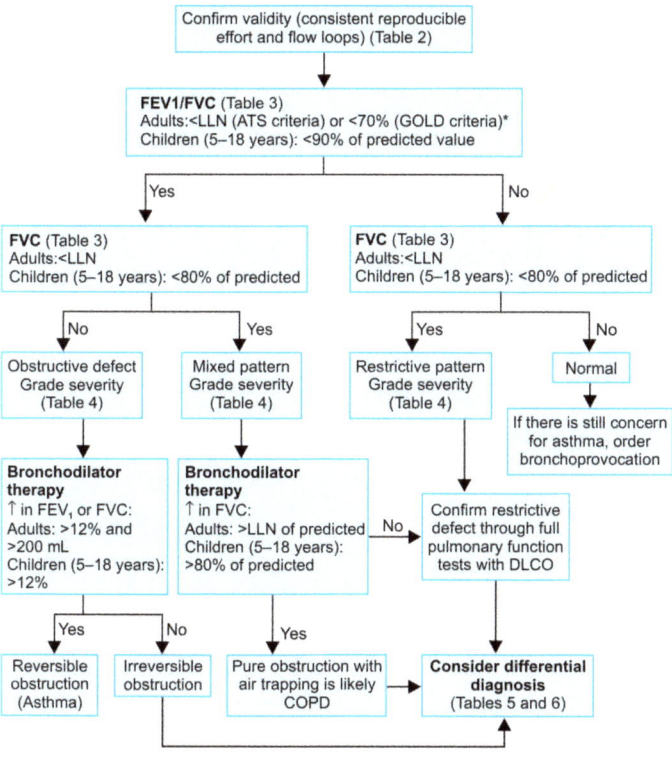

*70% criteria should be used for patients ≥65 years who have respiratory symptoms and are at risk of Chronic Obstructive Pulmonary Disease (COPD), i.e. current or previous smoker.
(ATS: American Thoracic Society; GOLD: Global Initiative for Chronic Obstructive Lung disease; DLCO: diffusing capacity of the lung for carbon monoxide; FEV1: forced expiratory volume in one second; FVC: forced vital capacity; LLN: lower limit of normal)
Source: Johnson JD, Theurer WM. A stepwise approach to the interpretation of pulmonary function tests. Am Fam Physician. 2014;89:359-66.

- Reactance (X_{rs}): It is the amount of recoil generated against the pressure wave, it depends upon inertance (I) of moving column and capacitance (Ca) of peripheral lung.
- Area of reactance (A_x): Area under the reactance curve.

Table 2: Quality control measure during spirometry.

Intraprocedure (Acceptable efforts)	Interprocedure
Adequate inspiration before starting to exhale	At least 3 acceptable trials
No hesitation or false start	FVC & FEV_1 reproducible: ≤0.15 L (≤0.1 L if FVC ≤1 L) variability between two largest efforts
No cough during early part of forced expiration	If reproducibility not met: repeat until 8 trials
No early termination of exhalation	FVC & FEV_1 values: take individual maximum
No artefact due to tongue in the mouthpiece	Best loop: In which FVC & FEV_1 sum is maximum
At least 6 sec of exhalation (3 sec in children)	
Good start (Back extrapolation <5% or <0.15 L)	

Table 3: Spirometry interpretation.

FVC	FEV_1/FVC ratio	Suggested diagnosis
5–18 years: ≥80% Adults: ≥LLN	5–18 years: ≥90% Adults: ≥LLN or ≥70%	Normal
5–18 years: ≥80% Adults: ≥LLN	5–18 years: <90% Adults: <LLN or <70%	Obstructive defect
5–18 years: <80% Adults: <LLN	5–18 years: ≥90% Adults: ≥LLN or ≥70%	Restrictive defect
5–18 years: <80% Adults: <LLN	5–18 years: <90% Adults: <LLN or <70%	Mixed pattern

Source: Johnson JD, Theurer WM. A stepwise approach to the interpretation of pulmonary function tests. Am Fam Physician. 2014;89:359-66.

Table 4: Grades for severity in children of a spirometry abnormality.

Severity	FEV_1 (% of predicted)	FVC (% of predicted)
Mild	>80%	70–80%
Moderate	60–80%	60–69%
Severe	<60%	<60%

Table 5: Differential diagnosis based on DLCO results.

DLCO results	Differential diagnosis
High DLCO	Asthma, left-to-right shunts, polycythemia, pulmonary hemorrhage
Normal DLCO with restriction	Kyphoscoliosis, morbid obesity, neuromuscular weakness, pleural effusion
Normal DLCO with obstruction	α_1-antitrypsin deficiency, asthma, bronchiectasis, chronic bronchitis
Low DLCO with restriction	Asbestosis, hypersensitivity pneumonitis, idiopathic pulmonary fibrosis, LCH, miliary TB, sarcoidosis, silicosis (late)
Low DLCO with obstruction	Cystic fibrosis, emphysema, silicosis (early)
Low DLCO with normal PFT	Chronic pulmonary emboli, CHF, connective tissue disease with pulmonary involvement, dermatomyositis, SLE, rheumatoid arthritis

(CHF: congestive heart failure; DLCO: carbon monoxide diffusing capacity; LCH: Langerhans cell histiocytosis; SLE: systemic lupus erythematosus; TB: tuberculosis)
Source: Johnson JD, Theurer WM. A stepwise approach to the interpretation of pulmonary function tests. Am Fam Physician. 2014;89:359-66.

Table 6: Common causes of obstructive and restrictive lung disease.

Obstructive	α_1–antitrypsin deficiency, asthma, bronchiectasis, bronchiolitis obliterans, chronic pulmonary obstructive disease, cystic fibrosis, silicosis (early)
Restrictive	Chest wall—ankylosing spondylitis, kyphosis, morbid obesity, scoliosis Drugs (adverse reaction)—amiodarone, methotrexate, nitrofurantoin Interstitial lung disease—asbestosis, berylliosis, eosinophilic pneumonia, hypersensitivity pneumonitis, idiopathic pulmonary fibrosis, sarcoidosis, silicosis (late) Neuromuscular disorders—amyotrophic lateral sclerosis, Guillain-Barré syndrome, muscular dystrophy

Indications

- Suspected airway obstruction or on asthma treatment now for follow-up, the patient who is unable for reliable spirometry

or normal spirometry results but unable to explain physical symptoms:
- <5 years
- Elderly person
- Physical and cognitive limitation
- Ventilated patients.

Interpretation of Parameters

- ↑R_5, ↑R_{20}, Normal R_5–R_{20} → central airway obstruction
- ↑R_5, Normal R_{20}, ↑R_5–R_{20} → peripheral airway obstruction
- ↑↑R_5, ↑R_{20}, ↑R_5–R_{20} → combined airway obstruction
- More negative X_5 and ↑Ax → peripheral disease (restrictive or obstructive, may indicate an asthma obstruction)
- Response to bronchodilator: ≥40% ↓Ax (for peripheral airways), ≥10% ↓R_{10} → Reversible obstruction
- Response to bronchoconstriction (methacholine challenge test): ≥50% ↓X_5 (more negative) → Reversible obstruction

Difference between Spirometry and Impulse Oscillometry System

Main differences in between two pulmonary function assessment techniques are highlighted in Table 7.

Exhaled Nitric Oxide

- Principle
  - Nitric oxide (NO) is an inert gas, which is generated from L-arginine through the action of an enzyme called NO synthase (NOS).
  - Low levels of NOS are continuously produced by human airway epithelial cells under normal conditions, which are upregulated by proinflammatory cytokines (IL-4 and IL-13) and stimuli after allergen exposure in atopic individuals.
- Measurement
  - Patient's lungs are filled to total vital capacity with air (free of NO), and then breath out at a steady rate for approximately

Table 7: Spirometry vs FOT/IOS.

Parameter	Spirometry	FOT/IOS
Main principle	Flow sensor/volume displacement helps measure flow rates and lung volumes	Forced oscillations of single FOT or impulses of multiple frequency sound waves (IOS) are pushed into the lungs as pressure waves to measure respiratory resistance and reactance
Main parameters	Volumes: FEV_1, FVC Flows: PEFR, $FEF_{25-75\%}$	Zrs, Rrs, Xrs, Fres, Ax
Patient cooperation required	+++	+
Type of breathing maneuver	Forced exhalation	Tidal breathing
Variability (Intra-subject)	3–5%	5–15%
Sensitivity to airway location • Central • Peripheral	 ++ +	 +++ +++
Cutoff for bronchodilator response	12–15% for FEV_1	↓40% for Ax OR ↓10% for R_{10}
Cutoff for bronchoconstrictor response	20% for FEV_1	↓50% for X_5
Insight into lung mechanics	+	+++
Standardized methodology	+++	++
Availability of robust reference values	+++	+

(FOT: forced oscillation technique; IOS: impulse oscillometry system; FEV_1: forced expiratory volume in 1 second; FVC: forced vital capacity; PEFR: peak expiratory flow rate; FEF 25-75%: forced expiratory flow at 25–75% of FVC; Zrs: respiratory impedance; Rrs: respiratory resistance; Xrs: respiratory reactance; Fres: resonant frequency; Ax: reactance area; R_5: respiratory reactance at 5 Hz; X_5: respiratory reactance at 5 Hz)

6 sec, the time necessary for the FeNO level to plateau, against a positive pressure.
- The standard flow rate used for FeNO estimation is 50 mL/sec.
- It can be used in patients as young as 4 years.

Table 8: Cutoff points for FeNO estimation for diagnosis of eosinophilic inflammation.

Pathophysiology	Adults	Children
Eosinophilic inflammation unlikely	<25 ppb	<20 ppb
Unclear, depends on clinical context	25–50 ppb	20–35 ppb
Eosinophilic inflammation likely, usually steroid responsive	>50 ppb	>35 ppb

Table 9: Factors affecting FeNO levels.

Decrease	Uncertain effect	Increase
Current smoking	Weight/BMI	Male gender
Past smoking	Menstrual cycle	Height
Bronchial provocation	Physical exercise	Allergen exposure
Dietary antioxidants	Spirometric maneuvers	Recent dietary intake of nitrate
Bacterial infections	Age (in adults)	Rhinovirus infection
Respiratory syncytial virus (RSV) and influenza virus	Diurnal variation	Holding one's breath between inhalation and exhalation maneuvers during test
		Air pollution; ozone or particulate matter

- Interpretation
  - Diagnostic cutoff levels for FeNO are depicted in Table 8. Various factors affecting FeNO estimation are enumerated in Table 9. Table 10 depicts asthma medication effects on FeNO levels.
- Clinical application
  - Detection of eosinophilic airway inflammation
  - Determining corticosteroid response
  - Unmasking of nonadherence to steroid therapy
  - Help in early detection of ongoing atopic inflammation in poor perceivers.

RADIOLOGICAL ASSESSMENT

Diagnosis of allergic conditions are mostly clinical; however, these may require radiological support sometimes. The common allergic

Table 10: Effect of long-term asthma treatment on FeNO levels.

Medications	Effect on FeNO levels
Corticosteroids (oral >> inhaled)	Marked decrease
Leukotriene receptor antagonists	Slight decrease
Omalizumab (anti-IgE receptor antibody)	Decrease
Chromones	No effect
Methylxanthines	No effect

conditions in which radiology may be helpful are rhinosinusitis, adenoid hypertrophy and asthma.

Rhinosinusitis

- X-ray: It is the commonly available modality for radioimaging the paranasal sinuses. Figures 2A to D demonstrate the normal and abnormal paranasal sinuses on plain occipitomental (Water's) view radiograph.
- Computed tomography (CT) scan: It is more useful in chronic sinusitis. Mostly a non-contrast CT (NCCT) scan suffices the need.
- Magnetic resonance imaging (MRI): MRI is routinely not required for sinus imaging. It might be required in case of suspected intracranial complications and extension of infection.
- Ultrasonography (USG): It is an upcoming modality with benefit of no radiation exposure and ready availability. Sonogram can depict 86% of infections when combined with conventional radiography.

Adenoid Hypertrophy

- X-ray: Radioimaging of extended neck (lateral view) provides adequate information about the adenoid enlargement. Figure 3A depicts a line diagram of normal nasopharyngeal passage. Figures 3A to C depict radiographic findings in X-ray soft tissue

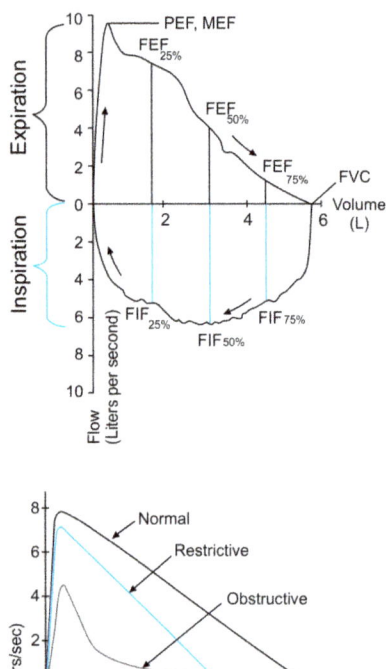

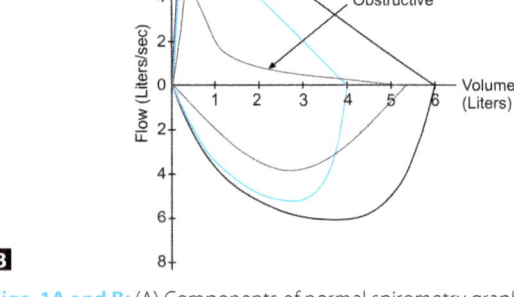

Figs. 1A and B: (A) Components of normal spirometry graph; (B) Obstructive and restrictive patterns compared with normal graph.

(PEF: peak expiratory flow; MEF: maximum expiratory flow; FVC: forced vital capacity; $FEF_{25\%}$, $FEF_{50\%}$, $FEF_{75\%}$: forced expiratory flow when 25%, 50% or 75% of the FVC has been expired respectively; $FIF_{75\%}$, $FIF_{50\%}$, $FIF_{25\%}$: forced inspiratory flow at 75%, 50% or 25% of FVC represents the flow rate at the 75%, 50% or 25% point relative to the total volume to be inhaled).

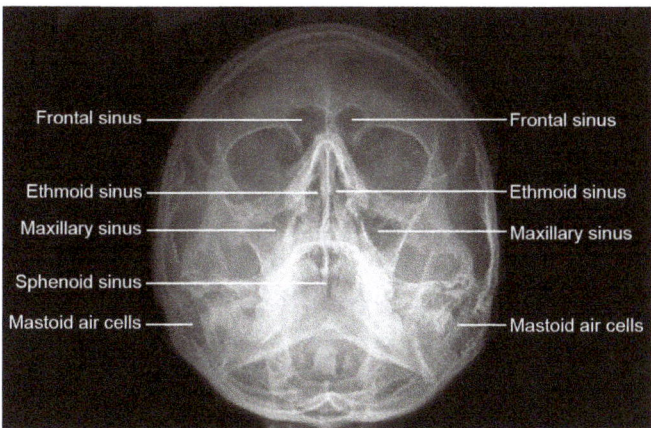

Fig. 2A: Plain radiograph of paranasal sinuses.

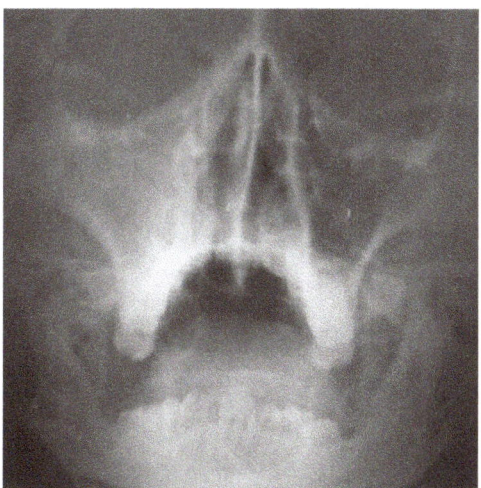

Fig. 2B: Right maxillary sinusitis; sinus if more opaque than ipsilateral orbit and contralateral sinus.

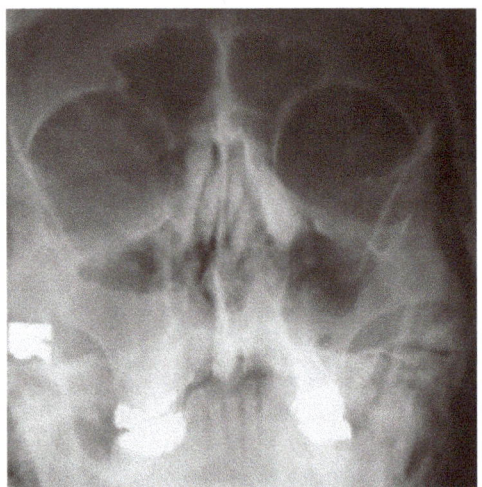

Fig. 2C: Acute sinusitis; Air fluid level in right maxillary sinus.

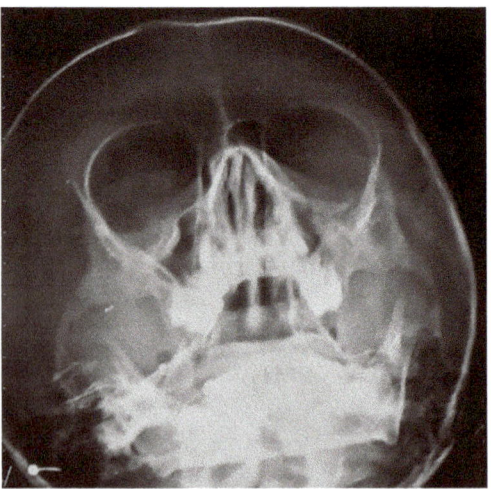

Fig. 2D: Mucosal thickening in maxillary sinuses.

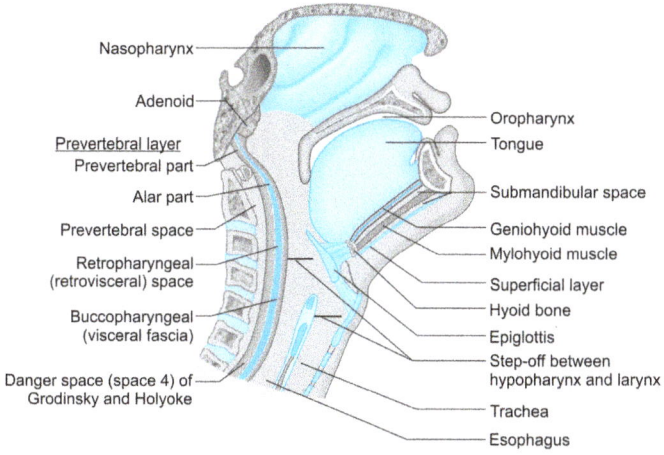

Fig. 3A: Line diagram of normal nasopharyngeal passage in lateral view of neck.

neck. Size of adenoid enlargement does not correlate with clinical severity in a given patient.

Asthma

There will be bilateral hyperinflation due to air trapping. X-ray usually helps in identifying mimickers of asthma. Figures 4A to E show common mimickers of asthma in children.

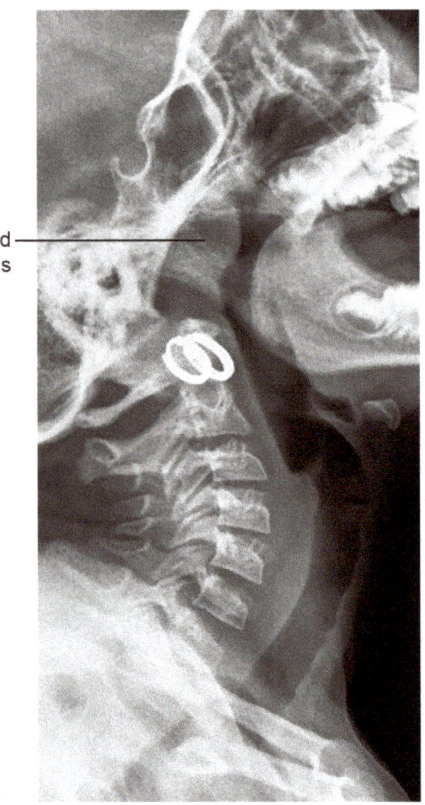

Fig. 3B: Adenoid hypertrophy in X-ray soft tissue neck—lateral view.

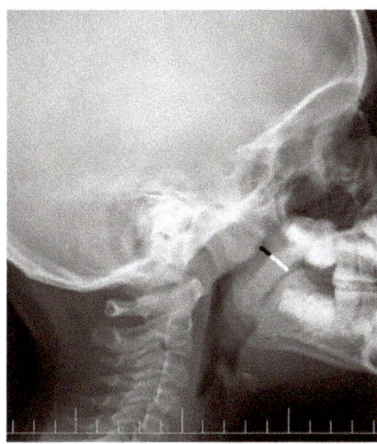

Fig. 3C: Cohen and Konak classification of adenoid hypertrophy by comparison of airway (black line) to soft palate (white line) ratio. Normal: Airway-to-soft-palate ratio ≥1; Mild-to-moderate hypertrophy: Ratio between 0.5 and 1; Severe hypertrophy: Ratio <0.5.
Source: Sharifkashani S, Dabirmoghaddam P, Kheirkhah M, et al. A new clinical scoring system for adenoid hypertrophy in children. Iranian J Otorhinolaryngol. 2015;27(1):55-61.

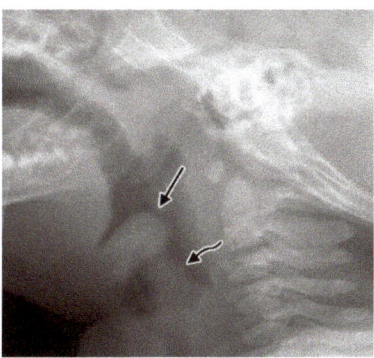

Fig. 4A: Epiglottitis: Swollen epiglottis; Hitchhiker's thumb (straight arrow) with thick aryepiglottic folds (curved arrow).

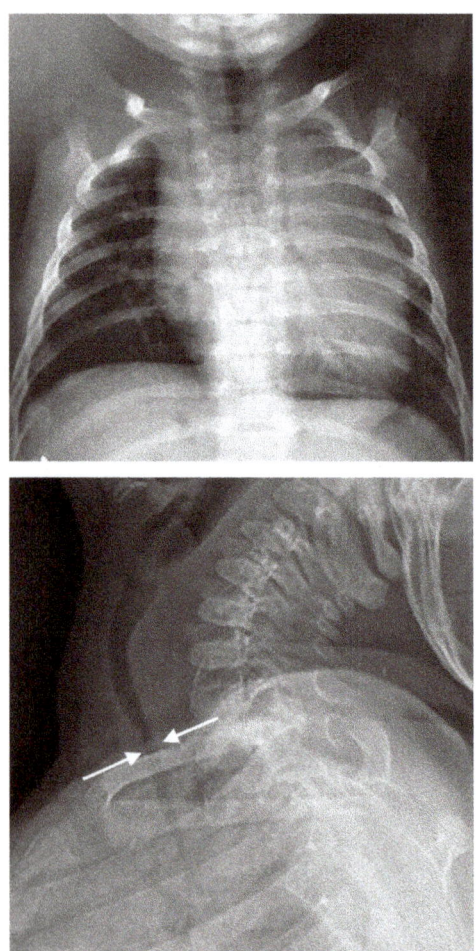

Fig. 4B: Tracheomalacia (anteroposterior and lateral view).

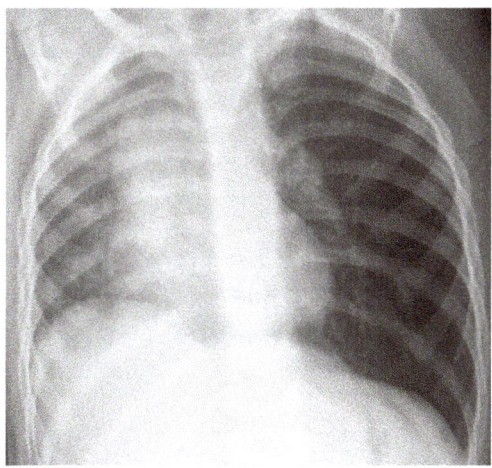

Fig. 4C: Left main bronchus foreign body; hyperinflation on left side.

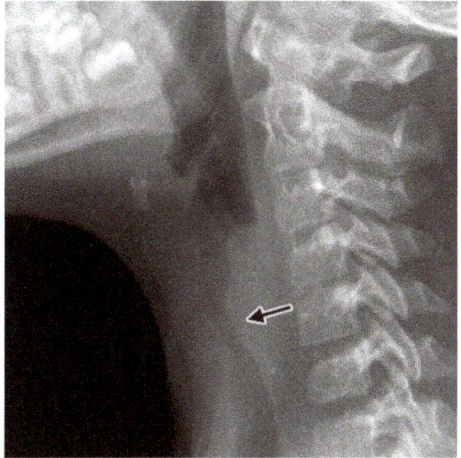

Fig. 4D: Bacterial tracheitis: Irregular narrowing of subglottic trachea.

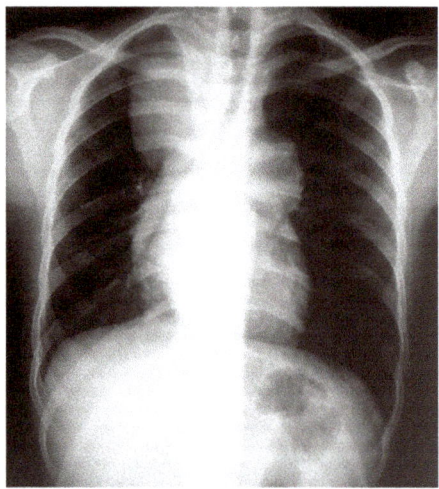

Fig. 4E: Extrinsic compression of airway by mediastinal mass.

SUGGESTED READING

1. Feres FN, Hermann JS, Sallum AC, et al. Radiographic adenoid evaluation: suggestion of referral parameters. J Pediatr (Rio J). 2014;90(3):279-85.
2. Fujioka M, Young LW, Girdany BR. Radiographic evaluation of adenoidal size in children: adenoidal-nasopharyngeal ratio. Am J Roentogen. 1979;133: 401-4.
3. Hoang JK, Eastwood JD, Tebbit CL, et al. Multiplanar sinus CT: a systemic approach to imaging before functional endoscopic sinus surgery. AJR Am J Roentgenol. 2010;194:W527-36.
4. Johnson JD, Theurer WM. A stepwise approach to the interpretation of pulmonary function tests. Am Fam Physician. 2014;89:359-66.
5. Momeni AK, Roberts CC, Chew FS. Imaging of chronic and exotic sinonasal disease: review. AJR Am J Roentgenol. 2007;189:S35-45.
6. Sharifkashani S, Dabirmoghaddam P, Kheirkhah M, et al. A new clinical scoring system for adenoid hypertrophy in children. Iran J Otorhinolaryng. 2015;78:55-61.

Newer Allergy Tests

INTRODUCTION

The conventional IgE-based allergy tests (skin prick and total or specific IgE) are insufficient for making correct allergy diagnosis in many clinical conditions. This could be due to other types of hypersensitivities apart from type I, nonimmunological mechanisms for certain allergic disorders, and diagnostic limitations of available techniques with significant false-positives and false-negatives. This creates a void in-between test results and clinical condition of the patient. Here, we are going to discuss some newer modalities and their potential in allergy testing.

NEWER AND ALTERNATE ALLERGY TESTS

- *Eosinophil count*: Eosinophilia is defined by temporary or permanent increase in circulating eosinophils more than $0.5 \times 10^9/L$. It can be generalized (blood eosinophilia) or localized (local tissue eosinophilia). Blood eosinophilia may be categorized as:
    - *Secondary reactive eosinophilia*: This is usually due to cytokine driven rise in eosinophil levels. The underlying causes could be "allergic" or "non-allergic" depending on the driving force. Allergic triggers cause activation of Th-2 pathway in response to an allergen exposure. Among the non-allergic causes, mostly are undetermined though a few might be mediated by IL-5 molecules like in "lymphoid variant of hypereosinophilic syndrome". Drug hypersensitivity, helminthiases (strongyloidiasis or toxocariasis), and other intestinal parasites (*Echinococcus*, filaria, schistosoma, etc.).

- *Primary neoplastic eosinophilia*: In this category, the usual causes are neoplastic with origin from stem cell, myeloid or eosinophils.
- *Hereditary eosinophilia*: Exact pathogenesis is unknown in this variant. There is some evidence of familial clustering present.
- *Due to immunologic disorders*: Immunodeficiency (DOCK8 deficiency, Omenn's syndrome, Hyper-IgE syndrome), autoimmune (sarcoidosis, inflammatory bowel disease, IgG4 disease and other connective tissue disorders) results in significant eosinophilia.
- *Miscellaneous*: Many causes of hypereosinophilia are attributed to radiation exposure, cholesterol emboli, hypoadrenalism, and IL-2 therapy.
- *Hypereosinophilia of undetermined significance*: This is usually a benign condition and cause of eosinophilia remains unknown with the currently available armamentarium of investigations.

Tissue hypereosinophilia may be defined as eosinophils more than 20% of all nucleated cells in a bone marrow aspirate, significantly increased tissue infiltration by eosinophils or extensive extracellular deposition of eosinophil-derived proteins in tissues.

Eosinophilia is commonly encountered in day-to-day practice. Though an important indicator of hematopoietic system activation due to varied etiologies, it is neither a sensitive or specific marker for allergic diseases.

- *Component resolved diagnostics*: Any particular allergenic substance can have many allergenic proteins, some of which have major allergenic potential and others minor. These allergenic components share structural homology with similar components in other allergens and giving false-positive results on crude allergen testing (both by skin prick or specific IgE based testing), a phenomenon of "cross reactivity".

Component resolved diagnostics (CRD) is the technique to detect specific IgE against individual allergen molecules or components using purified native or recombinant allergens. Using CRD, we can better diagnose, prognose, and grade the food allergy. Table 1 demonstrates various components of food allergens and their clinical significance.

- *Cytotoxic food testing (Bryan's test)*: The procedure consists of adding patient's serum (with white blood cells) to a dried

Table 1: Clinical characteristics of food allergen components.

Antigen	Components	Characteristics
Egg	Gal d 1 (ovomucoid)	Heat stable, no form of egg will be tolerated, delayed tolerance development
	Gal d 2 (ovalbumin)	Heat labile, boiled egg may be tolerated
Milk	Bos d 4 (α-lactoglobulin)	Heal labile, likely to tolerate milk after boiling for 15–20 minutes at >90°C
	Bos d 5 (β-lactoglobulin)	
	Bos d 8 (caseins)	Heat stable, will not tolerate any form of milk, high chances of prolonged allergy
Wheat	Gliadin	Associated with persistent wheat allergy, asthma development in children
	Omega-5 gliadin	Associated with immediate wheat hypersensitivity reaction
	Lipid transfer protein (LTP)	Associated with Baker's asthma, causes immediate symptoms
	Alpha-amylase inhibitors	Causes immediate symptoms
Soybean	Gly m 4 (Bet v 1 homolog)	Causes oral allergy syndrome and severe systemic reactions in birch allergic patients due to cross reactivity, heat labile allergen, tolerates fermented products
	Gly m 5 (7S globulin)	Causes severe allergic reactions
	Gly m 6 (11S globulin)	
	Gly m 8 (2S albumin)	Major allergen, best diagnostic marker for soybean allergy

Contd...

Contd...

Antigen	Components	Characteristics
Peanuts	Ara h 1 (7S globulin)	h 1,2 and 3 associated with severe reactions, h 2 is best diagnostic marker
	Ara h 2 (2S globulin)	
	Ara h 3 (11S globulin)	
	Ara h 6 (Bet v 1 homolog)	Cosensitization to h 2 and h 6 is associated with severe reactions
	Ara h 8 (Bet v 1 homolog)	No to very mild symptoms
	Ara h 9 (LTP)	Mild to severe symptoms
Hazelnut	Cor a 1 (Bet v 1 homolog)	Cross reactivity
	Cor a 9 (11S globulin)	Predicts clinical reactivity
	Cor a 14 (2S albumin)	
Cashew nut	Ana o 3 (2S albumin)	Highly predictive of cashew and pistachio allergy
Walnut	Jug r 1 (2S albumin)	Inherently allergic
	Jug r 2	Low clinical significance
	Jug r 3	Causes local symptoms
Brazil nut	Ber e 1 (2S albumin)	Predicts clinical reactivity
Sesame	Ses i 1 (2S albumin)	Best diagnostic marker
Buckwheat	Fag e 3 (7S globulin)	Improved diagnostic accuracy

food extract solution on a microscope slide. During a periodic examination of slide over next 2 hours, cytotoxic effects can be visualized in the white blood cells if patient is sensitive to that particular food item. There are many fallacies with this procedure like subjective interpretation and lack of correlation between test results and clinical allergy. The efficacy of Bryan's test has not been supported by scientific literature.

- *Provocation-neutralization*: This technique was used for testing sensitivity of food and environmental chemicals. Escalating doses of suspected substances are administered under the tongue or injected in the skin. If symptoms start developing, the test is considered positive, and then doses are further escalated till symptoms are neutralized. This neutralization process mimics the desensitization process but the subjective response makes this provocation-neutralization inferior.

- *Kinesiology*: This test works on the assumption that body muscles are sensitive to anything that is harmful to it. So, a potential food allergen causes weakness in the muscles of an allergic patient. There are occasional reports comparing results of applied kinesiology with serum IgE levels in patients with food allergy. This test is highly nonspecific and is not recommended.
- *Iridology*: The technique depends upon a belief that each part of the body is represented by a corresponding part of iris. Change in iris color, texture, and location of pigment flecks in eye determines health or disease in particular individual. This is an unproven technique.
- *Electrodermal/Vega testing*: An increased body's resistance to electric current, measured by a galvanometer, may be a sign of allergy once patient is exposed to certain food items. This logic is not supported by any scientific evidence.
- *Radionics (psionic medicine, dowsing)*: This is based on the claim that all living creatures on this earth are submerged in the electromagnetic energy field. Subtle changes in energy and vibrations from internal organs caused by a suspected food in sensitive individuals may suggest food allergy. This technique lacks scientific evidence.
- *Pulse testing reflexology*: This technique works on the hypothesis that sympathetic nervous system is stimulated during an allergic reaction causing a temporary increase in heart rate. This test has not shown any promising results in allergy diagnosis.
- *Hair analysis*: Various trace elements are measured from hair to determine nutritional deficiencies and excess. For allergy diagnosis, there is no role of this technique.
- *Lymphocyte subset analysis*: This technique is conventionally used for detecting suspected immunodeficiency or lymphoid malignancy. There have been recent claims of its use in detecting

chronic fatigue syndrome or environmental allergies, however, these claims have not been backed up by scientific evidence.
- *IgG/IgG4 testing*: These are indicative of protective response and may be of benefit for assessment of immunotherapy response.

SUGGESTED READING

1. ASCIA. (2007). ASCIA Position Statement—Unorthodox techniques for the diagnosis and treatment of allergy, asthma and immune disorders. [online] Available from https://www.allergy.org.au/hp/papers/unorthodox-techniques-for-diagnosis-and-treatment [Accessed December 2018].
2. Borres MP, Maruyama N, Sato S, et al. Recent advances in component resolved diagnosis in food allergy. Allergology International. 2016;65: 378-87.
3. Jewitt DL, Fein G, Greenberg MH. A double-blind study of symptom provocation to determine food sensitivity. N Engl J Med. 1990;323(7): 429-33.
4. Magnaval JF, Laurent G, Gaudre N, et al. A diagnostic protocol designed for determining allergic causes in patients with blood eosinophilia. Mil Med Res. 2017;4:15.
5. Singh V, Gomez VV, Swamy SG, et al. Approach to a case of eosinophilia. IJASM. 2009;53(2):58-64.
6. Statement on cytotoxic testing for food allergy (Bryan's test). Committee of Public Health. Bull NY Acad Med. 1988;64(1):117-9.
7. Williams KW, Ware J, Abiodun A, et al. Hypereosinophilia in children and adults: a retrospective comparison. J Allergy Clin Immunol Pract. 2016;4(5):941-7.

Management of Allergies

INTRODUCTION

Correct identification of allergen(s) should be associated with adequate preventive and curative measures. Dietary manipulations in infancy have been proposed as ways to alter Th1/Th2 balance with variable results. Maternal diet during pregnancy is an important area to be focused on. Despite various precautions, allergies are unavoidable for many with pharmacotherapy remains the only feasible alternative. Currently available drugs suppresses the allergic symptoms temporarily creating scope for long-term immune tolerance development with immunotherapy.

PREVENTION

Allergy prevention can be done at three levels:
- *Primary prevention*: It is recommended in individuals with high risk of allergy like familial history of atopy. Suggested steps for allergy control are:
    - Exclusive breastfeeding for 4-6 months
    - Hydrolyzed formula, rather than cow's milk, to be started for infants who are not breast fed (for any reasons)
    - Major allergenic foods (cow's milk, egg, soy, wheat, peanut, tree nuts, fish and shellfish) should be introduced at 4-6 months of age in a sequential manner at home
    - Probiotic (lactobacilli) or prebiotic (oligosaccharides influencing the intestinal microflora) supplements—inconclusive evidence
    - Any dietary avoidance, as an allergy preventive measure, during pregnancy is not recommended
    - Outdoor activities should be encouraged.

- *Secondary prevention*: Once the allergy has occurred in an individual, allergen exposure needs to be reduced in the environment. The preventive steps could be:
  - For indoor allergens:
    - Dusting should be reduced, wet mopping should be promoted
    - Vacuum cleaners are advocated
    - Air purifiers may be beneficial
    - Relative humidity should be reduced; dehumidifiers may be helpful
    - Beddings, mattresses, pillow covers, curtains should be washed periodically (at least once a week) and sun dried
    - Pets should be kept out of house, if possible
    - Pets should be regularly washed (at least once a week) and they should not be allowed in the bedrooms
    - Both indoor and outdoor smoking needs to be stopped
    - Mosquito coil, liquid or creams are not recommended. Only mosquito nets are advised.
  - For outdoor allergens:
    - Regional pollen calendars are helpful. Avoid going outdoors at the time of high pollen counts
    - Avoid going out on dusty surroundings
    - Avoid both active and passive smoking
    - Occupational exposure to relevant allergen needs to be avoided
    - Face mask (respirators) should be used in high polluted areas: N95 and N99.
- *Tertiary prevention*: This is meant to be done after onset of disease and targets for exacerbation prevention, improving disease control and reducing medication needs.
  - Allergen exposure should be reduced
  - Pollution (both indoor and outdoor) needs to be curtailed
  - Periodic functional assessment of patient needs to be done

- Controller and preventer therapy needs titration for better control with minimal side effects and improved quality of life.

Specific Preventive Measures

- House dust mite:
  - Special microweave covers for mattress, duvet and pillows
  - Regular washing of bedsheets, curtains, covers in hot water (>55°C) and sun drying
  - Foam carpets should be replaced by hard floorings
  - Regular vacuum cleaning
  - Replacement of fabric covers with leather or vinyl coverings
  - Replacement of curtains with blinds
  - Use of dehumidifiers to reduce the relative humidity (RH) and to keep RH in between 35-50%.
- House dust:
  - Avoid dusting
  - Allergic person should not visit the previously dusted area for at least 3-4 hours (average time taken by dust to settle)
  - Promote wet mopping
  - Use vacuum cleaners
  - Use of air purifiers: Purifiers with high efficiency particulate air (HEPA) filter efficiency, better minimum efficiency reporting value (MERV) rating (preferable 16-20) and high clean air delivery rate (CADR) factor should be preferred. Living room area and periodic cleaning of filters should be kept in mind. Ozone purifiers are not recommended.
- Pollens:
  - Pollen calendar of residential or occupational area should be used as a guide to delineate particular pollen/s as culprit allergen in an individual
  - Daily pollen count monitoring will be helpful
  - Avoid going outdoors on high pollen days
  - Respirator face mask should be used.

- Pets:
    - Ideally pets should be removed from the house
    - If pet cannot be removed, it should not be allowed in the living area or bed room
    - HEPA filter cleaners should be used to reduce dander levels
    - Weekly washing of pets is advised.
- Occupational allergens:
    - Proper precautions should be taken for contact exposure (rubber gloves to be used for chemical hypersensitivity)
    - Non-powdered or non-latex gloves use for latex allergy
    - Exhaust and HEPA filters should be implanted for removal of chemical fumes
    - May require occupational change in case of intractable allergies.
- Milk allergy:
    - Dairy products for both child and mother (in case of breast feeding) should be stopped
    - Exclusively breastfeeding should be promoted up to 6 months of age
    - After 6 months, partially or fully hydrolyzed milk formulas are recommended
    - Soya milk may be use, though 15% of milk allergic patients may be allergic to soya too.

Pharmacotherapy

Various pharmacological and nonpharmacological therapeutic measures have been previously discussed. The main aim should be use of optimal treatment with adequate disease control and minimal adverse effects. Pharmacotherapy can control the allergic phenomenon for a short duration but cannot modify the disease. For disease remission, body's allergenic tendency needs to be changed to nonallergenic, which is possible with immune teaching or immunotherapy.

Immunotherapy

Immunotherapy, also called as immune teaching, is a process of tolerance induction to specific allergens (Fig. 1). Minimum number of allergens (preferable <5) should be chosen based upon skin-prick test results and clinical relevance. Respective allergens are introduced in the body via various routes, in minimal concentration and gradually escalated to maintenance doses. These allergens can produce biochemical changes in the body but unable to produce allergic reaction by themselves. Immunotherapy targets conversion of allergic Th2 response to nonallergic Th1 response.

Early desensitization starts from day 1 of induction at tissue level (Fig. 2) with reduction in mast cell and basophil activities.

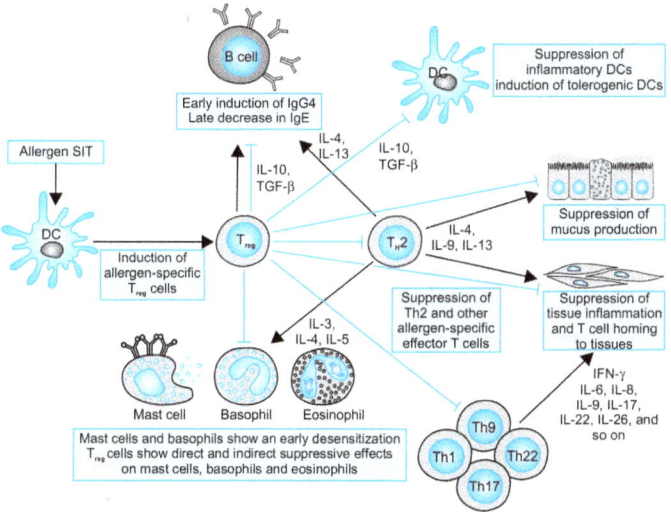

Fig. 1: Immunotherapy; mechanism of action. Immunotherapy causes reduction in IL-4 and IL-13, increase in IL-10 and TGF-β. By this process, it induced tolerogenic dendritic cells.

(SIT: specific immunotherapy; IL: interleukin; DC: dendritic cells; T_{reg}: T regulatory cells; Th: T helper cells; TGF: tissue growth factor; IFN: interferon)

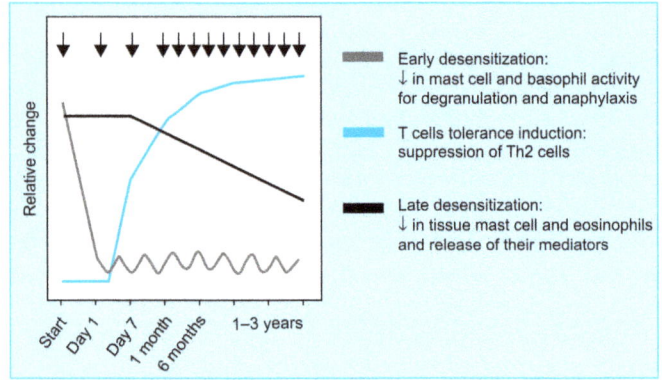

Fig. 2: Temporal response of immunotherapy to specific allergens.

Suppression of Th2 cells starts after a week and clinical response is usually evident by 6 months of continuous therapy with reduction in mast cells mediators. IgE levels might increase in early stages but later on IgG4 levels predominates with rise in IgG4:IgE ratio as a surrogate biochemical marker of successful immunotherapy response.

Failure of immunotherapy should be considered if there is no response after 1 year of continuous allergen targeted immunotherapy. Reduction of symptom and/or medication score at 1 year is considered to be treatment success. Once started, the minimum duration for which immunotherapy should be given is 3–5 years. There are several long-term prospective studies documenting beneficial effects of immunotherapy even after 2 decades of course completion.

The common routes of delivering immunotherapy are subcutaneous immunotherapy (SCIT) and sublingual immunotherapy (SLIT). Table 1 highlights the salient features of both types of routes. There is a situation of equipoise between both routes of administration as one seems to be more efficacious and other have better safety profile.

Table 1: Comparison of different routes of immunotherapy delivery.

Route	SCIT	SLIT
Ease of administration	Less	More
Personnel required for administration	Physician	Self/Family member
Frequency of visits required to health center	More	Less
Chances of anaphylaxis	Reported	Not reported
Chances of less severe systemic reactions	Less	Very less
Local side effects	Can occur	Can occur
Efficacy	More efficacious	Less efficacious
Safety profile	Less	More

(SCIT: subcutaneous immunotherapy; SLIT: sublingual immunotherapy)

Selection of Patients for Allergen Immunotherapy

- Allergic rhinitis: Best candidates
- Allergic asthma: Once the symptoms are adequately controlled with pharmacotherapy
- Insect hypersensitivity.

Age Limit for Immunotherapy

No absolute lower cutoff limit. Recommendations are for more than 3 years of age but reports for successful usage over 1 year are present in literature.

Prerequisites for Allergen Extracts

- Adequate doses of standardized allergen extracts
- Consider cross reactivity
- Avoid mixing extracts of strong proteolytic activity with susceptible extracts; Fungal and cockroach extracts have high proteolytic activity, so these should not be mixed with other susceptible allergen extracts

- Use glycerinated extracts of fungi & cockroaches to retain their allergenicity for prolonged period.

Schedule for Subcutaneous Immunotherapy

- **Rush:** It involves multiple injections over a single day or consecutive days. As there are more chances of severe systemic reactions including anaphylaxis, hence pretreatment with antihistamines is recommended. It usually requires hospitalization for initial few doses.
- **Cluster:** 2-3 injections are given per day with injection free days in between. It is not associated with serious reactions and still produces acceptable results.
- **Conventional:** It is started twice weekly and then doses and interval are gradually increased to weekly and then monthly. Results are best with negligible risk.

Allergoids

The molecular structure of allergens can be altered by chemical treatment with either glutaraldehyde or formalin. This reduces allergenicity but retains the immunogenicity. These are safer and maintenance doses can be achieved more rapidly.

Future of Immunotherapy

Allergoids have potential for safe, rapid and effective immunotherapy. There are early reports using oral immunotherapy for milk and egg allergy but no consensus has reached till date.

SUGGESTED READING

1. Cox L, Nelson H, Lockey R. Allergen Immunotherapy: A Practice Parameter. Third Update. J Allergy Clin Immunol. 2011;127:S1-S55.
2. Fleischer DM, Spergel JM, Assa'ad AH, et al. Primary prevention of allergic disease through nutritional interventions. J Allergy Clin Immunol: In Practice. 2013;1:29-36.
3. Frew AJ, Powell RJ, Corrigan CJ, et al. Efficacy and safety of specific immunotherapy with SQ allergen extract in treatment-resistant seasonal allergic rhinoconjunctivitis. J Allergy Clin Immunol. 2006;117:319-28.

4. Marinho S, Simpson A, Custovic A. Allergen avoidance in the secondary and tertiary prevention of allergic diseases: does it work? Prim Care Respir J. 2006;15(3):152-8.
5. Mavroudi A, Xinias I. Dietary interventions for primary allergy prevention in infants. Hippokratia. 2011;15(3):216-22.
6. Shamji MH, Durham SR. Mechanisms of allergen immunotherapy for inhaled allergens and predictive biomarkers. J Allergy Clin Immunol. 2017;140: 1485-98.

Complementary Medicine in Allergy

INTRODUCTION

Complementary and alternative medicine (CAM) is a group of medical and healthcare system, practices and products that are not a part of conventional medicine. These include herbal therapy, homeopathy, acupuncture, ayurveda and behavior modification techniques.

HOLISTIC APPROACH

It recognizes the emotional, mental, spiritual and physical elements of an individual and attempts to treat in whole. This approach is commonly used for chronic diseases like heart problems, diabetes, allergies and asthma. This approach helps through adequate nutrition, stress reduction and effective gentle remedies. It may include different systems of medicine like ayurveda, herbal drugs, homeopathy, naturopathy, siddha, unani and other alternative medicines.

Common Reasons and Beliefs for Complementary and Alternative Medicine Use

- Conventional medicines ineffective
- Side effects from conventional medicines
- Difficult to adhere to conventional therapy
- CAM is safer
- Desire to use natural products
- Disease with bad prognosis
- Recommendations from friends, family or media
- Ability to treat illness without seeing a physician.

Various Types of Complementary and Alternative Medicines

- *Herbals*: Several herbal therapies have been proposed in the literature (Table 1). Figures 1A to C show commonly available anti-asthma preparations.
- *Homeopathy*: It works on the principle of treatment with "similar." Smaller escalating doses of same substance is given to patient in order to modify the immune response. The commonly used remedies are onion (allergic rhinitis), eyebright, white arsenic, poison nut, wind flower, salt, goldenrod, house dust mite, Indian cockroach, potassium dichromate and histamine.
- *Acupuncture*: It works on the principle of redistribution of life energy. By using various needles at specific body points, flow of body energy is modified in the favorable direction.
- *Ayurveda*: It includes yoga, meditation, breathing exercises and herbal preparations. The main principle behind this system is "promotion of health" rather than "prevention of specific disease."
- *Behavior modification techniques*: It includes yoga and breathing retraining, especially useful for asthmatic patients.
- *Apitherapy*: Using periodic bee stings intentionally to treat specific inflammatory disorders for bronchitis and arthritis.
- *Halotherapy*: Using dry aerosol microparticles of salt and other minerals in chronic respiratory diseases with mucosal inflammation like asthma, sinusitis and rhinitis.
- *Magical potions*: Healing is claimed through medium of inspired concoctions of medicaments. These toxic herbs are foul-smelling mixtures and produce emesis or expectoration which was considered as equivalent to driving out evil spirits. Some interesting magical remedies are still used widely like swallowing newborn live mice, eating fried bat or consuming gecko (lizard) tails or earthworms.
- *Psychologic therapies*: Mesmerism, hypnotism, biofeedback mechanisms can change autonomic imbalance. Meditation

Table 1: Commonly used herbs in allergy and asthma.

Herb	Mechanism of action	Adverse effect noted
Allium cepa (onion)	Inhibits mast cell degranulation	Strong odor
Aloe arborescens	Bronchodilation	Electrolyte imbalance, abdominal cramp, pseudomelanosis coli
Atropa belladonna	Anticholinergic and bronchodilator action	Ataxia, hallucinations, extrapyramidal reactions, reduced bowel movements, photophobia, tachycardia, increased thirst and urinary retention
Bu-Zhong-Yi-Qi-Tang (traditional Chinese medicine)	Decreased capillary permeability; decreased eosinophils, CD4 cells, IL-4 and IL-5; inhibit Th2 cell response	None
Caffeine	Bronchodilator	Insomnia, GERD, hypertension
Coleus forskohlii	Bronchodilator	Hypokalemia, tremor
Datura stramonium (jimson weed)	Bronchodilator	Ataxia, hallucinations, extrapyramidal reactions, reduced bowel movements, photophobia, tachycardia, increased thirst and urinary retention
Echinacea	In vitro antiviral effects vs influenza	Anaphylaxis, bronchospasm, urticaria, angioedema, hepatitis, hypertension, acute renal failure, vasculitis
Eucalyptus	Cold/influenza remedy, mucokinetic, decongestant, cockroach repellent	Allergic reaction
Chamazulene (chamomile)	Leukotriene inhibitor	Botulism
Goldenseal (hydrazine)	Treatment of URI, diarrhea, conjunctivitis, acute otitis media, eczema	Nausea, vomiting, diarrhea, hypertension
Hi Chun (Korean)	Mast cell stabilizer, inhibits histamine release	

Contd...

Contd...

Herb	Mechanism of action	Adverse effect noted
Jisil (Korean)	Mast cell stabilizer, reduce IgE production	
Kutki/kuuro (Indian)	Mast cell stabilizer	
Licorice	Blocks histamine induced capillary permeability, inhibits PAF, antitussive	Hypokalemia, hyperaldosteronism
Ma huang (ephedra) Wu-hu-tang	Sympathomimetic activity, inhibits mast cell degranulation	Hypertension, tachycardia, palpitations, nervousness, headache, insomnia, dizziness, euphoria, nephrolithiasis, seizure, stroke, myocardial infarction
Menthol (mint)	Decongestant action	May be fatal
Minor Blue Dragon	Mast cell stabilizer	
Peppermint oil (mint)	Decongestant action, mast cell stabilizer	Cardiac arrhythmias
Sho-seiryu-to (Japanese)	Decrease IgE-mediated cutaneous reactions, complement inhibition, anticholinergic effect leads to drying of secretions	
Urtica dioica (nettle)	Used for treatment of allergic rhinitis	Contact urticaria with natural plant leaves, diarrhea, gastric irritation, edema, oliguria
Tylophora indica (India)	Bronchodilator	Nausea, vomiting and sore mouth
Saiboku-to (Japanese) Chaipo-tang (Chinese)	Increased endogenous cortisol levels	Pneumonia

can reduce wastage of energy and hence oxygen consumption. It can be achieved by relaxing, singing, chanting, listening to music, exercising and effective coughing.
- *Laser therapy*: It utilizes laser light to specific target tissues like endobronchial tissue, tympanic membrane, blood and skin.
- *Probiotics*: *Lactobacillus rhamnosus* has been used in infants and children for late induction of IL-10 and reduce allergic responses.

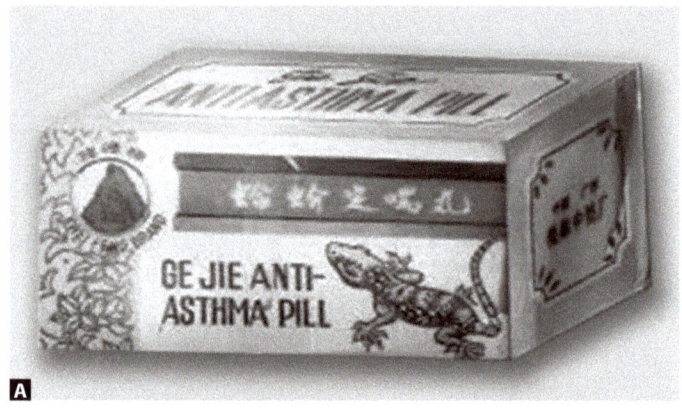
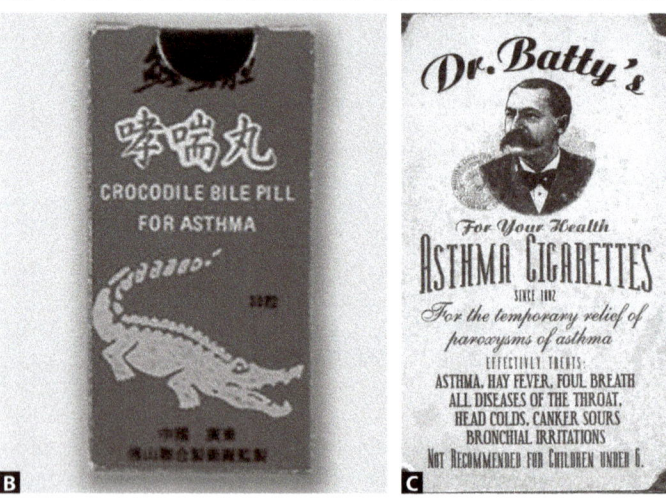

Figs. 1A to C: Available anti-asthma preparation. (A) Ge Jie anti-asthma pill contains apricot kernels, cinnabar, coptidis, ephedra, gecko lizard tail, licorice, ophiopogon and scutellaria; (B) Crocodile bile pill for asthma contains adenophora, asparagus, aster, calcium sulfate, crocodile bile, ephedra, gypsum, lily, ophiopogon, orange peel, peony, perilla, peucedanum, platycodon, scutellaria and trichosanthes; (C) Asthma cigarettes (Joy cigarettes) contains stramonium.
Source: Ziment I, Tashkin DP. Alternative medicine for allergy and asthma. J Allergy Clin Immunol. 2000;106(4):603-14.

Complementary and Alternative Medicine in Food Allergies

Researchers have tried many CAM therapies (Table 2) for food allergies. More scientific research and evidence are required before any final approval.

Ethical-legal Issues of Complementary and Alternative Medicine

The risks associated with CAM in form of direct toxicity and lack of beneficial evidence can put physicians at risk of liability for using CAM. Combining conventional therapy associated with CAM is an important issue and the answer needs to be individualized as per the current evidence:

Table 2: Proposed complementary and alternative medicine (CAM) use in food allergies.

CAM drug/technique	Mechanism of action
FAHF-2	• Blocks vascular leakage • Inhibits IgE production • Long-lasting beneficial effects on T and B cells in vivo
B-FAHF-2	• Dose-dependent inhibition of IgE production • In vitro suppression of Th2 cytokines • Enhancement of Th1 cytokines secretion
Berberine	• Inhibits IgE production • Suppression of IgE isotype switching
7,4'-dihydroxyflavone	• Inhibits GATA3 expression—reduces IL-4, IL-5 and IL-13
Ganoderic acid C1	• Inhibits TNF-α
Ganoderic acid B	• Inhibits TNF-α
Kakkonto	• Reduces Th1 cytokines (IFN-γ) and Th2 cytokines (IL-4, IL-5 and IL-10) • Increase Foxp3-positive cells in colonic mucosa
Acupuncture	• Reduces basophil activity
Probiotics	• Reduced peanut-specific IgE levels and skin prick test response with increased specific IgG4 levels • Downregulates Th2 responses

- Evidence for efficacy and safety present—acupuncture for chemotherapy-induced nausea
- Evidence for safety present but inconclusive for efficacy—homeopathy for rhinitis
- Evidence supports efficacy but inconclusive for safety—ginkgo for dementia
- Evidence indicates serious risk for safety and not useful—injections of unapproved substances, unknown interactions.

CONCLUSION

Complementary and alternative medicine is getting more and more popular for chronic ailments like allergies and asthma. Some of these might be helpful either alone or in combination with conventional therapies, however, more scientific evidence for their efficacy and safety is required before mass prescription.

SUGGESTED READING

1. Bielory L. Complementary and alternative medicine in the treatment of allergic and asthmatic disease. In: M. Mahmoudi (Ed). Chapter in Allergy and Asthma. 2016:531-52.
2. Land MH, Wang J. Complementary and alternative medicine use among allergy practices: results of a nationwide survey of allergists. J Allergy Clin Immunol Prac. 2018;6(1):95-8.
3. Li XM. Complementary and alternative medicine for treatment of food allergy. Immunol Allergy Clin N Am. 2018;38(1):103-24.
4. Ullman D, Frass M. A review of homeopathic research in the treatment of respiratory allergies. Altern Med Rev. 2010;15(1):48-58.
5. Ziment I, Tashkin DP. Alternative medicine for allergy and asthma. J Allergy Clin Immunol. 2000;106(4):603-14.

Myths and Beliefs about Allergies

Belief: Allergic disorders are due to weakened immunity of an individual

Fact: False

Explanation: Allergic reactions are an abnormal response of one's body to a harmless object. These could be mediated by various mechanisms. The most common allergic reactions are mediated by increased production of immunoglobulin E (IgE) after exposure to an allergen in a predisposed individual. Hence, allergies are not associated with weakened immunity rather these indicate an exaggerated abnormal immune response.

Belief: High IgE levels indicate allergy and normal IgE levels rule out allergy

Fact: False

Explanation: Allergic reactions can be mediated via various immunologic and nonimmunologic mechanisms; IgE-mediated hypersensitivity is only one of several types. Even in IgE-mediated hypersensitivity, the response to particular allergen might raise the specific IgE only but this may be insufficient to cause an effect on total IgE levels. So, a normal total IgE level does not rule out possibility of allergy.

On the other hand, IgE may be raised in many conditions apart from allergies like parasitic infections, viral infections (Epstein-Barr virus, cytomegalovirus, respiratory syncytial virus, human immunodeficiency virus), immunodeficiency states (Hyper-IgE, Wiskott-Aldrich, Di-George syndrome), neoplastic conditions (Hodgkin's disease, IgE myeloma), others (nephrotic syndrome, nephritis, liver disease, cystic fibrosis, Kawasaki disease, Guillain-

Barre syndrome), etc. So, high IgE levels alone should not be considered a marker of allergy.

Belief: Allergic disorders can never be cured

Fact: False

Explanation: In many of the IgE-mediated allergies, if culprit allergen is found, immunotherapy may be highly effective like insect hypersensitivity, allergens like house dust mite, and even certain pollens.

Belief: Allergies can affect only respiratory system

Fact: False

Explanation: Allergies can affect any body system and the symptomatology mostly depends upon route of exposure. Symptoms of rhinitis, conjunctivitis or asthma are usually caused due to allergen inhalation; urticaria and atopic dermatitis are caused due to skin exposure and allergen ingestion (systemic exposure) usually leads to angioedema and anaphylaxis. Important mind-body (psychosomatic) interactions are disturbed in case of prolonged and severe allergic states.

Belief: All allergies start in childhood

Fact: False

Explanation: Allergic symptoms can start at any age in a previously asymptomatic individual. People with family history of atopy usually get early symptoms. Also skin symptoms (eczema) predominate in children followed by asthma and allergic rhinitis, whereas, allergic rhinitis is the most common allergy in adults. The phenomenon of change of symptoms from dermatitis to asthma to rhinitis with age is called as 'allergy march'.

Belief: Hypersensitivity, allergy, and atopy are same

Fact: False

Explanation: Hypersensitivity is the phenomenon of reproducible signs and symptoms, initiated by exposure to defined stimulus that is tolerated by normal subjects. It could be mediated by various immunological or nonimmunological mechanisms. The most commonly used immunological mechanism is IgE mediated, commonly called allergy, others could be IgG mediated (anaphylaxis to dextran) and lymphocyte mediated (contact dermatitis). A personal or familial tendency to become sensitized and produce IgE antibodies in response to allergens is called atopy.

Belief: If you are allergic to one dog, you are allergic to all dogs
Fact: False

Explanation: Dog allergens are species specific so any dog could be allergenic to one person and hypo- or non-allergenic to another individual.

Belief: Regular washing of pets reduces allergies
Fact: True

Explanation: In a pet allergic individual, ideally pet should be removed from the surroundings. If pet removal is not possible due to any reason, keep pets outdoors. There should be at least 8 hours of pet free zone in the bedroom. Pet allergies are due to dander, skin, and body proteins in animal's urine, saliva, and skin. Do not allow pets on furniture to reduce dander levels. Regular vacuum cleaning of furniture and beddings is recommended. High efficiency particulate air filter (HEPA) (air purifiers) can help in dander removal from air. Washing of pets at least once a week is useful to reduce the dander levels.

Belief: If you are allergic to one cat, you are allergic to all cats
Fact: True

Explanation: Cats have universal allergens. If an individual is allergic to one cat, he or she will be allergic to most of the cats. Cat dander levels remain in the surroundings even 3–6 months after removal of cat from the place.

Belief: Rains reduces allergies
Fact: Partially true

Explanation: Tree pollen counts are higher during dry seasons. Counts are highest between 10 am and 4 pm on dry, hot, and windy days. Less moisture permits the pollen grains to reach farthest places when the wind blows. Light steady rain showers can wash pollen and reduces pollen allergy.

Grass and weed pollen counts are higher during rains. Water droplets can break the pollen clumps into individual pollens and assist in their dispersion. This happens more during sudden, heavy downpours. During rainy season, molds and dust mite concentration increases causing increase in symptoms in sensitive individuals.

To sum up, light and steady rain fall reduces pollen allergies whereas sudden and heavy rain may have deleterious effects on individuals with pollen allergies. Patients with mold or dust mite sensitization will have worsening of symptoms during and immediately after rainy season due to increase in humidity.

Belief: Neighbor's yard is the cause of your allergy

Fact: Partially true

Explanation: Pollens from tree, grass, and weeds can travel hundreds of kilometers with wind and can cause symptoms. Flora in the neighbors' yard might not be responsible for one's symptoms. A careful history about type of symptoms, seasonal and diurnal variation, aggravating and relieving factors, and environmental exposure assisted with targeted allergy testing will be helpful about pointing the culprit allergens.

Belief: Toxic black molds in bathroom are the culprit for my allergies

Fact: False

Explanation: Black mold (*Stachybotrys*) is commonly found in buildings and ceilings of washroom. It is very sticky and cannot travel via air so not likely to cause allergic symptoms. It can be cleaned with dilute bleach solution.

Belief: I have asthma, I cannot play or exercise

Fact: False

Explanation: You are allergic to some allergen but not to exercise or play. Exercise is the only trigger, which should be promoted in an asthmatic child. Patients should take preventer medications daily, may require controllers before unaccustomed exercise, breath through nose, and stay hydrated. Warming up for 10 minutes is helpful before the actual strenuous exercise or play.

Belief: Inhalers are habit forming, they are bad
Fact: False

Explanation: Anything which is not required, is bad for the body. Inhaled medicines have rapid and direct action on the inflamed airway mucosa. The symptomatic relief from original pathology may prompt an individual to take inhalers for a prolonged time, however, nebulizers and inhalers are not habit forming by themselves. On the contrary, a deserving patient if does not take his regular medications regularly (as advised by physician), the airway inflammation will worsen and compromise the quality and quantity of life. Any medication (oral or inhaled) should be taken under physician supervision with regular follow-up to optimize the treatment.

Belief: Air pollution increases allergic symptoms
Fact: True

Explanation: Air pollution and asthma have synergistic effect on asthma and allergies. Inhalable particulate matter (PM), due to their intrinsic electrostatic properties and porous surfaces, readily adhere to airborne allergens and promote their allergenicity. The direct effects of air pollution are inflammation and irritation of airways.

Major outdoor pollutants are produced from vehicular fuel combustion, construction and agricultural operations, power plants, and industries. Primary pollutants are carbon monoxide (CO), nitrogen dioxide (NO_2), sulfur dioxide (SO_2), and polycyclic aromatic hydrocarbons (PAHs). Ozone (O_3) is a secondary air pollutant as produced by reaction between NO_2 and volatile organic compounds (VOCs) in presence of heat and sunlight. Common indoor pollutants are CO, carbon dioxide (CO_2), NO_2, SO_2, VOCs, phthalates, formaldehyde, PM, and PAHs. These are produced by environmental tobacco smoke (ETS), biomass fuel, cleaning products, and biological allergens.

Belief: Size of particulate matter is directly related to type of allergic disease

Fact: True

Explanation: Particulate matter is a mixture of various particles (solid and liquid) which can be categorized into different categories as per their diameter (Fig. 1):

- PM_{10} (diameter ≤10 μm)—penetrate into upper respiratory tract (nose, throat, and larynx)
- $PM_{10\text{-}2.5}$ (diameter from 2.5–10 μm)—penetrate upper respiratory tract (nose, throat, and larynx)
- $PM_{2.5}$ (diameter ≤2.5 μm)—penetrate into tracheobronchial tract (trachea, bronchi, and bronchioles)
- $PM_{0.1}$ (diameter ≤0.1 μm)—penetrate into alveoli.

Studies suggests an important link between PM_{10} and allergic rhinitis whereas $PM_{2.5}$ is found to be associated with increased incidence of both rhinitis and asthma. $PM_{0.1}$ are associated with

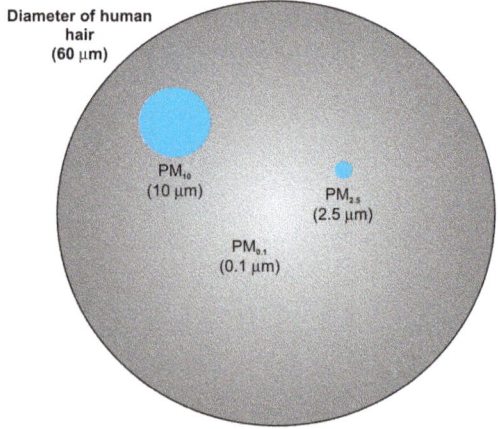

Fig. 1: Dimensional comparison of various particulate matter (PM) sizes with human hair.

Source: Baldacci S, Maio S, Cerrai S, et al. Allergy and asthma: effects of the exposure to particular matter and biological allergens. Respirator Med. 2015;109:1089-104.

subclinical molecular changes that manifest disease exacerbations and individual's predisposition toward symptoms. Improvement in respiratory mortality has been observed with 10 μg/m³ reduction of $PM_{2.5}$.

Belief: Living near heavy traffic roads causes more allergies

Fact: True

Explanation: People living in close proximity (within 100 meters) to heavy traffic density have more aeroallergies and reduced lung functions.

Belief: Air purifier can reduce my allergy

Fact: Partially true

Explanation: All air purifiers are not same. Most of the air cleaners remove particles, a few remove gases (and odors), and some do both of the things.

- *Particle removal*: Particles like dust and allergens are removed from air. These could be of two different types:
    - *Mechanical air cleaners*: Air is passed through a fibrous or metal filter with different sized pores to trap the particles. High efficiency or HEPA filters are used to remove most of the smaller particles without producing any ozone. These can be cleaned and reused.
    - *Electronic air cleaners*: Three different technologies (intentional ozone generators, electrostatic precipitators, and ionizers) are available. Ozone generators produce ozone in the living area, which is highly irritant and hence not recommended. Electrostatic precipitators collect charged particles from air whereas ionizers charge particles and let them deposit on the nearby materials (like carpet or walls). Ideally an air cleaner should produce no ozone or a maximum of 0.050 ppm.
- *Gas and chemical vapor removal*: Both the purchase and maintenance are costly. Gaseous pollutants are trapped and destroyed by activated charcoal or alumina coated with potassium permanganate. Filter needs to be replaced periodically.

- *Other technologies*: Photocatalytic oxidation (PCO) air cleaners use ultraviolet (UV) radiation and a photocatalyst, such as titanium dioxide to produce hydroxyl (OH) radicals for destruction of gaseous contaminants. Ultraviolet germicidal irradiation (UVGI) air cleaners use UV radiation to neutralize airborne biological contaminants.

During selection of an air purifier, following points should be kept in mind:

- Check the room size (in square feet of floor area) and select the appropriate purifier.
- Install the unit in the room where your family spend most of the time.
- Locate the unit away from doors, windows, and foot traffic.
- The unit should not be placed next to walls or corners so that air may easily reach the device for cleaning.
- A larger clean air delivery rate (CADR), measured in cubic feet per minute (cfm), should be chosen. Select an air cleaner that can replace the room air at least two or three times per hour. A minimum of 600 cfm should be chosen.

  Air flow rate needed (cfm) = $(A \times B \times C \times D)/E$

  A: Floor area of the room to be cleaned (square ft.)

  B: Ceiling height of room (ft.)

  C: Air exchange rate (AER) desired (per hour)—an AER of 0.5 air changes per hour (ACH) would be sufficient to remove moisture and odors whereas an AER of about 3 ACH would be appropriate for quickly removing pollutants from indoor air pollution like cooking or smoking

  D: Convert hours to minutes

  E: Cleaning efficiency of the air cleaner (on product specifications).
- Ozone generators and UV filtration-based cleaners should not be used.
- Fixed in-room air cleaner should be preferred than portable one.
- Higher minimum efficiency reporting value (MERV) filter should be chosen (Table 1).

Table 1: Minimum efficiency reporting value (MERV) ratings.

MERV RATING	Average particle size efficiency (PSE) in microns (μ) — % removal			PSE in μ (material)	Application
	0.3–1.0	1.0–3.0	3.0–10.0		
1–4			<20%	>10 (textile fibers, dust mites, dust, pollen)	Window AC units, minimal filtration
5			20–35	3–10 (cement dust, mold spores, dusting aids)	Industrial workplace, better residential, commercial
8			>70		
9		<50	>85	1–3 (Legionella, auto emissions, humidifier dust)	Hospital laboratories, better commercial, superior residential
12		>80	>90		
13	<75	>90	>90	0.3–1.0 (bacteria, droplet nuclei, tobacco smoke, insecticide dust)	Superior commercial, smoking lounge, hospital care, general surgery
16	>95	>95	>90		
17	≥99.97			<0.3 (HEPA/ULPA filters) (viruses, carbon dust, fine combustion smoke)	Clean rooms, carcinogenic and radioactive materials, orthopedic surgery
18	≥99.99				
19, 20	≥99.999				

(HEPA: high efficiency particulate air filter; ULPA: ultra-low particulate air filter)

- Need for filter changes should be clearly mentioned on the unit.
- Filter maintenance should be easy to perform.
- The noise created by the unit should allow for conversation at normal volumes.
- Ultraviolet air cleaners consume more power than mechanical cleaners.

- Prefer an air purifier that comes with activated carbon layer. This layer will absorb all harmful gases and chemicals present in the air.

Belief: I need to change my living place to hilly or desert area to reduce allergy

Fact: Partially true

Explanation: Under the sun, an individual could be allergic to anything including sun itself. Even if a person changes his living place, he or she might still suffer from allergic symptoms depending upon his or her allergen sensitization. Desert and hilly areas also have many potential allergens like grass and ragweed pollen. Change of habitat should be initially advised for a short period, if there is symptomatic benefit, an individual might consider long-term migration.

Belief: I am allergic to beautiful flowers

Fact: False

Explanation: Beautiful flowers attract insects and are insect pollinated (entomophilous) whereas dull lustreless flowers are wind pollinated (anemophilous). Hence beautiful flowers are usually nonallergenic. Allergies from flower bouquet could be due to attached pollens from fern or fragrance but not due to flower itself.

Belief: Pollen counts can predict bad allergy days

Fact: True

Explanation: Pollen meters can detect pollen counts on daily basis. These can be useful as the information revealed might warn the allergic patient to take necessary precautions (avoiding outdoors) on high count days.

Belief: Local honey can fight with allergies

Fact: Partially true

Explanation: Honey made in the local area, in the particular season, is likely to be contaminated with seasonal pollens. This might act as a form of immunotherapy to sensitized individuals for the same pollens but not for others. Though local honey might be beneficial to some people but quality and safety assurance is a big challenge.

Honey made in different geographical area or season is not likely to produce similar benefit.

Belief: I have been always allergic to penicillin

Fact: Partially true

Explanation: Actual drug allergy is much less prevalent than the perceived one. Only 10–20% of individuals with complaints of drug allergy have true allergy. Many people outgrow from drug allergy overtime.

Belief: My child is egg allergic, he cannot receive flu shot

Fact: False

Explanation: Egg allergic individuals may be safely vaccinated with the measles mumps rubella (MMR), the measles mumps rubella varicella (MMR-V) vaccines (which contains no egg protein), and the influenza vaccine (which may contain minute traces of egg protein). If there is documented reaction or anaphylaxis during MMR, MMR-V or influenza vaccine, the patient should be referred to an allergy specialist for further assessment before the next dose. Yellow fever and Q fever vaccines have higher egg proteins and egg allergic patients should be referred to allergy specialist for assessment and vaccination.

Belief: I feel weird after eating chocolate, am I allergic to chocolate?

Fact: False

Explanation: Chocolate contains cocoa, milk, and nuts. Milk allergy is quiet common in children followed by nuts in adolescents and adults. Cocoa allergy is very rare by itself. Try to identify the real allergenic culprit in chocolate and targeted avoidance will be more beneficial.

Belief: Children outgrow food allergies

Fact: Partially true

Explanation: Milk allergies are most common and the symptoms usually start in early infancy. Egg allergies are next to occur in 2nd year of life. Most of the children with either milk or egg allergy start tolerating these food items by 5–6 years of life. Rest of the food allergies start after 3 years of life and usually persist lifelong.

Belief: Peanut is the most common food allergy
Fact: False

Explanation: Milk is the most common food allergy followed by egg followed by peanut in children.

Belief: My child is cow's milk allergic, he can take buffalo's or goat's milk
Fact: False

Explanation: Cow's milk shares more than 80% structural homology with goat's, sheep's, and buffalo's milk. So a cow's milk allergic patient should not receive goat's, sheep's or buffalo's milk or milk products. The clinical reactivity of mare's, donkey's or camel's milk is very less in children with cow's milk protein allergy.

Belief: There are nondairy alternatives available for cow's milk allergic patients
Fact: True

Explanation: Fifteen percent of the milk allergic children might react to *soya* proteins. *Almond* and *coconut* milk, contain less than a quarter of the calories and less than half of fat as compared to cow' milk, are available alternate options. *Oat* milk has similar calories and half of protein content as compared to cow's milk. *Rice* milk is least allergenic with similar calories and less proteins to cow's milk. *Cashew* milk is another alternate, with significantly lesser calories and proteins, which can be easily made at home.

Belief: I am allergic to shellfish, I cannot undergo CT scan
Fact: False

Explanation: Shellfish allergy is due to protein and has no relationship with iodine. So contrast iodine dye have no relationship with shellfish allergy.

Belief: My child gets bloating sensation and abdominal cramps after milk intake, he is milk allergic
Fact: False

Explanation: He seems to be milk intolerant rather than milk allergic. Milk intolerance is due to carbohydrate component (lactose) and causes nonspecific gastrointestinal symptoms whereas milk allergy is due to milk proteins and usually causes skin, respiratory or gastrointestinal symptoms within 2 hours of ingestion though late reactions are also possible. Lactose intolerance is quantitative, children might tolerate small quantities of milk, whereas milk allergy is qualitative. Only lactose-containing milk needs to be reduced for a short time in intolerance whereas all milk products need to be stopped in case of true milk allergy.

Belief: Every food item is equally efficacious in causing allergies

Fact: False

Explanation: Though allergy is possible to any food item, there are eight food items responsible for 95% of food allergies. These are milk, egg, soy, peanut, tree nuts, wheat, fish, and shellfish.

Belief: Fortified and processed foods causes allergy, one should consume only natural food items

Fact: False

Explanation: Fortification and processing causes addition of certain vitamins and minerals, whereas, most of the allergies are due to allergenic proteins. Hence fortified and processed food items are equally allergenic to natural or organic foods.

Belief: Allergies disturb mind-body relationship

Fact: True

Explanation: Allergic disorders have a significant impact on quality of life, school and/or work performance of patients, with financial and social effects on family members and caregivers. All these factors increases the stress level in patient and caregivers affecting mind-body relationship. There are postulated hypothesis about cross-talk between brain mast cells and microglia. Resurgence in neurological symptoms have been noticed during allergic exacerbations in children with behavioral disorders.

Belief: Allergies are not life-threatening

Fact: False

Explanation: Uncontrolled allergic reaction in a sensitized patient could be life-threatening in form of anaphylaxis. Anaphylaxis should be suspected early if 2 or more of the following symptoms occur to a likely allergen (within minutes or several hours of exposure):

- Involvement of skin-mucosal tissue—generalized hives, swollen lips-tongue-uvula
- Respiratory compromise—sudden onset cough, breathlessness, fast breathing, hoarseness of voice, sudden change in quality or quantity of voice
- Reduced BP or associated symptoms of end-organ dysfunction—cool and calm peripheries, peripheral or central cyanosis, feeble or bounding pulses, giddiness, and postural hypotension
- Persistent gastrointestinal symptoms—painful abdominal cramps and vomiting.

Intramuscular epinephrine should be given immediately and urgent healthcare referral should be sought. These patients should be prescribed home epinephrine for emergency administration.

Belief: Allergy testing is waste of time and money

Fact: False

Explanation: A patient with recurrent or persistent symptoms should be tested for suspected allergies. Skin prick test, by an expert, is much more reliable, economical, and clinically relevant than any of the other blood test. It is considered to be "test of choice for aeroallergens" whereas oral challenge test is "gold standard for food allergies". An allergen panel should be carefully selected with limited number of allergens. Detection of relevant positive allergens will help in instituting specific allergen avoidance measures and immunotherapy in selected cases.

Belief: Costly blood allergy panels detects many allergies

Fact: False

Explanation: Blood allergy panels can detect immunological hypersensitivity to a group of allergens that may not be clinically relevant. These can be falsely positive in case of high total IgE levels.

Belief: Allergy testing should be done for all allergic patients

Fact: False

Explanation: Testing is indicated in patients with recurrent or persistent symptoms. Patients, in whom there is frequent requirement of reliever medications despite the regular use of controller medications or in whom controller medications cannot be tapered or stopped are the right candidates for allergy testing.

Belief: Skin prick test is dangerous

Fact: False

Explanation: Though there is a theoretical risk of severe reaction during skin prick test, no serious reaction or anaphylaxis has been reported in literature. As precautionary measure, skin prick test should be done in settings with availability of all the resuscitation facilities.

Belief: Skin prick test is painful

Fact: False

Explanation: Skin prick test is epicutaneous test, in which special lancets are used to prick a maximum depth of 1 mm only that lies in epidermis only. All blood vessels and pain fibers are in deep dermal layers. So this test is painless and blood less, if performed by an expert. The test may also be called as "Skin Touch test" to reduce the apprehension of children and their caregivers.

Belief: Skin prick test is better than any blood allergy tests

Fact: True

Explanation: Blood allergy test detects only IgE production whereas skin prick test mimics the original clinical reaction in a controlled manner. The sensitivity is far superior than any blood test. Blood specific allergy panels are recommended in following conditions:

- Extremes of ages—where skin prick test is usually not recommended like below 6 months and above 65 years of age
- Unhealthy skin—where no healthy skin is available, due to severe eczema, for prick test
- Patient on long-term (>10 days) oral steroids and other immunosuppressants
- Patient on antihistaminics and these cannot be stopped as in chronic urticaria
- *After anaphylaxis:* Skin prick test should be done with a minimum of 4 weeks interval after anaphylaxis as mast cell

mediators (including histamine) will take some time for regeneration after an anaphylactic episode
- Patient or caregivers are unwilling for skin prick tests.

Belief: Skin prick test cannot be done when patient is on antiallergic medications

Fact: Partially true

Explanation: The following medications should be stopped for desired duration before skin prick testing:
- H_1 blockers—48 hours
- Astemizole—60 days
- Ketotifen—5 days
- Tricyclic antidepressants—2 weeks
- Long-term steroids (>10 days)—2 weeks
- Long-term topical steroids—2-3 weeks.

Belief: One should be testing for maximum possible allergens at one time

Fact: False

Explanation: "Less is more" should be the rule. One should try to narrow down to only few allergens (preferably 6-8) with focused history and relevant physical examination.

Belief: Inhalers are better than nebulizers

Fact: True

Explanation: Most of the medicine through nebulizers is dispersed in air and does not take part in therapeutic inhalation of drugs. Use of inhalers (with correct techniques and spacers) is definitely better than any other form of drug delivery.

Belief: Allergy testing is unsafe in children

Fact: False

Explanation: It is as safe in children as in adults. The minimum recommended age for skin prick test is 4 months.

Belief: Skin prick tests are costly and more time consuming

Fact: False

Explanation: Skin prick test are much cheaper than corresponding blood tests. It takes only 15-20 minutes from test to result for skin prick test whereas minimum 24–48 hours are required for the blood tests.

Belief: Outdoor allergies are more common than indoor

Fact: False

Explanation: Indoor allergens originate from house dust mites, furred pets, cockroaches, molds, plants, and rodents. Huge use of biomass for heating, cooking, and lighting becomes the major source for indoor PM exposure. Outdoor allergens arise from mainly plants, fungi, molds, and yeast. Air pollution has an additive effect on biological allergens. Environmental Tobacco Smoke (ETS) by parents increases the risk of lower respiratory infections in infants.

Belief: Allergies runs in families

Fact: True

Explanation: One atopic parent increases the chances of persistent allergy in children to 33% whereas both parents increases this chance to 66%.

Belief: It may be a good practice to combine bronchodilators (asthalin or levolin) with steroids (budesonide) in the same nebulizing chamber

Fact: True

Explanation: Various types of permissible mixtures for nebulization are depicted in Table 2.

Mixture are compatible, if preservative-free solutions (no benzalkonium chloride) are used.

Table 2: Admixture advices for commonly used drug solution or suspension in nebulizers.

	Albuterol	Ipratropium	Cromolyn	Budesonide
Albuterol	-	Possible	Possible	Possible
Ipratropium	Possible	-	Possible	Possible
Cromolyn	Possible	Possible	-	Possible
Budesonide	Possible	Possible	Possible	-

Source: Kamin W, Schwabe A, Kramer I. Inhalation solutions—which one are allowed to be mixed? Physicochemical compatibility of drug solutions in nebulizers. J Cystic Fibrosis. 2006:205-13.

Belief: Montelukast-Levocetirizine combination is better than either drug alone

Fact: Partially true

Explanation: The combination of two drugs is better than either alone. Montelukast sodium is alkaline stable and levocetirizine dihydrochloride is acid stable. In case of matrix tablet, both the drugs would be in contact and make it unstable during the shelf life of the formulation. A bilayer tablet improves the stability of both the drugs in combination. In the absence of bilayer tablet, both the drugs should be prescribed independently.

Belief: Any type of facemask can prevent from pollution and respiratory allergies

Fact: False

Explanation: Three types of face masks are commonly available:
- Simple flat mask (surgical mask)—simple filter against PM
- Dust and particulate mask (respirator)—better protection from fine suspended PM and microorganisms. N-95 and N-99 are best to combat pollution and allergies. N-95 respirator masks are able to filter out 95% of PM ($PM_{2.5}$) while N-99 filters 99% of PM
- Gas mask—protection against chemical fumes.

Masks available in India:
- Cambridge masks are triple layer masks available in India. These remove 99% of PM_{10}, $PM_{2.5}$, and $PM_{0.3}$ pollutants. They also have a layer of activated carbon filter to remove bacteria, viruses, and gaseous pollutants
- Vogmask antipollution masks—these are N-99 rated
- Respro—N-99 rated
- Totobobo—N-95 rated.

Belief: Smoking in patient's surroundings can aggravate allergies

Fact: True

Explanation: Both active and passive smoking can trigger the allergic symptoms in a sensitized individual. Parents or caregivers, who are doing outdoor smoking, carry small smoke particles home on their clothes making contact feasible with allergic children and other family members.

Belief: Mosquito coils and mats are effective ways of prevention for an allergic child

Fact: False

Explanation: These produce toxic fumes and can worsen allergic symptoms.

Belief: Common cold can cause allergy

Fact: False

Explanation: People with allergies are more prone to catching cold. Cold is due to viral infections. It can precipitate allergic symptoms in an already sensitized individual.

Belief: Drug allergies are very common

Fact: False

Explanation: Real drug allergies are very rare. One needs to take detailed history about sequence of events and do directed allergen testing before labeling someone with drug allergy.

Belief: Allergies can happen to anyone

Fact: True

Explanation: Under this sun, anything can cause allergy to anyone.

Belief: Immunotherapies (allergy shots) are waste of money

Fact: False

Explanation: Immunotherapy, under supervision of a trained allergy specialist, for selected group of allergens can give excellent results. It converts allergenic Th2 response to nonallergenic Th1 immune response. Limited number of relevant allergens should be chosen for selecting immunotherapy. Monoallergen therapy is the best followed by oligoallergen (<5) therapy. Polyallergen (>5) immunotherapy is usually not effective due to extract dilution and hence subtherapeutic doses.

Belief: Yoga and physical exercise reduce allergies

Fact: True

Explanation: Yoga and physical exercises improve respiratory muscle endurance and reduce the work of breathing, thus help in asthma symptoms.

Belief: Alternative medicines like Homeopathy or Ayurveda can cure allergies

Fact: Partially true

Explanation: There are limited drugs from complementary and alternative medicine (CAM) which have shown promising results in treatment of allergies. Many therapies have significant side effects. More robust scientific data are required before considering CAM as a good therapeutic option.

Belief: Immunotherapy works good for food allergies

Fact: False

Explanation: There have been several trials of oral immunotherapy in certain food allergies but with limited success. Currently, there is no role of immunotherapy for food allergies.

Belief: Immunotherapy should be given for all allergens to which patient is sensitive

Fact: False

Explanation: It should be given to only clinically relevant limited number of allergens. Monoallergen therapy is the best followed by oligoallergen (<5) therapy. Polyallergen (>5) immunotherapy is usually not effective due to extract dilution and hence subtherapeutic doses.

Belief: Celiac disease is a type of wheat allergy

Fact: False

Explanation: Celiac disease is gluten intolerance and it is IgA mediated. True wheat allergy is IgE mediated.

Belief: Specific covers are available to avoid house dust mites

Fact: True

Explanation: House dust mite covers are made from microwave fabric. The pore size must be less than 8 microns to be effective for dust mite prevention. These covers are very thin and light weight but cost is limiting factor.

Belief: Intravenous hydrocortisone and pheniramine (avil) are the drug of choice in case of anaphylaxis

Fact: False

Explanation: Intramuscular epinephrine is the drug of choice in case of suspected or proven anaphylaxis.

Belief: Intramuscular epinephrine should be given by a healthcare personnel, in healthcare settings, in case of anaphylaxis

Fact: False

Explanation: Intramuscular epinephrine should be given as soon as possible in case of anaphylaxis by the affected individual himself or herself or the nearest caregiver. Requirement of a healthcare personnel or setting is not mandatory for epinephrine injection.

Belief: My child is allergic to curd and banana

Fact: Partially true

Explanation: Any child allergic to milk will be allergic to curd also. Banana allergy is not very common, though possible. An estimated 0.1-1.2% of the population experience severe banana allergy. The perceived symptoms after curd intake are mostly due to cold temperature rather than curd itself.

Belief: A very high total or specific IgE level is directly proportional to severity of allergic symptoms

Fact: False

Explanation: The numbers are not directly proportional to presence or severity of allergic symptoms.

Belief: Vaccination can protect against allergies

Fact: Partially true

Explanation: Vaccination (pneumococcal, Flu) decreases the likelihood of a serious infection. Frequent respiratory infections worsen a patient's allergy or asthma symptoms.

Belief: Vaginal delivery is better than cesarean section for allergy prevention

Fact: True

Explanation: Babies are exposed to healthy vaginal flora during vaginal delivery which has a healthy interaction on induction of immunological tolerance and thus reduces the chances of allergies as compared to cesarean section.

Belief: Ayurvedic products (like Chyawanprash) will reduce allergies

Fact: Partially true

Explanation: Following Ayurveda strategies have been reported to reduce allergies:

- Using a neti pot daily, with a weak saline solution and distilled water, to loosen up the kapha
- Putting little sesame oil spiked with eucalyptus or camphor in each nostril after neti pot
- Trikatu (combination of black pepper, long pepper, and ginger) to improve digestion
- Kapha-reduced diet—fresh, organic vegetables
- Using warm spices like ginger, cinnamon, black pepper, turmeric, cumin, and cayenne during cooking
- Ginger tea
- Triphala tablets at night
- Daily exercise for at least 30 minutes.

Allergy: Future Perspective

Allergic disorders are on the rising trend. We need to be better equipped with latest modalities to deal with these problems. Following lacunas need to be fulfilled in near future for better management of deserving patients.

- Greater awareness of allergic manifestations among general population is needed. This can be achieved by regular public awareness programs, media help, and one-to-one basis education.
- *Education of healthcare providers*: This is a very important area as current medical curriculum in India does not have any formal training schedule for allergic disorders. Healthcare providers need to be educated via various educational activities. Government at both state and national level should ensure better education regarding allergic disorders.
- Measures for primary allergy prevention should be introduced in individuals with family history of atopy.
- Better diagnostic facilities should be available. Standardized allergen extracts for skin prick test are desired. Component resolved diagnostics needs to be utilized in places where there is high probability of cross-reactivity.
- Regional pollen calendars need to be made and periodically updated.
- Daily pollen counts need to be monitored and should be in easy domain of general public.
- More effective avoidance measures should be introduced.
- Safe and more effective ways of immunotherapy need to be introduced.

- Effective food allergen immunotherapy needs to be developed.
- Standardized protocols for allergy diagnosis and management need to be devised on national paltform.
- More dedicated asthma and allergy centers are required to cater rising need of patients.
- Quality research and studies are required to better understand the disease process and their effective therapy.

Annexures

ANNEXURE I: ALGORITHMIC APPROACHES

Flowchart 1: Multimodel approach for allergic disorders.

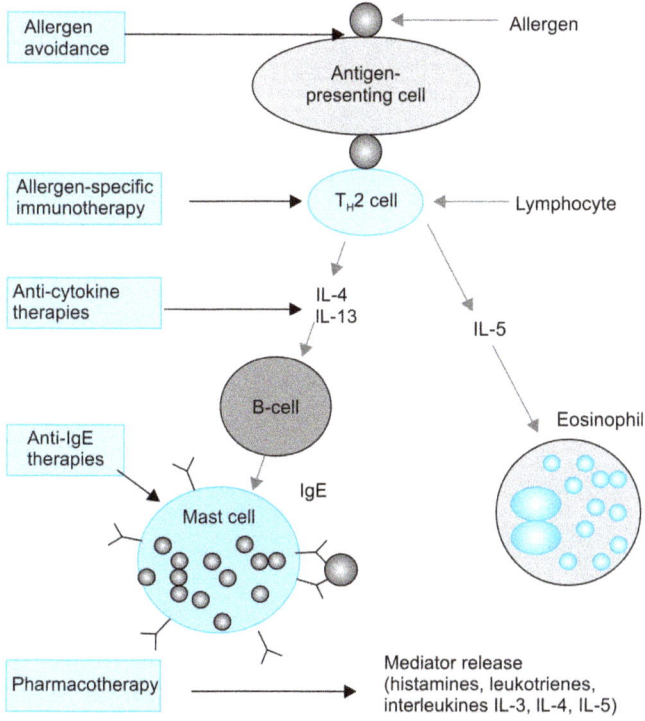

338 *Allergy in a Nutshell: A Handbook*

Flowchart 2: Approach to a child with allergic symptoms.

```
                    History and physical examination
                              │
                ┌─────────────┴─────────────┐
          Mild symptoms           Persistent/worsening symptoms
                │                           │
       • Eliminate or avoid cause    • Screening with test
       • Treat with antihistamines   • Eliminate or avoid cause
                │                    • Treat with antihistamine
                └─────────────┬─────────────┘
                         Symptoms decrease?
                    Yes ┌────┴────┐ No
                        │         │
              Continue management  Further testing and treatment
                                        │
                                    Suspected
          ┌─────────────────────────────┼─────────────────────────────┐
   Atopic dermatitis              Food sensitivity              Allergic rhinits/asthma
          │                             │                             │
   • Treat for 1 month           • Test for common             • Treat with nasal spray
     (Triamcinolone,               foods                         (Antihistamine/steroids)
     Tacrolimus)                 • Elimination of offending    • Treat asthma as per
   • Skin care advice              food for 3 months             guidelines
          │                             │                             │
   Symptoms decrease            Symptoms decrease              Symptoms decrease
   Yes ↓      ↓ No              Yes ↓        ↓ No              Yes ↓       ↓ No
  Continue  Refer to            Continue                      Continue    Test for
  treatment allergy             elimination                   treatment   aeroallergens
            specialist          for 3 years
                                Retest                              No ← Is test result
                                    │                                    negative?
                                Is test                                      ↓ Yes
                                result  → No                          • Environment
                                negative?                                control
                                    ↓ Yes                             • Medication
                                Oral food                                    │
                                challenge                             Symptoms decrease
                                preferably                            Yes ↓
                                by allergy                            Continue
                                specialist                            treatment
                                                                      ↑ No
```

TEST- IgE specific
• Serum-in-vitro
• Skin prick-in-vivo

Refer to allergy specialist

Flowchart 3: Approach to a child with suspected milk allergy.

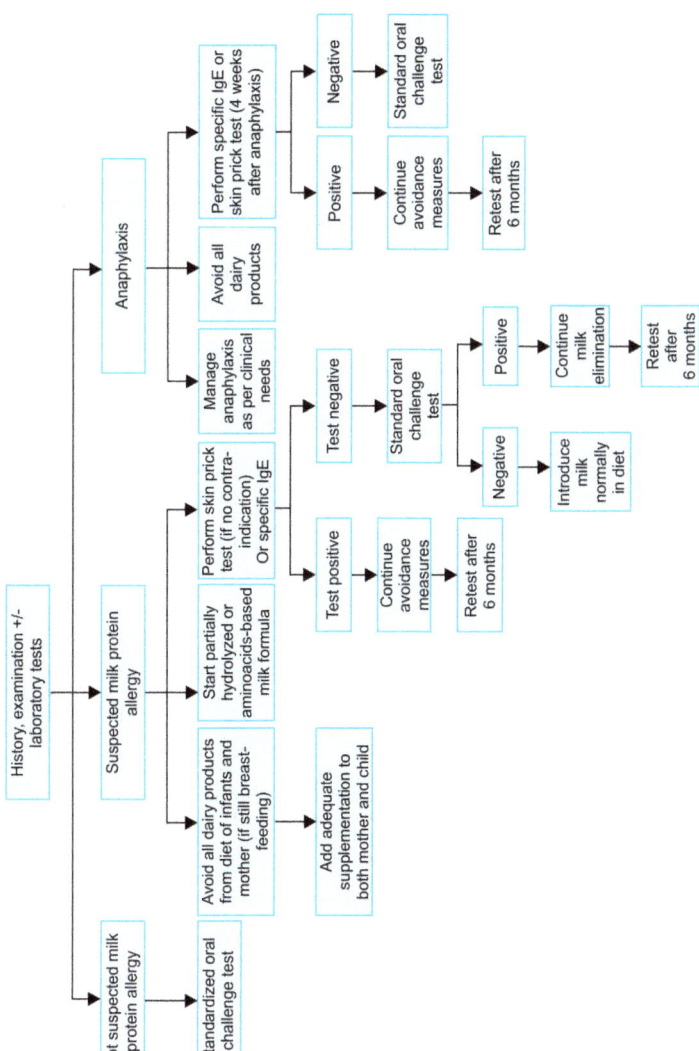

Flowchart 4: Approach to a patient with suspected adverse food reaction.

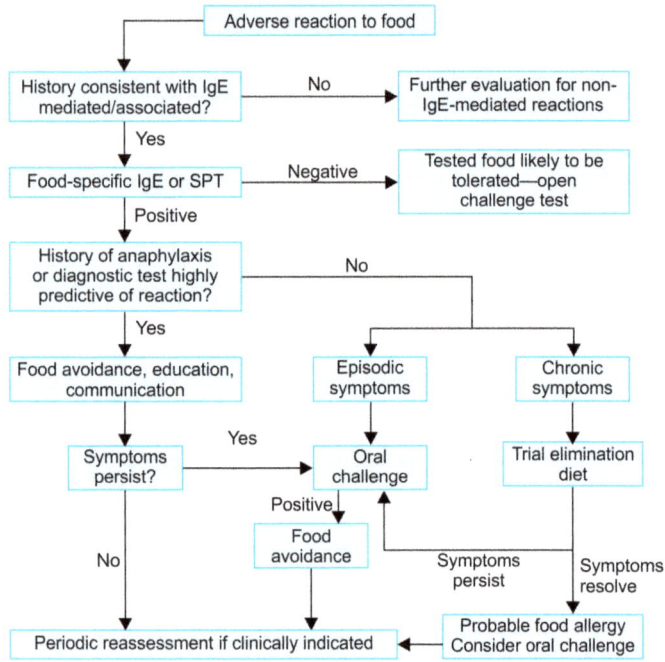

Source: Chapman JA, Bernstein L, Lee RE, et al. Food allergy: a practice parameter. Ann Allergy Asthma Immunol. 2004;S1-S68.

Flowchart 5: Immunotherapy (IT) algorithm.

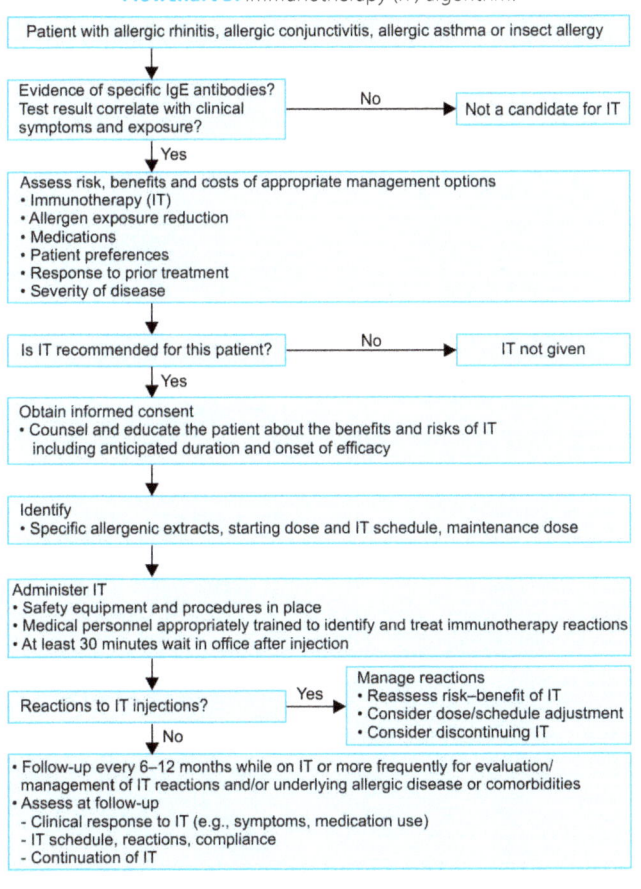

Flowchart 6: Approach to a child with hypereosinophilia (HE).

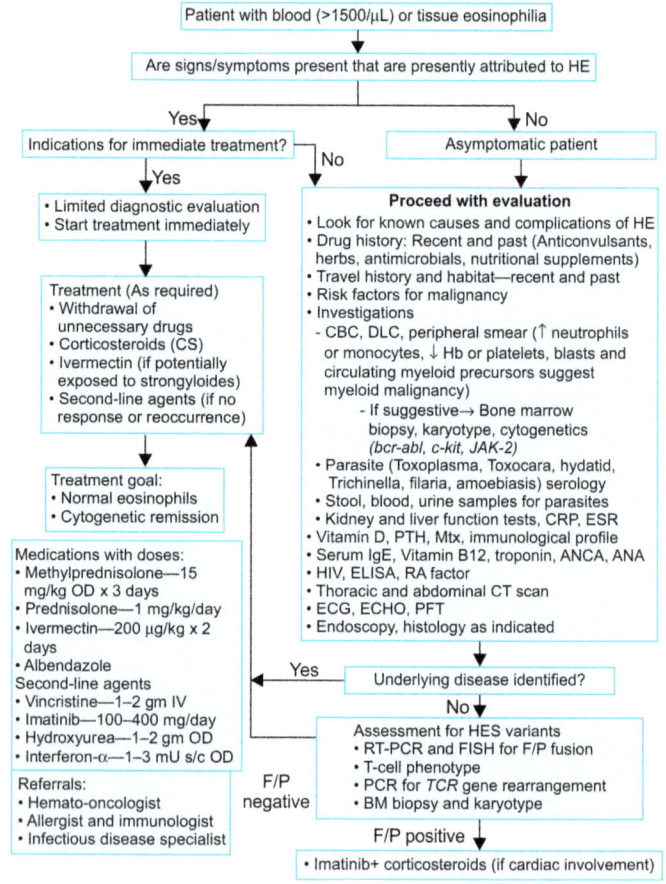

(ANCA: antineutrophil cytoplasmic antibodies; CBC: complete blood count; DLC: differential blood count; ECG: electrocardiography; ELISA: enzyme-linked immunosorbent assay; FISH: fluorescence in situ hybridization; HIV: human immunodeficiency virus; PFT: pulmonary function test; PTH: parathyroid hormone; RT-PCR: reverse transcription polymerase chain reaction; HES: hypereosinophilic syndrome)

Source: Modified from Roufosse F, Weller PF. Practical approach to the patient with hypereosinophilia. J Allergy Clin Immunol. 2010;126:39-44.

Flowchart 7: Approach to a child with atopic dermatitis.

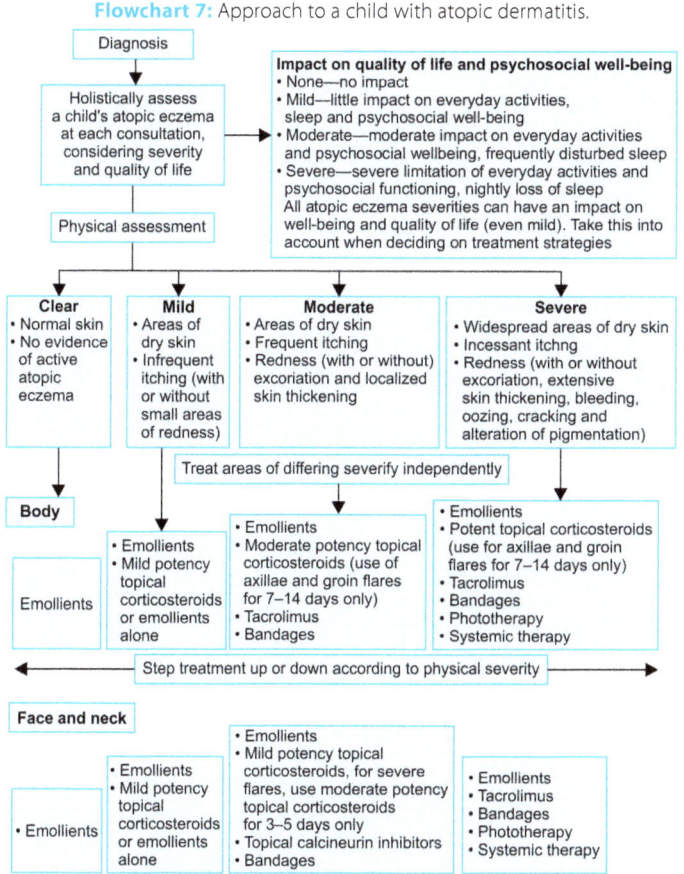

Flowchart 8: Approach to a patient with suspected insect hypersensitivity.

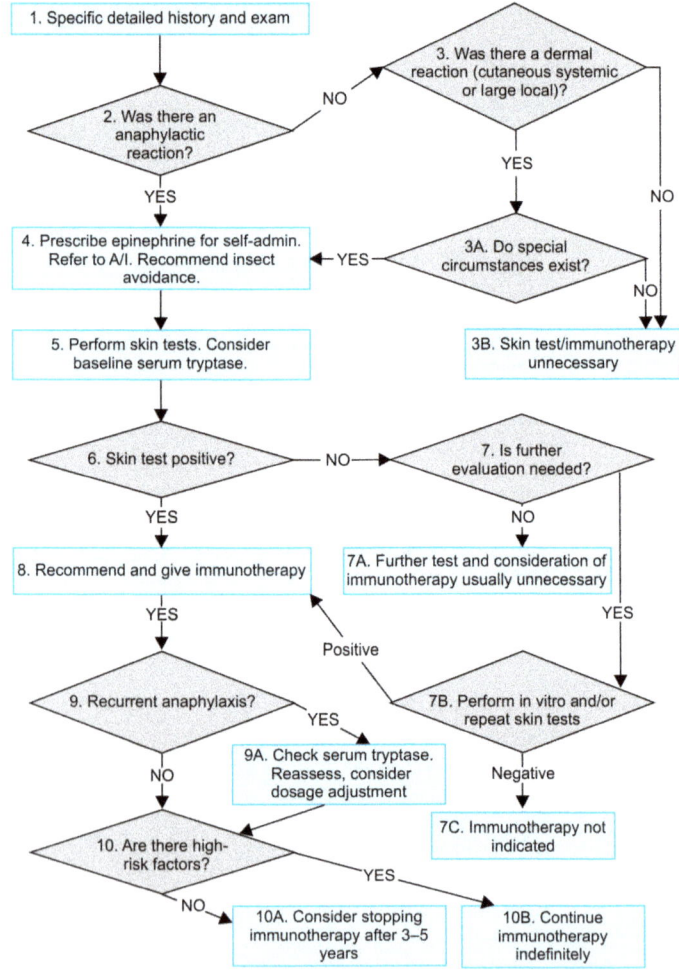

Source: BK Golden D, Demain J, Freeman T, et al. Stinging insect hypersensitivity. A practice parameter update 2016. Ann Allergy Asthma Immunol. 2017;118:28-54.

Box 1: High total IgE levels—differentials.

- Atopic diseases:
    - Allergic rhinitis
    - Asthma
    - Dermatitis
- Parasitic diseases:
    - Cestodes (*Echinococcus*)
    - Trematodes (*Schistosoma*)
    - Nematodes
    - Ascaris
    - Strongyloides
    - *Ancylostoma*
    - Capillaria
    - *Toxocara*
- Infections:
    - Systemic candidiasis
    - Epstein-Barr virus
    - Cytomegalovirus
    - Bronchopulmonary aspergillosis
    - Leprosy
    - Respiratory syncytial virus
    - HIV-1
- Various immunodeficiency states, including:
    - Hyper-IgE syndrome
    - Wiskott-Aldrich
    - DiGeorge
    - Nezelof
- Neoplastic diseases:
    - Hodgkin's disease
    - IgE myeloma
    - Post-bone marrow-transplant
    - Bronchial carcinoma
- Cutaneous diseases:
    - Bullous pemphigoid
    - Chronic acral dermatitis
    - Streptococcal erythema nodosum
- Other diseases:
    - Nephrotic syndrome
    - Nephritis
    - Liver disease
    - Cystic fibrosis
    - Kawasaki disease
    - Guillain-Barre syndrome

*Allergen-specific IgE levels are likely to be falsely high if total serum IgE >300 IU/mL.
*Skin prick test will be more reliable test for detecting hypersensitivity with clinical correlation.

Box 2: Approach to a child with anaphylaxis.

Immediate measures:
- Allergen: Remove the inciting allergen, if possible
- Airway: Assess airway, breathing, circulation. If needed, support the airway (non-invasive/invasive)
- Cardiopulmonary resuscitation: Start chest compression, in case of arrest or heart rate less than 60 min
- Epinephrine intramuscular: <10 kg–0.01 mL/kg, 10–30 kg–0.15 mL, ≥30 kg–0.3 mL of 1:1,000 strength (Undiluted preparation)
- Call for help
- Position of comfort—recombinant—adult & adolescents, supine—children, left lateral—pregnant
- Oxygen: 8–10 L/min through non-rebreathing face mask, monitor with pulse oximetry
- Epinephrine intramuscular: Repeat every 5–15 minutes up to 3 doses, if no response
- Activate EMS—if no response to first dose of epinephrine or if compromised mentation, airway or hemodynamics
- Intravenous (IV) fluids: 5–10 mL/kg of normal saline–up to 30 mL/kg in case of hypotension

Additional measures:
- Salbutamol: 2.5–5 mg of nebulized salbutamol in 3 mL of saline if bronchoconstriction, repeat in 15 minutes if required
- Glucagon: 1–5 mg of glucagon intravenously slowly over 15 minutes if patient is on β-blockers and not responding to epinephrine
- Epinephrine infusion: If inappropriate response to previous epinephrine and IV fluids
- Intraosseous access: If no IV access obtained and patient is in refractory anaphylaxis

Refractory anaphylaxis:
- Advanced airway management
- Vasopressors: Consider adding dopamine after epinephrine

Optional treatment: Efficacy not proven
- H_1-antihistamine: 1 mg/kg in children (Maximum 50 mg)
- Corticosteroids: 1–2 mg/kg up to 125 mg/dose of methylprednisolone, for prevention of delayed reactions

Observation and monitoring:
- In hospital—8 hours
- In office—until full recovery + additional 30–60 minutes for all patients who do not require hospitalization

Discharge management:
- Education—about home recognition and treatment of anaphylaxis
- Auto-injectable epinephrine—prescribe 2 doses to patients who experienced anaphylactic reaction or those who are at risk of severe anaphylaxis
- Anaphylaxis emergency action plan

Source: Modified from Lieberman P, Nicklas RA, Randolph C, et al. Anaphylaxis—a practice parameter update 2015. Ann Allergy Asthma Immunol. 2015.

Box 3: Approach to a patient with chronic urticaria.

Patient with chronic urticaria (Hives > 6 weeks)
- Detailed history
- Baseline investigations: Complete blood count, liver function test, kidney function test, C-reactive protein, erythrocyte sedimentation rate, urine routine
- Selected investigations:
  - Vasculitis: Ig, antinuclear factor, immune complex, skin biopsy
  - Infections: Serologic studies for: hepatitis C virus, hepatitis B virus, hepatitis A virus, Epstein-Barr virus, *Mycoplasma pneumoniae*, Cultures, fecal antigen of *Helicobacter pylori* or urea breath test
  - Allergic: IgE (Total or specific), skin tests, eosinophil count, challenge test, elimination diet, tryptase
  - Hereditary angioedema: C3, C4, C1 esterase inhibitor
  - Physical: Methacholine test, running test, ice cube test, UV and visible light exposure, dermatographism, pressure test, and warm water immersion test
  - Autoimmune chronic urticaria: Autologous serum skin test (ASST), basophil histamine release test (BHRT)

Management
- Level I
  - Detection (Skin prick test or specific IgE for relevant allergens) and elimination of possible eliciting factor
  - Non-sedating second-generation H_1 antihistamines (nsAH)
- Level II (If symptoms persist after 2 weeks of level I therapy)
  - Updosing of nsAH ($\times$ up to 4 times)
  - Add another 2nd-generation H_1 antihistaminic agent
  - Add H_2 antagonist
- Level III (If symptoms persist after 4 weeks of level II therapy)
  - Add leukotriene antagonist or change nsAH
  - Add 1st-generation antihistaminic at bedtime
- Level IV (If symptoms persist after 2–4 weeks of level III therapy)
  - Immunomodulators, $H_1 + H_2$ blocker, anti-IgE antibody
  - Thyroxine supplements—If hypothyroid or anti-thyroid antibody positive
  - Vitamin D
  - Plasmapheresis
  - Autologous whole blood injection–In adults with refractory chronic urticaria

During exacerbations, systemic steroid for 3–7 days in all levels.

ANNEXURE II: PHARMACOTHERAPY

Table 1: Allergic rhinoconjunctivitis.

Drug	Dose	Monitor for
Intranasal or intraocular H_1 blockers		
Azelastine puff	6 months-5 years—1 puff per nostril BD Adults—1–2 puffs per nostril BD	• Nose pain, bitter taste, fever, headache, sore throat, cough, nasal ulceration
Azelastine eye drop	≥3 years—1 drop in affected eye BD	
Intranasal steroids		
Beclomethasone	50–100 μg/nostril BD	• Effect starts after 6–12 hours • Maximal effect after few days • Irritation, headache, nose bleed, rhinorrhea, nasal mucosa ulcer, nasal septum perforation, dryness, burning
Budesonide	6–12 yrs—128 μg/nostril OD ≥12 yrs—256 μg/nostril OD	
Flunisolide	6–14 yrs—25 μg/nostril TDS ≥14 yrs—50 μg/nostril BD-TDS	
Fluticasone propionate	4–12 yrs—50 μg/nostril OD ≥12 yrs—100 μg/nostril OD	
Fluticasone furoate	2–12 yrs—27.5 μg/nostril OD ≥12 yrs—55 μg/nostril OD	
Mometasone furoate	2–12 yrs—50 μg/nostril OD ≥12 yrs—100 μg/nostril OD	
Triamcinolone	6–12 yrs—55 μg/nostril OD ≥12 yrs—110 μg/nostril OD	
Ciclesonide	≥6 yrs—100 μg/nostril OD	
Intranasal anticholinergics		
Ipratropium	≥5–12 yrs—2 pufs/nostril TDS	• Headache, dry nose, nose bleed, bad taste
Oral decongestants		
Ephedrine	≥12 yrs—12.5 to 25 mg QID	• Cautious in heart disease • Nervousness, restlessness, dizziness, headache, fear, anxiety, loss of appetite, tremors, hallucinations
Pseudoephedrine	2–6 yrs—5–30 mg PRN q 6 hourly 6–12 yrs—30 mg PRN q 6 hourly ≥12 yrs—60 mg PRN q 6 hourly	

Contd...

Contd...

Drug	Dose	Monitor for
Intranasal decongestants		
Epinephrine	PRN	• Act more rapidly than oral • Limit duration to <10 days to avoid rhinitis medicamentosa
Naphazoline	≥12 yrs—1–2 pufs/nostril PRN q 6 hourly	
Oxymetazoline	≥6 yrs—2–3 pufs/nostril PRN q 12 hourly	
Xylometazoline	1–2 puff/nostril PRN q 8 hourly	
Phenylephrine	2–6 yrs—2–3 drops (0.0125%)/nostril PRN q 4 hourly ≥6 yrs—2–3 pufs (1%)/nostril PRN q 4 hourly	
Tetrahydrozoline	≥6 yrs—2–4 drops/nostril PRN q 3 hourly	
Local chromone		
Cromoglycate	≥2 yrs—1 puff/nostril q 6 hourly ≥4 yrs—1–2 drops/eye q 4 hourly	• Intraocular more effective than intranasal • Excellent safety
Nedocromil	1 puff/nostril q 6 hourly 1 drop/eye q every 6 hourly	• Unpleasant taste, headache, conjunctivitis

Table 2: Angioedema.

Drug	Dose	Monitor for
Tranexamic acid (Drug of choice)	10 mg/kg TDS oral (Alternate day or twice weekly) Max dose/day—3 g	• Diarrhea
C1-inhibitor (INH) concentrate (Human)	20 U/kg (in acute attacks)	• Slow IV injection • Watch for anaphylaxis
rC1-INH (recombinant)	50 U/kg weekly (for long-term prophylaxis)	• Used for ≥13 years • Do not use if allergic to rabbit • Contraindicated in pregnancy and lactation
Fresh frozen plasma	For acute attacks and short-term prophylaxis	

Table 3: Asthma.

Drug	Dose	Monitor for
Short-acting β_2 agonists		
Salbutamol	• MDI 100 µg/dose—2–4 puffs PRN; may be repeated thrice at 20 minutes intervals and then 1–4 hourly as needed • DPI Rotacap 200 µg/dose—1–2 Rotacap as needed • Neb respirator solution 5 mg/mL—0.15 mg/kg (minimum 1.25 mg for <6 months; 2.5 mg for 6 months–6 yrs; 5 mg for >6 yrs of age). • For continuous nebulization 10 mg/10 mL saline via jet nebulizer • Neb respule (2.5 mg in 2.5 or 3 mL)—use equivalent dose • Syp 2 mg/5 mL and Tab 2 mg, 4 mg, 8 mg—0.15 mg/kg/dose 3–4 times a day	• Tachycardia, tremors, headache, hypokalemia, hyperglycemia • Inhaled route minimizes systemic adverse effects
Levosalbutamol	• Neb respule 0.31 mg/2.5 mL, 0.63 mg/2.5 mL, 1.25 mg/2.5 mL—0.075 mg/kg	
Terbutaline	• Neb solution 10 mg/mL—2.5 mg in dilution • Syp 1.5 mg/5 mL and Tab 2.5 mg, 5 mg—0.075 mg/kg/dose TDS • Inj. 0.5 mg/mL—0.01 mg/kg subcutaneously once; bolus 5–10 µg/kg over 10 minutes followed by 0.1–10 µg/kg/min	
Nonselective β_2 agonists		
Adrenaline	• Inj. 1 mg/mL (1:1,000 solution)—0.01 mg/kg subcutaneously, may be repeated up to 3 times every 20 minutes	• Tachycardia, hyperglycemia
Anticholinergics		
Ipratropium bromide	• MDI 20 µg/dose, 40 µg/dose—80–160 µg thrice at 20 minutes interval and then every 6–8 hourly as needed • DPI Rotacap 40 µg/dose—1–2 Rotacap as needed • Neb solution 0.25 mg/mL—0.5 mL <1 yr, 1 mL >1 yr every 20 minutes for 3 doses, then every 6–8 hourly for 24 hours • Neb respule 0.5 mg/2 mL—use equivalent doses	• Dry mouth, increased wheezing sometimes, blurred vision if sprayed in eyes, fever (atropine effect)

Contd...

Contd...

Drug	Dose	Monitor for
Systemic corticosteroids		
Prednisolone	• Tab 5 mg, 10 mg, 20 mg, 40 mg and Syp 5 mg/5 mL, 15 mg/5 mL—1 mg/kg/day (max. 20 mg/day under 2 yrs, 30 mg/day for 2–5 yrs and 40 mg for ≥6 yrs) for 3–7 days	• Side effects rare with short-term use • Increased appetite, hyperglycemia, fluid retention, hypertension, mood alteration, growth retardation
Hydrocortisone	• Inj. 100 mg/vial—4–5 mg/kg every 6 hourly	
Methyl-prednisolone	• Inj. 40 mg, 125 mg, 500 mg, 1 g—1 mg/kg every 6 hourly	
Inhaled corticosteroids		
Beclomethasone dipropionate	• MDI 100, 200 μg/puff—100–400 μg BD • DPI Rotacap 100, 200, 400 μg/dose—100–400 μg BD	• Cough, dysphonia, oral thrush, oropharyngeal deposition • In high doses, systemic side effects like adrenal suppression, growth suppression, skin thinning and cataract
Budesonide	• MDI 100, 200 μg/dose—100–400 μg BD • DPI Rotacap 100, 200, 400 μg/dose—100–400 μg BD • Neb solution 0.5 mg/2 mL, 1 mg/2 mL—0.5–1 mg BD	
Fluticasone propionate	• MDI 125, 250 μg/dose—100–200 μg BD • DPI Rotacap 100, 250, 500 μg/dose—50–200 μg BD • Neb respule 0.5 mg/2 mL, 2 mg/2 mL—1 mg BD	
Ciclesonide	• MDI 80/160 μg/dose—1–2 puffs OD	
Inhaled corticosteroids + Long-acting β_2 agonist		
Fluticasone + Salmeterol	• MDI (50 + 25, 125 + 25, 250 + 25 μg/dose)—1–2 puffs BD • DPI Accuhaler (100 + 50, 250 + 50, 500 + 50 μg/dose)—1 puff BD • DPI Rotacaps (100 + 50, 250 + 50, 500 + 50 μg/dose)—1 Rotacap BD	• Similar to inhaled steroids and shortacting β_2 agonists
Budesonide-Formoterol	• MDI (100/200/400 + 6 μg/dose)—1 puff BD • DPI Rotacap (100/200/400 + 12 μg/dose)—1 Rotacap BD	

Contd...

Contd...

Drug	Dose	Monitor for
Leukotriene receptor antagonists		
Montelukast	• 4 mg granules, 4 mg, 5 mg, 10 mg dispersible tablets—4 mg for 6 months–5 yrs, 5 mg for 6–14 yrs, and 10 mg for >14 yrs OD	• Uncommon • Headache, nightmares, stomach pain, hypersensitivity reactions, mood changes
Methylxanthines		
Aminophylline	• Inj. 250 mg/mL—5 mg/kg diluted in 5% dextrose slow IV as bolus followed by 0.5–1 mg/kg/hr as continuous infusion in 5% dextrose	• Serious toxicity at serum level >20 µg/mL • Nausea, headache, tachycardia, insomnia, drowsiness, seizures
Theophylline	• Tab 100 mg, 200 mg, 300 mg, 450 mg; Syp 50 mg/5 mL—to be used after age of 1 yr	
Other drug		
Magnesium sulfate	• Inj. 25% (250 mg/mL), 50% (500 mg/mL)—25–50 mg/kg in normal saline infused over 30 minutes	• Tachycardia, hypotension, muscle weakness

(DPI: dry powder inhaler; MDI: metered dose inhaler)

Table 4: Topical steroid potency chart.

Class of potency	Drugs
I (Super potent)	• Clobetasol propionate (0.05%) cream, ointment • Betamethasone dipropionate (0.05%) ointment • Halobetasol propionate (0.05%) ointment
II (Potent)	• Betamethasone dipropionate (0.05%) lotion • Mometasone furoate (0.1) ointment • Desoximetasone (0.25%) cream, ointment
III (Upper mid-strength)	• Fluticasone propionate (0.05%) ointment • Betamethasone valerate (0.1%) cream
IV (Mid-strength)	• Mometasone furoate (0.1%) cream • Triamcinolone (0.1%) ointment
V (Lower mid-strength)	• Fluticasone propionate (0.05%) cream • Desonide (0.05%) lotion

Contd...

Contd...

Class of potency	Drugs
VI (Mild)	• Aclometasonedipropionate (0.05%) cream, ointment • Desonide (0.05%) gel • Clobetasone butyrate (0.05%) cream • Fluocinolone acetonide (0.025%) ointment, shampoo
VII (Least potent)	• Hydrocortisone acetate (0.5%, 1%, and 2.5%) lotion, ointment

Source: Modified from Sayaseng KY. Vernon P. Pathophysiology and Management of mild to moderate Pediatric Atopic Dermatitis. J Pediatr Health Care. 2018;32:S2-S12.

Table 5: Urticaria.

Drug	Dose	Monitor for
1st-generation H_1 antihistamines		
Hydroxyzine	2 mg/kg/day 6–8 hourly	• Renal and liver dysfunction • Contraindicated in pregnancy and lactation
Diphenhydramine	5 mg/kg/day 6–8 hourly	• Contraindicated in pregnancy and lactation
Chlorpheniramine	2–5 yrs—1 mg 4–6 hourly 6–11 yrs—2 mg 4–6 hourly ≥12 yrs—4 mg 4–6 hourly	• Caution in asthma
Promethazine	0.1 mg/kg 6 hourly oral (Max 12.5 mg/dose)	• Dry mouth, dizziness, constipation
Cyprohepatidine	0.25 mg/kg/day 8–12 hrly (Max 12 mg in children and 16 mg in adolescent) 2–6 yrs—2 mg 8–12 hrly 7–14 yrs—4 mg 8–12 hrly	• Drowsiness, weight gain, dry mouth
2nd-generation H_1 antihistamines		
Cetirizine	6 months–5 yrs—2.5–5 mg OD 6–11 yrs—5–10 mg OD ≥12 yrs—10 mg OD	• Dry mouth, drowsiness, tinnitus, constipation
Levocetirizine	≥6 yrs—5 mg OD	• Same as cetirizine
Loratadine	2–9 yrs—5 mg OD 6-10 yr—10 mg OD	• Sleepiness, diarrhea, headache, liver dysfunction

Contd...

Contd...

Drug	Dose	Monitor for
Fexofenadine	≥12 yrs—60 mg BD or 120–180 mg OD	• Headache, drowsiness, menstrual cramps
Leukotriene receptor antagonist (LTRA)		
Montelukast	1–5 yrs—4 mg OD 6–14 yrs—5 mg OD ≥12 yrs—10 mg OD	• Headache, mood changes, tremors, skin rash, tiredness
H_2 antihistaminic		
Ranitidine	4–8 mg/kg/day divided in 2 doses	• Headache, constipation
$H_1 + H_2$ blockers		
Doxepin	25–50 mg HS *or* 10–25 mg 3–4 times per day	• Constipation, dry mouth, sedation
Immunomodulators		
Cyclosporine	1.5–2.5 mg/kg/day	• Hypotension, renal function
Tacrolimus	0.05–0.07 mg/kg BD × 4 weeks → ↓ to half × 6 weeks	• Abdominal pain, diarrhea, headache
Dapsone	25–100 mg/day	• Hemolysis, methemoglobin
Intravenous immunoglobulin	2 g/kg (over 5 days) every 4–6 weeks	• Headache, dizziness, aseptic meningitis
Anti-IgE antibody		
Omalizumab	150–300 mg subcutaneously every 4 weeks	• Pruritus, joint pain, wheeze, hypotension
Steroids		
Prednisolone	1–2 mg/kg/day	• Anxiety, dizziness, headache, depression, weight gain, weakness

Index

Page numbers followed by *b* refer to box, *f* refer to figure,
fc refer to flowchart, and *t* refer to table

A

Abdominal pain 169
    crampy 148
    spasmodic 186
Acacia arabica 41, 61
Acacia auriculiformis 32
Acacia mangium 32
Acetaminophen 110
Acquired immunodeficiency
    syndrome 95
Acrodermatitis enteropathica 192
Actinia 7
Activate emergency medical
    system 153
Acupuncture 307
Acute asthma flare-up,
    management of 125
Adenoid hypertrophy 90, 281, 286*f*
    Cohen and Konak
    classification of 287*f*
Adenopathy, regional 272
Adenophora 310*f*
Adrenaline 152, 350
    dosages chart 152
Adverse drug reactions 228
    management 235
    types of 228
Aeroallergens 85
    avoidance measures for 60

Aeroallergy 86
Aerobiology 31
Ageratum conyzoides 41, 43, 61
Ailanthus excelsa 41, 44, 61
Air
    pollutants 190
    pollution, components of 13
Airborne
    particles 34
    pollen 213
        grains 31
Air-O-cell sampling 36
Airway 152
    diseases, allergic 272
    edema 149
    extrinsic compression of 290*f*
Albizia lebbeck 44, 62
Albuterol 329
Allergen 12, 17, 18*f*, 28, 42, 80, 152
    ailanthus 42
    alnus 42
    alternaria 43
    argemone 42
    artemisia 42
    ascospores 43
    aspergilli 43
    avoidance 218
    azadirachta 42
    borassus 42
    brassica 42

- *candida* 43
- *cassia* 42
- *casuarina* 42
- *cedrus* 42
- *chenopodium album* 42
- *cladosporium* 43
- *cocos* 42
- cross-reactive 171*t*
- *curvularia* 43
- *cynodon* 42
- *dodonaea* 42
- exposures 248
- helminthosporium 43
- *holoptelea* 42
- identification of 255, 297
- immunotherapy 29, 197, 303
- indoor 298
- inhalant 60
- major 77
- *mallotus* 42
- *morus* 42
- *mucor* 43
- *nigrospora* 43
- occupational 300
- outdoor 298
- *parthenium* 42
- *pennisetum* 42
- *phoenix* 42
- *phoma* 43
- *prosopis* 42
- *salvadora* 42
- smuts 43
- *sorghum* 42
- specific immunotherapy 218
- specific therapy 176
- *syzygium* 42
- types of 220
- uredospores 43
- *xanthium* 42

Allergenic foods, major 297
Allergenic pathway, selection of 21
Allergic conditions, diagnosis of 280
Allergic conjunctivitis 90, 213
- diagnosis of 216
- treatment 218
- types of 213

Allergic contact dermatitis 203*f*
Allergic dermatitis 203*t*
Allergic disease 1, 13, 78, 136, 213, 248
- basis of 16
- types of 318

Allergic disorders 3, 11, 77, 252, 257, 313, 314, 325, 335, 335, 337*fc*
- diagnosis of 248
- hypothesis for 4*fc*
- quantum of 2
- signs of 253

Allergic fungal rhinosinusitis 102
- pathophysiology of 102*f*

Allergic hive 16
Allergic inflammation 23
Allergic manifestations 18, 335
Allergic march 250
Allergic reaction 25, 144, 145, 147, 226, 231, 234, 256, 313
- adverse 10
- IgE-mediated 219
- inflammatory 77
- severe 173
- time course of 25*f*
- various phases of 26*f*

Allergic rhinitis 16, 77, 78, 84, 89*t*, 91, 91*fc*, 94, 98, 101, 118, 122, 136, 190, 221, 251, 272, 303, 307
- allergen avoidance 86
- classification of 82, 83*f*
- diagnosis 84
- early versus late reaction 81
- laboratory diagnosis 84

nasal clearance 86
pathophysiology 80
pharmacological treatment 86
prevalence of 2*f*
treatment 86
triggers of 80
Allergic rhinoconjunctivitis 348*t*
Allergic salute 254
Allergic shiners 84, 253
Allergic status 224
Allergic symptoms 248, 338*fc*
severity of 333
Allergic triggers 291
Allergoids 304
Allergology 17
Allergy 9, 10, 11*f*, 12*f*, 16, 17, 31, 213, 248, 308*t*, 314, 315, 333, 335
aggravate 330
and anaphylaxis over last century, prevalence of 10*f*
causes of 319, 331
complementary medicine in 306
current concept of 11*f*
diagnosis of 257, 270, 273, 295
gastrointestinal 160
history of 4, 250
immunology 16, 30*f*
immunotherapy 301
importance of cofactors 250
management of 297
march 314
mediators 256
medical history 248
myths and beliefs about 313
ocular 216, 217*t*
original idea of 9*f*
outdoor 329
pets reduces 315
pharmacotherapy 300
phenomenon of 6
physical exercise reduce 331
pollution 330
prevention 297, 333
primary prevention 297
public health issue 1
rains reduces 315
respiratory 13, 77, 78, 330
secondary prevention 298
skin testing 259, 260*t*, 262, 263*f*
correlation of 266
factors influencing 264
lancets and multi-test devices for 264*f*
specific preventive measures 299
spectrum 11
tertiary prevention 298
testing 117, 255, 270, 272, 326, 328
basis of 255
different modalities of 255
functional assessment 274
laboratory tests 256
radiological assessment 280
structural assessment 272
Alnus nitida 44, 62
Alpha 1-adrenergic receptors 151
Alpha-lactalbumin 160
Alternaria 40
Amaranthus spinosus 41, 45, 62
American Academy of Pediatrics 175
American Thoracic Society 275
Aminoalkyl ethers 88
Aminophylline 352
Amoxicillin 100, 110
Analgesics 110
Anaphylactic reactions 148
severity of 174*t*

Anaphylaxis 6, 7, 16, 18, 130, 143, 145, 147*f*, 152*t*, 157, 158, 173, 252, 332, 346*b*
  acute management 152
  causes of 143
  diagnostic criteria 148
  differential diagnosis 149
  emergency 157
  immunoglobulin E
    dependent 144
    independent 144
  immunological mechanisms of 144
  long-term management 156
  management 151
  severe 248
Andersen 6-stage sampler 38*f*
Anemophilous 32, 46
Anesthetics, local 231
Angioedema 169, 184, 189*fc*, 221, 249, 252, 349*t*
  ACE inhibitor-induced 186
  acquired 186, 187
  acute attacks of 184
  classification 185
  diagnosis 186
  hereditary 182, 185, 187
  histaminergic 185
  management 187
  pathophysiology 184
Angiotensin-converting enzyme 145, 189
  inhibitors 251
Anogeissus pendula 41
Antiallergic 218
  agents, multi-model 218
  medications 328
Antibiotics 100*t*
Antibody 18, 24
  dependent cellular cytotoxicity 22
  isotypes 146

Anticholinergic
  agents 87, 350
  intranasal 348
Antigen 24
  antibody immune complexes 24
  presenting cells 21, 22
  selection of 262
Antihistamines 28, 88, 88*t*, 197
  intranasal 87
  oral 87
  second-generation 87
Antihistaminic agents 173
Antihistaminic medications 179
Anti-IgE antibody 89, 281, 354
Antineutrophil cytoplasmic antibodies 342
Anxiety 130
Aortic aneurysm 268
Apitherapy 307
Argemone mexicana 41, 45, 63
Arrhythmia 87
Artemisia
  scoparia 41
  vulgaris 45, 63
Arthritis, comorbid 132
Arthus reaction 24
Ascospores 40
Aspergilli-penicilli spores 40
Aspergillus 34, 40
Asphodelus tenuifolius 41, 46, 63
Aspirin 231
  challenge 132
  desensitization 236
  exacerbated respiratory disease 114, 132, 236
    diagnosis 236
    management 236
Astemizole 88
Asthma 13, 78, 92, 103, 112, 114, 125, 126*fc*, 132, 133*t*, 135, 136, 138, 190, 221,

250-252, 257, 272, 285, 308t, 314, 316, 350t
action plan 129
allergic 112, 117, 303
assessment 118
atypical 272
biomarker based 114
cessation of 131
childhood 2
complications of 129
control 114f
development of 160
diagnosis 273
differential diagnosis of 120t, 137
exacerbation 125t
features of 133t
late-onset 114
management 121, 130, 138, 140f
    steps of 122f
managing comorbidities 130
nonallergic 112
nonpharmacological interventions 127
occupational 128, 131
perimenstrual 131
phenotypes 112, 114f
    characteristics 115t
primary prevention of 141
related death 129
selected cohort of 236
severe 89
steps of 121
subtypes of 129
supportive tests 117
symptom 118
treatment
    long-term 281t
    stepping down 127
    stepping up 127
with fixed airflow limitation 114
with obesity 114
Astringents 99
Atopic dermatitis 136, 160, 181, 188, 191, 199fc, 343fc
    diagnosis of 191
    differential diagnosis 192
    pathophysiology of 188, 190f
Atopic diseases 250, 251, 345
Atopic patch test 266
Atopy 17, 314, 315
Atrophic rhinitis 79
Azadirachta indica 46, 64
Azatadine 88
Azelastine 87, 88
    eye drop 348
    puff 348
Azithromycin 100, 110

B

Balsam of Peru 206
Basophils 89
Bauhinia variegata 41
Beclomethasone 348
    dipropionate 87, 123, 139, 351
Beta 1-adrenergic receptors 151
Beta agonists, long-acting 122
Beta-lactoglobulin 160
Betula utilis 46, 64
Bharband 45
Bhojpatra 46
Blood
    allergy 326
        tests 327
    eosinophilia 291
Body's allergenic tendency 300
Bony erosion 103
Borassus flabellifer 47, 64
Bothriochloa pertusa 41

Bowel disease, inflammatory 7, 8, 292
Bradykinin 28, 184
    mediated reactions 185
    release 187
Brahmadandi 45
Brain 24
Brassica campestris 47, 65
Breast-fed infant 161
Breath, shortness of 136
Brompheniramine 88
Bronchial challenge test 268
Bronchitis, eosinophilic 117
Bronchoconstriction, exercise induced 114
Bronchoscopy 273
Bronchospasm 148
Bryan's test 268, 293, 294
Budesonide 123, 329, 348, 351
    formoterol 351
    nebulized 139
Bullous pemphigoid 181
Burden of allergic diseases over last five decades 1*f*
Burkard spore trap 36*f*

C

Cannabis sativa 41, 47, 65
Carbinoxamine 88
Carbohydrate determinant, cross-reactive 171
Carbon monoxide diffusing capacity 275, 277
Carcinoid syndrome 149, 232
Carica papaya 33
Cassia fistula 48, 65
Cassia occidentalis 41
Cassia siamea 41
Casuarina equisetifolia 41, 48, 66
Catamenial asthma 131
CD4+ T helper cell differentiation 21*f*
Cedrus deodara 32, 41, 49, 66
Cefdinir 110
Cefixime 100
Cefpodoxime 100, 110
Ceftriaxone 110
Cefuroxime 100, 110
Celiac disease 332
Cenchrus ciliaris 41, 48, 66
Cetirizine 88, 353
Challenge test 223
Charcot-Leyden crystals 103
Chemokine ligand 26
Chemosis 214*f*
Chenopodium album 41, 67
Chenopodium murale 41
Children outgrow food allergy 323
Chlorofluorocarbon propellant 123
Chlorpheniramine 88, 353
Choanal atresia 80
Choline 231
Chromones 281
    local 87
Chronic obstructive pulmonary disease 128, 133*t*, 135*t*
Churg-Strauss syndrome 95
Ciclesonide 123, 139, 348, 351
Ciprofloxacin 100, 110, 231
Cladosporium 40
Clarithromycin 100, 110
Clavulanate 110
Clemastine 88
Clindamycin 100, 110
Cobalt dichloride 206
Cobblestone-like appearance 215*f*
Cocos nucifera 41, 49, 67
Cohen and Konak classification 287*f*

Collapse, causes of 149
Colophony 206
Complementary medicine 306, 311, 311*t*
Complete blood count 126, 342
Component resolved diagnostic tests 259
Computed tomography 105
Conjunctiva, swollen 84
Conjunctival challenge test 216
Conjunctival inflammation, types of 214
Conjunctivitis 257, 314
    medicamentosa 218
    perennial allergic 213
    vernal 215*f*
Contact allergy 216
Contact dermatitis 192, 200, 219
    acute irritant 201
    allergic 201, 202
    chronic 201
    common causes 208
    diagnostic tests 205
    irritant 201, 203*t*
    management 209
    patch testing 205
    pathophysiology 201
    photoaggravated 201
    photoallergic 201
    phototoxic 201
    prevention 211
    prognosis 211
    protein 201
    subjective irritancy 201
    systemic 201
    types 201
Contact urticaria 221
Coriandrum sativum 50, 67
Corticosteroids 218, 281
    inhaled 122, 123*t*, 139*t*, 140, 351
    intranasal 87
    systemic 351
    topical 195
Cosmetics and skin care products 209
Cough 136
    chronic 272
    persistent 169
Cow's milk 167
    protein allergy 160, 162, 164, 165, 165*fc*, 166
        signs of 162*t*
        symptoms of 162*t*
Cromoglycate 349
Cromolyn 329
    sodium 28
Crude allergen
    extracts 258
    testing 292
Culprit allergen 250
Curvularia 40
Cyclizines 88
Cyclosporine 354
Cylindrica 52
Cynodon dactylon 41, 50, 68
Cyproheptadine 88, 353
Cystic fibrosis 94, 137
Cytokines 28
Cytomegalovirus 313
Cytotoxic food testing 268, 293

D

Dapsone 354
Daytime somnolence 91
Decongestants
    intranasal 349
    oral 348
Dendritic cells 26, 203, 301, 301*f*
Dennie-Morgan lines 254
Depression 91, 130

Dermal reaction 241
Dermatitis 257
    irritant 219
Dexchlorpheniramine 88
Diabetes 92
Dibenzocycloheptenes 88
Dichanthium annulatum 41
Dietary antioxidants 280
Differential blood count 342
Di-George syndrome 313
Diphenhydramine 88, 353
Distress, respiratory 169
Dodonaea viscosa 50, 68
Dolichandrone platycalyx 33
Double-blind placebo control food challenge 163
Down syndrome 107
Doxepin 354
Drechslera 40
Drug 80
    allergy 233, 331
        differential diagnosis of 232
        IgE-mediated 232
    class 89
    desensitization 235
    interactions 228
    provocation test 235
    rash with eosinophilia and systemic
        signs 233
        symptoms 230
    reaction 192, 229
        immunologic 230*t*
Dry powder inhaler 123
Dysbiotic microflora 8*f*
Dyskinesia, primary ciliary 137
Dysplasia, bronchopulmonary 137
Dyspnea 148, 153

E

Earache 272
Edema, angioneurotic 184
Electrodermal/vega testing 269, 295
Electronic air cleaners 319
End-organ dysfunction, symptoms of 148
Enzyme-linked immunosorbent assay-based test 270
Eosinophil
    chemotactic factor-a 27
    count 291
Eosinophilia 103, 116, 291
    causes of 292
    hereditary 292
    primary neoplastic 292
    secondary reactive 291
    syndrome 79
Eosinophilic inflammation, diagnosis of 280*t*
Eosinophilic mucin containing fungus 103
Eosinophils 89, 116, 214
    proliferation of 80
Ephedrine 348
Epicoccum 40
Epicutaneous allergy skin testing, technique of 261
Epidermis 260
Epiglottis, swollen 287*f*
Epiglottitis 287*f*
Epinephrine 152, 152*t*, 173*b*, 349
    infusion 155
    intramuscular 155*f*, 333
Epistaxis 272
Epstein-Barr virus 182, 231, 257, 313
Eragrostis tenella 41
Erythema 169
    multiforme 181

Erythromycin 100
Esophagitis, eosinophilic 11
Ethanolamines 88
Ethylenediamine 88
　　dihydrochloride 206
Eustachian tube dysfunction 90
Exanthematous pustulosis, acute generalized 230
Eye 1, 24
　　allergic disease of 213
　　chronic inflammation of 214
Eyelid skin, sandpaper-like texture of 216f

F

Facemask, types of 330
Facial pain 272
Familial cold autoinflammatory syndrome 181
Fatigue 91
Fexofenadine 88, 354
Filaria 291
Filtration technique 34
Fingertip units 194
Fixed drug eruptions 181
Flexible rhinolaryngoscopy 257
Flu shot 323
Flunisolide 87, 348
Fluorescence in situ hybridization 342
Flushing syndromes 149
Fluticasone
　　furoate 123, 348
　　propionate 87, 123, 139, 348, 351
Food allergen 2, 60, 60t
　　components 293t
Food allergy 130, 160, 167, 257, 311t, 332
　　alternative medicine in 311
　　component-resolved diagnostics 171
　　diagnosis of 169, 223
　　emerging therapeutics 176
　　epidemiology 168
　　prevention 175
　　retesting 174
　　treatment 172
Food challenge 267
　　test 163
Food molecules
　　high-risk 171t
　　low-risk 171t
Food protein-induced enterocolitis syndrome 162
Forced expiratory flow 115, 279, 282
Forced oscillation technique 279
Forced vital capacity 275, 279, 282
Fresh frozen plasma 349
Fungal allergens 43t
　　localized distribution of 40
Fungal flora
　　indoor 40
　　outdoor 40
Fungus, culture positive for 103

G

Gastroesophageal reflux 137
　　disease 79, 205, 130
Gastrointestinal symptoms, persistent 148
Gastrointestinal system 257
Gastrointestinal tract 24
Gene-host influences 145
Genetic
　　and immune-mediated disorders 28
　　polymorphisms, role of 228
Giant papillary conjunctivitis 213
Global Economic Burden of Asthma and Rhinitis 3t

Global initiative for asthma guidelines 272
Glomerulonephritis 24
Glove use test 223
Glucagon 155
Glucose-6-phosphate dehydrogenase 229
Graft-versus-host disease, acute 233
Group of medical and healthcare system 306
Gynandropsis gynandra 51, 69

H

Haemophilus influenza 93, 107
Hair analysis 270, 295
Halotherapy 307
Harboring food allergy 169
Hay fever 16, 259
Headache 272
Heart disease
    congenital 137
    coronary 92
Heart failure, congestive 277
Heiner syndrome 160
Helicobacter pylori 5, 182
Helminthosporium 40
Heparin 27
Hepatitis
    A 5, 233
    B 233
    C 233
    C virus 182
Heptanes 88
Herbs
    allium cepa (onion) 308
    atropa belladonna 308
    caffeine 308
    chaipo-tang (Chinese) 309
    chamazulene (chamomile) 308
    coleus forskohlii 308
    datura stramonium (jimson weed) 308
    echinacea 308
    eucalyptus 308
    goldenseal (hydrazine) 308
    hi chun (Korean) 308
    jisil (Korean) 309
    kutki/kuuro (Indian) 309
    licorice 309
    ma huang (ephedra) 309
    menthol (mint) 309
    minor blue dragon 309
    peppermint oil (mint) 309
    saiboku-to (Japanese) 309
    sho-seiryu-to (Japanese) 309
    tylophora indica (India) 309
    urtica dioica (nettle) 309
Heropogon contortus 41
Hevea brasiliensis tree 218
Histamine 27, 150, 184
    challenge test 268
Hitchhiker's thumb 287*f*
Hoarse voice 169
Hodgkin's disease 313
Holoptelea integrifolia 41, 51, 69
Hormones, role of 147
Horner syndrome 98
Horner-Trantas dots 215*f*
Host-allergen interaction 20
House dust mite 262, 299
Human immunodeficiency virus 231, 313, 342
Hydrocortisone 110, 351
    intravenous 332
Hydrofluoroalkane propellant 123, 139
Hydroxyzine 88, 353
Hymenoptera venoms 244
Hyperemia 218

Hypereosinophilia 292, 342*fc*
Hypereosinophilic syndrome 291
Hyper-IgE syndrome 292, 313
Hyperresponsiveness 82
Hypersensitive disorders 5
Hypersensitivity 11*f*, 17, 219
    diagnosis of 256
    reactions 11, 21, 23*f*
        types of 21, 22*f*
    syndrome, drug induced 229, 230
Hypertrophy
    mild-to-moderate 287*f*
    severe 287*f*
Hypothermia 145
Hypotonia 148

I

Ibuprofen 110
Ichthyosis vulgaris 192
Immotile cilia syndrome 94
Immune
    reactions 161*t*
    system 6, 28
Immunity
    adaptive 204, 204*t*
    innate 204*t*
Immunoglobulin 18, 26, 78
    E 22, 23, 122, 165, 230
        mediated allergic reaction, classification of severity of 249*t*
        serum 190
    G 230
    intravenous 354
    M 230
Immunologic disorders 292
Immunologic drug reactions, types of 235
Immunology 9

Immunotherapy 90, 341*fc*
    age limit for 303
    delivery 303*t*
    failure of 302
    future of 304
    oral 176
    specific 301
    subcutaneous 90, 302-304
    sublingual 90, 302, 303
Impaction technique 34
Imperata cylindrica 41, 70
Impulse oscillometry system 278, 279
In vitro test 257
In vivo test 85, 259
Infections 345
    bacterial 280
    parasitic 313
    secondary 93
    severe 101
Inflammation
    eosinophilic 114
    neurogenic 82
Inflammatory disorder 104
Influenza virus 280
Innate immune system 19
Insect
    bites 233
    habits of 240*t*
    hypersensitivity 241, 242*fc*, 344*fc*
    identification of 238
    stings 233
    venom allergy 238
Interferon 26
Interleukin 26, 203, 301
Internal nose, anatomy of 93*f*
Intestinal microbiota 8*f*
Intradermal skin tests 261*t*
Ipratropium 329, 348
    bromide 350

Iridology 269, 295
Isoniazid 231
Itch-flush 148
Itchy skin lesions 179

K

Kante bhaji 45
Kantewali chaulai 45
Kartagener syndrome 94, 95
Kasagaha 48
Kawasaki disease 233, 313
Keratoconjunctivitis
    atopic 214
    vernal 214
Ketotifen 28
Kinesiology 269, 295

L

Lactobacillus rhamnosus 309
Langerhans cell histiocytosis 277
Laser therapy 309
Latex allergens, types of 220
Latex allergy 218, 222*fc*, 223
    clinical manifestations 221
    diagnosis of 222
    treatment 224
    types of 219
    unresolved issues 228
Latex-fruit allergy syndrome 221
    diagnosis of 224*fc*
    treatment of 224*fc*
Leprosy 24
Leukocytes 268
Leukotriene 28
    receptor antagonist 86, 89, 122, 281, 352, 354
Levocetirizine 353
Levofloxacin 100
Levosalbutamol 350
Lipopolysaccharides 20

Lipoteichoic acid 20
Liver disease 313
Local tissue eosinophilia 291
Lolium perenne 52, 70
Loratadine 88, 353
Lung 24
    disease
        chronic obstructive 275
        obstructive 134
    function test 135
Lupus erythematosus, subacute cutaneous 181
Lymphocytes 19, 89
    subset analysis 295

M

Magnesium sulfate 352
Major histocompatibility complex 26
Mallotus philippensis 41, 53, 70
Mangifera indica 53, 71
Mast cell 23, 29, 80, 179, 214
    activation 158, 213
    degranulation 234
    mediators of 89
    stabilizers 218
Mastocytosis, systemic 151, 181
Maxillary sinuses 284*f*
Maximum expiratory flow 282
Mediastinal mass 290*f*
Medicines
    ayurveda 307
    herbals 307
    homeopathy 307
Melia azedarach 53, 71
Methacholine 268
Methdilazine 88
Methyl-prednisolone 351
Methylxanthines 281, 352
Metronidazole 100
Microflora hypothesis 5

Milk allergy 160, 300, 339*fc*
    clinical presentation 161
    diagnosis 161
    investigations 162
    pathophysiology 160
    prevention 166
    re-evaluation 166
    treatment 164
Milk beverages 166
Mimosa invisa 32
Mini-allergen test 259
Minimum efficiency reporting value ratings 321*t*
Mometasone furoate 87, 123, 139, 348
Monocytes 89
Montelukast 236, 352, 354
Moraxella catarrhalis 94, 107
Morus alba 54, 71
Muckle-Wells syndrome 181
Mucociliary dysfunction 94
Mucocutaneous junction 249
Mycoplasma pneumoniae 182
Myelodysplastic syndromes 151

N

Naphazoline 349
Nasal
    air sampler 37
    congestion 169
    crease 84
    endoscopy 85, 272
    eosinophilia 85
    itching 79
    mucosa 81
        swelling of 84
    obstruction 78, 84, 272
    polyposis 90
    provocation test 85, 268
    pruritus 84
Nasopharyngitis 106
Nedocromil 349
    sodium 123
Neomycin 110, 206
Neoplastic diseases 345
Nephrotic syndrome 313
Netherton syndrome 192
Neurological syndromes 149
Neurospora 40
Neutrophil 24, 214
    chemotactic factor-A 27
Newer and alternate allergy tests 291
Nickel sulfate 206
Nigrospora 40
Nitric oxide, fractional exhaled 114, 117, 278
Nonallergic disorders 249
Non-breast-fed babies 164
Non-immunologic drug reactions, types of 235
Nonsteroidal anti-inflammatory drugs 128, 218, 229-231, 250
Normal spirometry graph 282*f*
Nose 1, 24
Nutritional deficiencies 192

O

Obstructive lung disease, causes of 277*t*
Ofloxacin 110
Old friend hypothesis 5, 7*fc*
Olopatadine 218
    nasal sprays 87
Omalizumab 29, 124, 144, 257, 281, 354
Omenn's syndrome 292
Open-patch testing 208
Opiates 231

Opioids 234
Oral corticosteroids, short course of 127
Oral food challenge 163, 172
Otitis media 104, 110*t*, 111, 112, 113*fc*, 257
  acute 106, 109
  chronic 272
    suppurative 109
  clinical features 108
  complication 111
  diagnosis 109
  investigations 108
  pathogenesis 107
  predisposing factors 106
  recurrent 109, 272
  stages 108
  treatment 109
  with effusion 90
Oxymetazoline 99, 349

P

Palynology 31
Paraben mix 206
Paranasal sinuses, anatomical location of 92*f*
Parasites, gastrointestinal 233
Parasitic diseases 345
Parthenium hysterophorus 54, 72
Paspalum distichum 41
Patch test 223, 266
  reaction scoring 208*t*
Peak expiratory flow 282
  rate 257, 279
Pediatric allergy 13
Peeling skin disorder 192
Penicillin 323
Penicillium 34, 40
Pennisetum typhoides 41, 54, 72
Periodic fever syndromes 251
Phalaris minor 41

Phenindamine 88
Pheniramine 332
Phenothiazines 88
Phenylephrine 99, 349
Phoenix sylvestris 41, 55, 72
Phosphodiesterase 4 inhibitors 196
Photopatch testing 207
Phototherapy 197
Phthalazinone 88
Pinus
  pollens of 32
  strobus 55, 73
Piperazines 88
Piperidines 88
Plantago major 41
Plasma kallikrein, inhibitor of 187
Platelet-activating factors 27, 28
Poa annua 41, 55, 73
Pollen 60, 299
  allergens 41
    cross-reactive 59
  calendar 36
  grains 31
Polychondritis, relapsing 80
Polymyxin B 110
Polypogon monspeliensis 41
Positive bronchial challenge test 117
Positive exercise challenge test 117
Potassium
  clavulanate 100
  dichromate 206
Prednisolone 351, 354
Pressurized metered dose inhaler 139
Prick devices 262
  types of 262
Prick-prick test 223, 224, 261
Principal collection methods 33
Probiotics 197, 309

Promethazine 88, 353
Prosopis juliflora 41, 56, 73
Prostaglandins 28
Protamine 231
Protease 27
    activated receptor 20
Protective microbiota, loss of 6*fc*
Protein 18*f*
    allergenic 292
    allergens 259
    eosinophilic cationic 116
Provocation neutralization 269, 294
Provocation test 266
Pruritic urticarial papules 181
Pruritus 169, 218
Pseudoallergic reactions 231, 231*t*
Pseudoephedrine 348
Pseudomonas 110
Psionic medicine 295
Psoriasis 233
    infantile 192
Psychologic therapies 307
Pulse test 270
    reflexology 295
Putranjiva roxburghii 41
Pyrilamine 88

Q

Quercus incana 41
Quincke's edema 184
Quinolones 234

R

Radioallergosorbent test 258
Radiocontrast media 231
Radionics 295
Ranitidine 354
Red flag signs 125
Red man syndrome 149
Reduces pollen allergy 315
Reflexology 270
Refractory anaphylaxis 156
Respiratory
    infections, acute 13
    syncytial virus 107, 280, 313
    system 1, 257
    tract 77
Restrictive lung disease, causes of 277*t*
Resuscitation, cardiopulmonary 152
Rheumatic disease 236
Rheumatoid arthritis 24, 257
Rhinitis 13, 106, 130, 250, 252, 272, 314
    anatomic abnormalities causing 99
    drug induced 79
    evaluation of 251
    exercise induced 79
    gustatory 79
    hormone-induced 79
    infectious 79, 98
    medicamentosa 98
    mimic symptoms of 79
    nonallergic 79, 94, 98
    occupational 79
    pattern of 83*t*
    perennial nonallergic 79
    reflux-induced 79
    secondary 98
    vasomotor 79
Rhinoconjunctivitis 13
Rhinorrhea
    persistent 272
    watery 78, 84
Rhinosinusitis 90, 281
    acute bacterial 101
    chronic 101
Rhinovirus 93, 107

Rhizopus 40
Ricinus communis 41, 56, 74
Rotorod sampler model 37*f*
Rubbing test 223

S

Saccharomyces 40
Salbutamol 153, 350
Salicylate intolerance 250
Salix caprea 57, 74
Salvadora persica 41
Samter's triad 236
Sarcoidosis 292
Satyanashi 45
Scabies 192
Scarring, conjunctival 214
Schistosoma 291
Schnitzler's syndrome 181
Scleral injection 84
Sclerosis, multiple 7
Seasonal allergic conjunctivitis 213, 214*f*
Seborrheic dermatitis 192
Sensitivity 17
Sensitization 22
Serological tests 268
Serotonin 27
Serum tryptase 150
Sickness, serum 24
Sieve impactors 37
Single nucleotide polymorphisms 7*fc*
Sinus 1
 contralateral 283*f*
 paranasal 283*f*
Sinusitis 89, 92-94, 100*t*, 105*fc*, 130, 257, 272
 acute 93, 99, 284*f*
 anatomy 92
 chronic 94, 96, 99
 complications of 97
 diagnosis 95
 diagnostic criteria 96
 imaging 97
 management 104
 pathophysiology 93
 physical examination 96
 right maxillary 283*f*
 subacute 96
 treatment 99
Sjogren's syndrome 79
Skin 24
 allergies 179
 care 197
  after flare maintenance therapy 198
  bathing practices 197
  dilute bleach baths 197
  moisturizing agents 197
 damage 202
 diseases, occupational 200
 inflammation, types of 200
 irritation 202
 lesions 203
 prick test 85, 117, 170, 259, 261, 265*f*, 327, 328
  interpretation of 262
  number of 262
 touch test 261, 265*f*, 327
  interpretation of 262
Sneezing 79, 84
Sodium cromoglycate 123
Sorghum vulgare 41, 57, 74
Spirometry 257, 274
 abnormality 276*t*
 interpretation 276*t*
 systematic interpretation of 275*fc*
Spore trap slit impactors 34
Sporotrichum 40
Stachybotrys 316
Staphylococcus aureus 94, 188

Stem cell factor 26
Steroids 28, 354
   intranasal 348
   long-term 265
      topical 265
   short-term 265
   systemic 196
Stevens-Johnson syndrome 229, 233
Still's disease 233
Stinging insect, types of 238
Streptococcal infection 233
Streptococcus pneumoniae 93, 107
Stridor 148, 169
Strongyloidiasis 291
Suaeda fruticosa 41, 57, 75
Subglottic trachea, irregular narrowing of 289f
Sulfamethoxazole 100
Sulfisoxazole 100
Superficial skin layer 260
Swelling, conjunctival 214f
Swollen lips-tongue-uvula 148
Syncope 148
Systemic lupus erythematosus 24, 277
Systemic venom allergic reaction 246
Syzygium cumini 57, 75

T

T helper cells 301
T regulatory cells 301
Tacrolimus 354
Terbutaline 350
Tetanus vaccine 236
Tetrahydrozoline 349
Theophylline 352
Thiopurine methyltransferase 229
Thyroid autoantibodies 183
Tissue
   growth factor 301
   swelling 149
Topical calcineurin inhibitors 196
Topical steroid potency chart 195t, 352t
Toxic black molds 316
Toxic epidermal necrolysis 233
Toxocariasis 291
Toxoplasma gondii 5
Tracheitis, bacterial 289f
Tracheomalacia 137, 288f
Tranexamic acid 349
Triamcinolone 348
   acetonide 87, 123, 139
Trimeprazine 88
Trimethoprim 100
Tripelennamine 88
Triprolidine 88
True food allergy 2
Tryptase 150
Tuberculosis 137, 277
Tumor necrosis factor 26, 203

U

Upper airways 273t
Upper respiratory infection 89
Uromyces 40
Urticaria 169, 179, 249, 252, 353t
   acute 160, 180, 183
   chronic 180, 183, 347, 347b
   classification 180
   diagnosis 186
   diagnostic evaluation 181
   differentials of 180
   management 183
   pathophysiology 179
   treatment of 183
Ustilago 40

V

Vancomycin 231, 234
Vascular ring 137
Vasculitis 180
    necrotizing 24
Venom hypersensitivity testing 244*t*
Venom immunotherapy 157
    injections 245
Vilayati jhau 48
Vilayati mehndi 50
Vipomas 149
Viral infection 233, 313
Vomiting 169

W

Wegener's granulomatosis 80
Wheat allergy, types of 332
Wheeze 132, 136, 148, 169
Wiskott-Aldrich syndrome 313

X

Xanthium strumarium 41, 58, 75
Xylometazoline 99, 349

Y

Young syndrome 95

Z

Zafirlukast 236
Zea mays 58, 76
Zileuton 236

www.ingramcontent.com/pod-product-compliance
Lightning Source LLC
Chambersburg PA
CBHW040515220526
45473CB00012B/2873